MEDICAL ETHICS AND THE FAITH FACTOR

A CRITICAL ISSUES IN BIOETHICS SERIES BOOK FROM

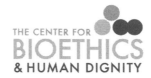

THE CENTER FOR
BIOETHICS
& HUMAN DIGNITY

Exploring the nexus of biomedicine, biotechnology,
and our common humanity.

This volume continues the Center's second book series, CRITICAL ISSUES IN
BIOETHICS. Each of these volumes features one or two authors bringing
Christian perspectives into dialogue with other perspectives that are partic-
ularly influential today.

This series is a project of The Center for Bioethics & Human Dignity,
an international bioethics research center of Trinity International University. The Center endeavors to bring Christian perspectives to bear on the
pressing bioethical issues of our day. It pursues this task by developing print,
electronic, audio, and video resources, as well as hosting conferences, educational opportunities, and other strategic events throughout the world. Additionally, the Center provides numerous online resources for an international
network of individuals interested in bioethical matters.

For more information on membership in the Center or its various resources, including present or future books in the Critical Issues in Bioethics
Series or books from our Horizons in Bioethics Series, contact the Center at:

The Center for Bioethics & Human Dignity
Trinity International University
2065 Half Day Road
Deerfield, IL 60015 USA
Phone: (847) 317-8180
Fax: (847) 317-8101
Email: info@cbhd.org
Website: www.cbhd.org

MEDICAL ETHICS AND THE FAITH FACTOR

*A Handbook for Clergy
and Health-Care Professionals*

Robert D. Orr, M.D., C.M.

WILLIAM B. EERDMANS PUBLISHING COMPANY
GRAND RAPIDS, MICHIGAN / CAMBRIDGE, U.K.

Published 2009 by

Wm. B. Eerdmans Publishing Co.

2140 Oak Industrial Drive N.E., Grand Rapids, Michigan 49505 /
P.O. Box 163, Cambridge CB3 9PU U.K.

Printed in the United States of America

15 14 13   7 6 5 4 3 2

Library of Congress Cataloging-in-Publication Data

Orr, Robert D. (Robert David), 1941-
    Medical ethics and the faith factor: a handbook for clergy and
       health-care professionals / Robert D. Orr.
          p.   cm.   — (Horizon in bioethics series)
      (A critical issues in bioethics series book)
    Includes bibliographical references and index.
    ISBN 978-0-8028-6404-8 (pbk.: alk. paper)
    1. Medical ethics — Religious aspects — Christianity.   I. Title.

R724.07445 2009
172.2 — dc22

                    2009027389

www.eerdmans.com

Contents

PART IV

Series Editors' Foreword

We live in an age when scientific knowledge has provided human beings with an unprecedented ability to manipulate life and death. In the West there has been a cultural shift from a so-called Judeo-Christian consensus to fragmented secular assumptions about the nature of human life, community, and "reproduction" as well as the practice of medicine and scientific research. There is little doubt that these changes in science and culture have fueled the controversies surrounding abortion, physician-assisted suicide, genetic engineering, the patient-doctor relationship, reproductive technologies, cloning, and the allocation of health-care resources, to name just a few.

Bioethics is the interdisciplinary study of these and other issues of life and health. It involves an attempt to discover normative guidelines built on sound moral foundations.

The purpose of this series is to bring thoughtful and biblically informed Christian voices in bioethics into dialogue with other voices that are influential today. As Christians we believe that human persons are made in the image of God and for that reason their lives are sacred. We also believe that God's entire creation was made for a purpose, and we discover this purpose from the Holy Scripture as well as philosophical reflections on the nature of things. Because we live in a pluralist society, we believe that it is our responsibility to explain why all people should take Christian perspectives into account. Such is the case not least because these perspectives have shaped so much of Western culture, especially its assumptions about human dignity. Accordingly, the books in this series will be useful to those who do not share our theological commitments. They can be read side by side with books espousing secular or other perspectives and are ideal for bioethics courses in nontheological as well as theological settings.

Because bioethics is theoretical as well as practical, the authors in this series are committed to providing a principled case for their perspectives as well as suggestions and insights on how scientists and/or health-care practitioners may employ these principles in a laboratory and/or clinical setting. In addition, we believe that pastors, students, professors, and others will profit from these books. C. S. Lewis warned of a future in which "Man's final conquest has proved to be the abolition of Man." The purpose of this series is to help forestall or even prevent such a future.

DENNIS HOLLINGER
President and Professor of Christian Ethics
Gordon-Conwell Theological Seminary

FRANCIS J. BECKWITH
Associate Professor of Philosophy and
Church-State Studies
Baylor University

Preface

Chaplains, pastors, priests, rabbis, and other people of faith, along with health-care professionals, frequently interact with individuals and families who are facing life-threatening illness, chronic illness, or disability. The conversations stimulated by such life events and conditions may include crucial questions of faith, God's will, the meaning of life and death, and eternity. Many believers are prepared for and comfortable with such discussions.

However, these conversations often include questions that make clergy and other people of faith distinctly uncomfortable — questions they are not typically prepared to answer. Such as: "Should we use a feeding tube for Mom?" "Is it OK if I stop dialysis and die?" "What should we do for our baby who is about to be born with life-threatening anomalies?" "Dear God, what should we do?"

These questions of ethics are usually first posed to physicians and other health-care professionals. Physicians are usually able to address the "Can we?" questions, which are generally questions of fact, laced significantly with matters of experience and training, often focused on the fine art of prognosis. But the "Can we?" questions are often insufficient, and answers to these questions are often inadequate.

Increasingly we must address the "Should we?" questions. Just because we *can* use a ventilator to postpone death for a few more hours or days in a man dying of lung cancer, *should* we? Are there other considerations — patient comfort, social interactions, spiritual matters — that might help to answer the various questions? Not infrequently different individuals answer the "Should we?" questions differently, based on their own experience or values. Health-care professionals are increasingly encouraging patients and families to discuss these "Should we?" questions with an ethics committee or a specialist in clinical ethics, who is often referred to as an ethics consultant, a clinical ethicist, or simply an ethicist.

Clinical ethics is a relatively new discipline within medicine, generated primarily by such "Should we?" questions. Those who serve as ethics consultants may be clinicians (physicians, nurses, social workers) with additional training in ethics. Or they may be individuals whose primary training is in another field (philosophy, law, theology) who have in addition some experience in or exposure to clinical medicine.

The ethicist, in an attempt to resolve conflict or bring clarity to the ambiguous questions, will often inquire about the personal and religious beliefs of the patient. This often leads to a recommendation to discuss the difficult value-laden question with the patient's clergyperson or other spiritual adviser. Many clergy are not fully informed on such ethical questions. Indeed, health-care professionals themselves cannot be expected to keep abreast on all the ethical nuances relevant to such value-laden decisions. Their devotion, after all, is primarily to the "Can we?" questions.

This book is intended to help fill the information gap so that clergy and health-care professionals can become more comfortable with these questions in clinical ethics. The core message of the book is that questions in clinical ethics are not beyond the purview of religious leaders or health-care personnel. In fact, they are manageable if you know the medical facts; if you know the principles of Scripture and of clinical ethics; if you know the values of the patient and his or her family; and in the Christian tradition, if you rely on the leading of the Holy Spirit.

It is not my intention that each reader will serve as an ethics consultant. Rather, my hope is that the reader will become somewhat familiar with the clinical issues, will recognize the moral questions raised by those issues, and will then be able to apply religious or spiritual tenets from his or her own tradition to the pertinent questions. If this is accomplished, I believe the reader will then be of great assistance to patients, families, and clinicians.

I am a Christian, and my faith is important to me. Some of the patients and families I have interacted with share my faith and beliefs. Some, however, are Christians whose teaching or beliefs are somewhat different from my own. And a significant percentage of the situations where I have been involved in ethics discussions, including many of the cases reported in this book, involve people from different faith traditions or different cultures.

I believe the clinical information and the principles and precepts of clinical ethics presented here are equally applicable in all these situations. I do not expect the reader to agree with each recommendation made in every case discussed. But I hope the discussion that ensues will help clergy and chaplains, students and clinicians, professionals and laypersons as they delve into dilemmas in clinical ethics.

The introduction tells a personal story about treatment decisions for a dear friend, decisions that were exceedingly difficult but at the same time remarkably easy.

Part I will look at the foundations of contemporary clinical ethics. Chapter 1, entitled "An Ethical Foundation," gives a brief overview of treatment decision-making, including the role of ethics consultations. Principles, precepts, and precedents of clinical ethics are described, including patient autonomy; surrogate decision-making for patients who have lost the capacity to make decisions; the use of advance directives; do-not-resuscitate orders; dealing with uncertainty; the understanding that there is no difference between withholding and withdrawing treatment; conflict resolution; and more. Chapter 2, "A Theological Foundation," outlines an approach to decision making in clinical ethics that is consistent with teaching in the three monotheistic faith traditions, including discussion of God's creation and sovereignty; the sanctity of human life; quality of life; free will; dominion and stewardship; boundaries; caring for others; miracles; and more.

Part II will look at some of the more common issues encountered when a patient's life is threatened by failure of one or more organ systems. Chapters 3 through 8 focus on different clinical issues that raise questions about what should be done when a patient encounters failure of his or her heart, lungs, kidneys, gastrointestinal tract, brain, or mind. Of course, not all dilemmas in clinical ethics are about life-threatening issues. Woven into these chapters are also cases of nonlethal conditions in these organ systems that often lead to ethics consultation.

Each of these chapters includes background information about the condition or treatment modality that will increase a nonprofessional's understanding of the issues. In addition, each includes some discussion of how personal values, professional standards, legal precedents, and biblical perspectives may influence decisions in these cases. The bulk of each chapter consists of several case discussions, each with a story, discussion (ethical analysis), recommendations, follow-up, and comments.

Part III (chapter 9) is about specific ethical dilemmas that arise because of differing cultural or religious beliefs. An attempt is made in each case to understand the values and beliefs of the various individuals involved, and to identify common ground that might allow resolution of the dilemma or conflict. When compromise is not possible, the patient's values and beliefs are generally given top priority.

Part IV includes five chapters that focus on ethical issues encountered in patients of a specific age or condition (neonatal issues, other pediatric issues, pregnancy), or patients faced with decisions about the use of specific technologies (assisted reproductive technology, transplantation).

In part V, the chapter entitled "The Priesthood of Believers" explores ways that family members, clergy, counselors, and friends can assist patients and families as they struggle with these difficult decisions, emphasizing the priesthood of believers and the importance of prayer for God's wisdom and peace.

The story in the introduction is true. Dave's family has given me permission to share the story with pastors, students, and other people of faith in an effort to make a bit easier the journey through complicated dilemmas in clinical ethics. The other stories in this book are also true or they are based on actual cases, sometimes representing a synthesis of two or more stories. However, names and some of the nonpertinent details have been changed to protect the identity of those involved.

It may be tempting to think that the resolution of these cases represents "the answer," since the reports are written by a person of faith. Let me refute that notion right at the outset. I do not claim any particular wisdom in these cases. I do believe that most were resolved in a manner consistent with religious principles as understood by the individuals involved at the time. Some readers may disagree with the recommendations or with the resolution of the issue. In fact, I personally disagree with the choices made by some of the patients, families, and professionals; I try to point these out in the "Follow-Up" or "Comment" sections of the case reports. My purpose in offering these examples is to show that biblical principles, personal values, and denominational tenets play a vitally important role in the resolution of difficult ethical dilemmas at the bedside.

Most of these consultations were done in secular hospitals. Some of the patients were people of faith; some said they were not. Some of the health-care professionals involved in their care were also people of faith, but some were not. These reports were written for the benefit of professionals, patients, and families, regardless of their faith traditions. You will find few, if any, theological terms or scriptural references in the text of the consultations. But the discussions and recommendations are designed to fit within professional and personal boundaries of acceptable practice.

At the end of most chapters I have listed other cases in the book that address similar conditions or treatment modalities. These may be reviewed to expand the discussion of that chapter. I have also included a few references at the end of most chapters that might be of value for readers particularly interested in that subject. Most of the references come from the secular literature without specific focus on the faith factor. Most of the information in these references is of high quality and representative of contemporary secular clinical ethics. Some of the information or opinions, however, are not consistent with the theological foundations addressed in chapter 2 of this book, and some may even be in direct opposition. Such references are included to give the reader a better understanding of the depth and scope of modern clinical ethics.

The glossary in appendix 1 is intended to define terms used in the text that may not be familiar to readers. The first time terms that are defined in the glossary, or their cognates, are used in a chapter or a case study, they are printed in the text in boldface type. Some unusual terms that are used only once or only in one chapter may not appear in the glossary but are instead defined in the text or in a footnote.

The case index in appendix 2 is a cross-reference tool to help readers find cases with similar issues in various chapters. For example, while all cases in chapter 6 will be about the use or nonuse of artificially administered fluids and nutrition, the issue in a particular feeding tube case may be the interpretation of a written advance directive, or resolution of conflict between family members, or a question of futility, or caring for someone with severe cognitive impairment, or a host of other issues. The case index will allow the reader to find similar discussions and analyses in cases involving differing diagnoses or treatment modalities, thus offering broader assistance.

This book is intended to be a reference book. While I would not discourage reading it from cover to cover, my expectation is that users will read chapters 1, 2, and 15 for a foundation and thereafter peruse or read chapters that are focused on specific clinical issues. Alternatively or in addition, the reader may find cases listed in the case index focused on a specific problem. For this reason, many of the discussions in the case studies will be repetitive or redundant since a reader may be reading only that one case.

It is my hope that the content and format of these discussions will assist people of faith as they seek satisfactory resolution of difficult ethical dilemmas. Perhaps they will gain a better understanding of the clinical situation. Even more important, I hope they will gain an understanding of the moral dilemma in light of the personal and religious beliefs of the patient, family, and professional. Most important of all, I hope the reader will come to a greater reliance on the leading of the Divine in the given situation.

God bless.

Acknowledgments

The idea of this book has been in the back of my mind for several years. I had difficulty, however, finding the blocks of time needed to review cases and organize them into a meaningful format. I was granted a significant gift in this regard by the C. S. Lewis Foundation, based in Redlands, California. I was invited to live for several months at the Kilns, C. S. Lewis's home in Oxford, England, which has been lovingly restored by Foundation volunteers to its 1930s-1940s condition, much as it was when Lewis lived there from 1930 until his death in 1963.

During my three months as scholar in residence at the Kilns, I spent most of my time writing. I chose to read or reread many of Lewis's works during my nonwriting hours. What a joy to contemplate the "Joy" he discussed at length.

In thinking about my hubris — a nonclergyperson writing for clergy and other people of faith about matters of both clinical and spiritual importance — I came across the following words from Lewis that at least partially absolve me:

> People say "The Church ought to give us a lead." That is true if they mean it in the right way, but false if they mean it in the wrong way. By the Church they ought to mean the whole body of practising Christians. And when they say that the Church should give us a lead, they ought to mean that some Christians — those who happen to have the right talents — should be economists and statesmen, and that all economists and statesmen should be Christians, and that their whole efforts in politics and economics should be directed to putting "Do as you would be done by" into action. If that happened, and if others were really ready to

take it, then we should find the Christian solution for our own social problems pretty quickly. But, of course, when they ask for a lead from the Church most people mean they want the clergy to put out a political programme. That is silly. The clergy are those particular people within the whole Church who have been specially trained and set aside to look after what concerns us as creatures who are going to live for ever: and we are asking them to do quite a different job for which they have not been trained. The job is really on us, on the layman. The application of Christian principles, say, to trade unionism or education, must come from Christian trade unionists and Christian schoolmasters: just as Christian literature comes from Christian novelists and dramatists — not from the bench of bishops getting together and trying to write plays and novels in their spare time. (From "Social Morality," chapter 3 in *Mere Christianity* [New York: Harper Collins, 2001], pp. 83-84)

Similarly, I believe, the application of religious principles to clinical ethics must come from people of faith who are experienced in clinical ethics.

I am also indebted to professional colleagues Gail Cashman, R.N., Dennis de Leon, M.D., M.B.A., Leigh Genesen, R.N., Robert Macauley, M.D., S.T.M., and Ronald Perkin, M.D., M.A. for allowing me to include in this book a few cases in which they did the actual consultations. In each case, I was involved in contemporaneous or retrospective review of their ethical analyses. These are all people of faith who are exceptionally competent and dedicated to analysis of ethical dilemmas at the bedside in a manner consistent with the standards of clinical ethics and their understanding of the role of faith in these matters. I have been very pleased and privileged to be on clinical ethics consultation teams with these fine clinical ethicists.

Many other professional colleagues participated in the review of these cases at Clinical Ethics Case Conferences held weekly at the University of Chicago Hospitals, Loma Linda University Medical Center, and Fletcher Allen Health Care at the University of Vermont. Insightful questions, practical comments, thoughtful criticism, affirmation, and doses of good humor have made these meetings the highlight of my professional career in clinical ethics. To each of them, my sincere thanks.

In addition, I received helpful comments on earlier drafts of the book from Dr. Macauley and Rev. Jeffery Jensen.

Introduction

It was one of those life-defining events that becomes indelible in your memory. I had just returned from a Saturday morning council meeting of the Vermont Medical Society and my wife, Joyce, met me at the door. I could tell from the look on her face that she had terribly bad news: "Dave Pollock is critically ill in Vienna."

Dave and I had been friends since college, more than forty years earlier. Our families had been very close for many years. I was his family physician and racquetball competitor for eight years when our families lived in the same community. Joyce worked as his office manager for those eight years. He had been involved in international ministry with missionary families for twenty-five years and was in Vienna to speak at a conference of Christian educators. The news was now fourth-hand, so I had to hope some of the details were wrong: sudden abdominal pain; hospitalization; gallstone blocking his bile duct causing pancreatitis; stone successfully removed; unexplained cardiac arrest thirty-six hours later; successful resuscitation, but now, another twelve hours later, Dave was unconscious, in the intensive care unit (ICU), on life support.

What a mixture of responses. The optimistic doctor in me said, "Well, since he is on a ventilator, the doctors have probably given him heavy sedation and he'll awaken when it wears off." The cautious clinical ethicist in me said, "This does not sound good. Betty Lou and their three children will probably have some difficult decisions to make in the next few days." The friend in me said, "I've got to get to Vienna."

It took about forty-eight hours for me to rearrange my schedule and get to Dave's bedside. I cried as I hugged his family and especially as I held Dave's flaccid hand. We spent the next six days praying, talking with doctors and nurses, waiting for test results. The five of us talked, reminisced, laughed, and cried. We vacillated between hope and despair. "Our God is a great God. He can do what is humanly unexplainable." "Dear God, what should we do?" "It is very, very rare for someone with this amount of brain damage after a cardiac arrest to have any meaningful recovery." "We can always hope." I shared with them Václav Havel's concept of hope: "Hope is not the conviction that things will turn out well, but the certainty that things make sense, regardless of how they turn out."[1] We began our grief process.

What was my role in this situation? As a physician I explained to Dave's family the mechanism of brain injury from lack of oxygen and how this has a much worse outlook than brain injury from trauma. I was the intermediary and spokesperson between the family and the intensive care team and the neurologist. As a clinical ethicist I talked with the family about Dave's personal values and previous conversations about his wishes in the event of overwhelming illness. He had clearly and repeatedly said he did not want to survive with the aid of machines or tubes if he would be permanently unable to interact with his loved ones. I also helped them understand how medical decision making was somewhat different in Europe than in the United States. As a friend I kept denying this was really happening, hoping I would awaken from this horrible dream at any moment.

Of the nearly fifteen hundred ethics consultations I have been involved with in my second career as a clinical ethicist, this was the most difficult. Knowing I was so emotionally involved that objectivity would be difficult, I alerted my closest professional colleague before I left Vermont that I would probably be on the phone asking for his help.

At the same time, this was one of the easiest ethics consultations I have done. The medical facts were clear and unambiguous — there was virtually no possibility that Dave would recover to a level of function he would find acceptable. He had made his personal preferences known both in writing and in conversations with his wife and each of their three children. The standards of medical ethics, though somewhat different in Austria, had fairly clear boundaries of permissible options. And the five of us standing around Dave's bed were united in one Spirit, knowing he was poised to enter God's presence.

Nine days after his cardiac arrest, he did just that. His condition deteriorated suddenly, and God made the decision the five of us were dreading. God took Dave home on Resurrection Sunday 2004.

1. Václav Havel, *Disturbing the Peace* (New York: Vintage Books, 1991).

PART I

CHAPTER 1

An Ethical Foundation

Medical ethics involves the application of moral guidance to issues that arise in the practice of medicine. Medical ethicists address issues like abortion, euthanasia, research with human subjects, cloning, access to health care, allocation of resources, and many others. Clinical ethics,[1] on the other hand, is the identification, analysis, and resolution of ethical dilemmas that arise in the care of individual patients. It is case-based rather than issue-based. But what standards do ethicists use in making recommendations, either about issues or about individual cases?

There are at least three sources for standards in medical/clinical ethics: the medical profession, theology, and law.

The oldest and most revered standards in the medical profession were set forth in the Oath of Hippocrates (ca. 450 B.C.E.). This oath was really a minority view when introduced, but over the next several centuries it, along with the other writings of Hippocrates, came to be considered *the* foundation for medical ethics, focusing primarily on physician virtue and competence. One Roman Catholic medical historian has posited that this strand of physician competence was woven with the strand of compassion taught by Jesus Christ to form the braided ethos of medicine for hundreds of years.[2] In this ethos the physician dominated the doctor-patient relationship and was expected to make decisions that were in the patient's best interest. In the second half of the twentieth century, however, this physi-

---

1. A more accurate subtitle for this book would be *Clinical Ethics and the Faith Factor.* I instead used the more familiar term "medical ethics" in the title since "clinical ethics" might not catch the eye of the reader for whom this book is intended.

2. Albert Jonsen, *The New Medicine and the Old Ethic* (Cambridge: Harvard University Press, 1992).

cian dominance was challenged and more dilemmas were encountered, raising questions about what should be done for patients.

Questions about what should be done for individual patients were first voiced by theologians in the 1960s and 1970s — questions about surgery for handicapped newborns, the use of **ventilators**, abortion. This emergence came about at this time in history for several reasons. Probably most important was the rapid advances in medical technology. Individuals began to ask, "Just because something can be done, does that mean it should be done?" Rules of conduct had to be developed and applied to new technologies. And new technology was very expensive, so huge and growing questions were raised about the cost of care and its distribution. Perhaps the most prominent early example of expensive new technology was the development of dialysis for chronic kidney failure in the 1960s. In addition, this was a period of great social upheaval in North America. Major advances were made in individual rights, minority rights, consumer rights, and even patient rights, so the trump card for medical decisions gradually seemed to pass from the physician to the patient.

During this period of early development of clinical ethics, theologians asked questions and gave opinions based on their own Catholic, Protestant, Jewish, or Islamic traditions. They helped establish some of the foundations of what came to be called contemporary clinical ethics.[3] But they did not always agree with each other. And even when they did agree, people who followed a secular instead of a theistic tradition sometimes disagreed with their conclusions.

The focus of clinical ethics gradually shifted from people who relied primarily on their faith for moral decisions to people who used primarily secular reasoning in such situations. Philosophers, attorneys, judges, experts in health policy, and others became increasingly influential and did much to solidify the emerging discipline. And of course, clinicians were part of the discussions: physicians, nurses, social workers, chaplains, and others.

When conflicts were encountered in specific cases, physicians and pa-

---

3. To help in my chosen task, scholars more familiar than I with this history have pointed out that there is broader agreement on ethics than on theology. For example, Peter Kreeft wrote in *Between Heaven and Hell* (Downers Grove, Ill.: InterVarsity, 1982), p. 111: "Now Christian ethics is not as elitist, as distinctive, as Christian theology. Love fits the egalitarian religion of the modern world much better than faith does. . . . Nearly everyone admits the claims of love, at least in principle if not in practice; but only believers admit the claims of faith."

tients occasionally turned to the court system for resolution. A body of case law slowly developed whereby legal precedents became established that could be used as guidance in future similar cases. If an individual case was decided in a local court, that decision applied only to that case. If the case was appealed to a higher court, however, the decision then set a precedent for the jurisdiction of that court. Thus a state supreme court decision would apply to future conflicts in that state; a U.S. Supreme Court decision would set precedent for the entire country.

In addition to case law established by court decisions and precedents, some issues were taken up by state legislatures. Many states constructed laws about issues like **advance directives**, brain death, organ donation, and surrogate decision-making.

Thus the legal system, both through case law and statutory law, has played a prominent role in establishing precedent and in setting boundaries for acceptable medical practice. Unfortunately, some clinicians and some families look primarily to the law for answers when they encounter specific dilemmas. But as a decisional standard, we must recognize that the law is the lowest common denominator for our society. Other standards are more nuanced and more sensitive to common morality. Alexandr Solzhenitsyn told the graduating class from Harvard in 1978: "A society that is based on the letter of the law and never reaches any higher is taking small advantage of the high level of human possibilities. The letter of the law is too cold and formal to have a beneficial influence on society. Whenever the tissue of life is woven of legalistic relations, there is an atmosphere of mediocrity, paralyzing man's noblest impulses."[4]

One of the reasons that analysis and recommendations in clinical ethics seem so "gray" is that the standard to which we appeal is often not codified, that is, it is not defined in law, but relies on common morality. One author has insightfully suggested that ethics is about "obedience to the unenforceable."[5]

Since the genesis of contemporary clinical ethics in the 1960s and 1970s, the theological voice sadly has become marginalized, ignored, or even ridiculed. People of faith must understand medical tradition and the law, but they must also be knowledgeable about standards of conduct es-

4. A. Solzhenitsyn, "A World Split Apart" (delivered June 8, 1978), reprinted in *Harvard* magazine, 1978, and available online at http://www.columbia.edu/cu/augustine/arch/ solzhenitsyn/harvard/1978.html.

5. R. M. Kidder, *How Good People Make Tough Choices* (New York: Simon and Schuster, Fireside Books, 1996), p. 66.

poused by their own tradition and limits within which they should make decisions.

In the remainder of this chapter we will look at some of the professional and legal standards that have evolved, and in chapter 2 we will look at some of the theological standards.

Principles of Medical Ethics

Some professionals who work in medical or clinical ethics focus on foundational principles. Though this is not the primary approach of this book, it is important for readers to be familiar with the terminology. It is well accepted that there are four foundational principles:

1. Nonmaleficence — from the Hippocratic writings we have retained the maxim "First of all, do no harm." This remains an important principle, though it is well recognized that virtually no treatment options are free from potentially harmful side effects.
2. Beneficence — we should do what is in the patient's **best interests**.
3. Autonomy — patients have a right to make their own decisions about medical treatment.
4. Justice — we should treat patients without favoritism or discrimination. Thus, if two patients have a similar condition, we should offer the same recommendations and treatments to them rather than giving preference to one or the other based on status or our potentially biased assessment of them.

As important as these principles are, in many situations two principles come into conflict, and the method of principlism gives no guidance on how to set priorities. For example, it is occasionally justifiable to override a patient's autonomy for the patient's benefit by treating him or her involuntarily.

In addition, other principles besides these four must be considered. Though some may be subsumed under one of these four (e.g., respect for the sanctity of life may be considered part of nonmaleficence), others are not easily categorized. For example, the concept of faithfulness is occasionally mentioned, more often in the literature of nursing ethics. This concept of continuing obligation to a specific patient is very important. Once a health-care professional takes on the professional responsibility to provide care for a patient, he or she has a continuing obligation to not abandon the patient.

Decision-Making Authority

The practice of medicine often seems like an ongoing series of decisions about what to do. Sometimes those decisions raise ethical dilemmas. Should the elderly woman with **dementia** be taken to the intensive care unit (ICU) for potentially lifesaving treatment, or not? Should the man with mental illness be hospitalized and treated over his objection, or not? Should the severely premature newborn be subjected to painful procedures that have a very small chance of saving his life, or not? Who has the authority to make the decision: the patient, or the physician, or a **surrogate** (sometimes called a proxy) for the patient?

As mentioned above, prior to the 1960s physicians were rather paternalistic, that is, they assumed or were given the authority to make major decisions. Some readers may remember Dr. Kildare and Dr. Welby from television in the 1950s and 1960s, both rather clear examples of the paternalistic physician. But in more recent times, patients have rightly claimed the authority to be involved, or even to hold the trump card, in such decisions.

Informed Consent

It is now a well-established standard that diagnostic testing may not be done and treatment may not be given without the informed consent of the patient or his or her surrogate. But this has not always been the case. For centuries, it was assumed that physicians practicing in the Anglo-American tradition would seek the consent of their patients for any intervention, but only in the last one hundred years has the concept of *informed* consent been developed. Through legal challenges to the paternalistic stance of physicians, there has gradually been constructed the legal doctrine that the physician must give adequate information to the patient about the proposed intervention prior to the patient giving consent.

Valid informed consent can occur only when a competent decision-maker (whether patient or surrogate) has been given adequate information about the decision to be made, and is allowed to make the decision voluntarily, without coercion.

7

There are, of course, emergency situations where physicians are expected to provide lifesaving treatment without prior consent, and urgent situations where there is not time to give full disclosure of "adequate information." But apart from these unusual situations, the clinician is expected to provide the following information: the reason for the intervention (whether diagnostic test or treatment); the benefits, risks, and burdens of the intervention; alternative options and their benefits, risks, and burdens; the likely outcome without the intervention; and his or her recommendation. Of course, opinions differ about what information is pertinent, or as the attorneys argue, what is "material." But after receiving this information, the patient or surrogate then decides for or against the proposed intervention.

This exercise of patient autonomy, that is, self-determination, is foundational in medicine and in clinical ethics. A physician may certainly try to persuade a reluctant patient, but in doing so must not withhold or distort information given to the patient to "convince" him or her.

Capacity and Competence

It seems intuitive when we say that the decision-maker must be competent, but in reality, application of this concept leads to many dilemmas in clinical ethics. Competence is fairly easy to define but not so easy to determine. On paper, a person is competent if he or she knows a decision must be made, understands the (adequate) information provided, and is able to use reasoning to assess that information to make a decision that is consistent with his or her values and goals.

Actually, there are two words commonly used for this concept: competence and capacity (or, **decision-making capacity**). Though often used interchangeably, they are not the same. Competence is a global concept — the person is competent or not — and is most applicable in the legal setting. A judge is most commonly the one who makes a decision about the patient's competence. Decision-making capacity, on the other hand, is a clinical concept, and it acknowledges that capacity is task-specific (e.g., a person may be capable of consenting to hospital admission but not capable of deciding about undergoing risky surgery), and it may fluctuate (e.g., a person may be capable of making a treatment decision now but may be incapable tomorrow due to changes in the clinical situation, use of drugs to treat symptoms, etc.).

Advance Directives

The term "advance directive" usually refers to a written document prepared and signed by persons with capacity, explaining to their physician and family what they want done in situations when they do not have capacity. There are other less commonly used advance directives such as video or audio recordings. Written advance directives come in two basic types, though in recent years they have often been combined into a single document.

A living will is an advance directive that reveals what kinds of treatments a person would or would not want to have in given circumstances. Most are worded to limit treatment and include several vague terms, for example, "If I am terminally ill and imminently dying with no reasonable expectation of recovery, I want to avoid burdensome life-prolonging treatment and receive only those measures directed at ensuring my comfort." Others include specific desires for treatment: all treatment necessary to sustain a life regardless of its quality. These are good statements of a person's philosophy but are seldom very helpful in making specific decisions. What did that person mean by "imminently dying" — hours, days, weeks? What is the person's understanding of a "reasonable expectation of recovery" — 20 percent, 10 percent, 5 percent? What would the person consider burdensome? In an attempt to be more precise, some people include specific instructions: no resuscitation, no ventilator, no dialysis, etc. Written statements for full treatment are usually less ambiguous than are those for **limitation of treatment**.

The primary problem with living will–type advance directives is that the condition encountered is often not included in the wording. Or the person may refuse an option while writing about a theoretical situation that, in fact, the person might accept when faced with the reality of that situation. For example, many patients say they wouldn't want to be on a "breathing machine" (ventilator). But when asked if they were to develop a severe pneumonia leading to respiratory failure, and the physician felt that use of a ventilator for two to five days would allow antibiotics to clear the pneumonia so that they could return to the same status as before the pneumonia, many say, "Well, of course I would want the ventilator then!" What they had envisioned when they wrote that they did not want to be on a ventilator was long-term ventilator support.

The other type of advance directive is the durable power of attorney for health care, sometimes called a proxy document. In this type the person designates someone he or she would trust to make treatment decisions if the patient should lose capacity. The person writing the document is usually called the principal, and the person designated to make the decisions is referred to as the principal's **agent**. In addition to naming the agent, the principal may or may not give other written instructions about treatment wishes. In fact, probably more important than signing the document is the actual conversation between the patient and the agent. Does the decision-maker appointed understand the personal and/or religious values that might guide such decisions? Does the agent know whether the patient would want resuscitation, and if so in what circumstances?

Though the concept of advance directives is supported by most clinicians, patients, clergy, and others, only about 20 percent of the North American adult population has signed such a form. Failure to do so is often due to denial of or unwillingness to contemplate future serious medical events, or sometimes to a discomfort with the formal legal nature of the document.

Surrogacy

When a patient lacks the capacity to make a treatment decision, informed consent is still required, but it must be given by a surrogate or proxy. If the patient has named an agent in a durable power of attorney for health care, that person has nearly the same authority as the patient. However, for the 80 percent of adults who do not have an advance directive, for most adults with developmental disability, and for most children, the clinician must identify the appropriate surrogate decision-maker.

By tradition, clinicians have granted this surrogacy to the "next of kin." This most often means a spouse, parents of a child, adult children of elderly patients, etc. However, the concept of next of kin is most often not explicitly defined. The idea is that the person who knows the patient best, and is familiar with his or her values or wishes, is in the best position to make decisions that would be consistent with what the patient would choose if he or she were able. Sadly, but not surprisingly, research has shown that the performance record of such surrogates is poor, minimally better than chance.

Some states have passed surrogacy laws that set out a hierarchy of individuals, based on relationship, who have the legal authority to make decisions for an individual who has lost capacity and has left no written instructions. This is sometimes helpful, but on occasion the person who appears at the top of the hierarchy doesn't know the patient's values or even has another agenda. There is quite often a more appropriate surrogate than the one legally designated.

Standards Used for Surrogate Decision-Making

Once a surrogate is identified, whether as a designated agent, as a state-authorized surrogate, or as next of kin, he or she is expected to use **substituted judgment** in reaching a decision. Some people misunderstand this concept and think the surrogate is to substitute his or her judgment for that of the patient. Rather, it means the surrogate is to substitute a process to arrive at the decision that the patient would make, based on the patient's written or verbal expressed wishes, or an understanding of his or her values. Without being familiar with the term "substituted judgment," the wife of a man who had experienced a devastating stroke articulated the concept clearly when she said, "If it were my choice, I would want him to stay alive in the ICU or nursing home for as long as possible, even if he couldn't recognize anyone or do anything for himself. But I know that he would not want to live like that. He would want to stop the ventilator and accept the fact that he will not survive."

Only when there is no way to identify the patient's wishes or values do we drop to the lower best interest standard. When we have no personal guidance, we try to make decisions that are in the best interest of the patient, recognizing that this is a very poor substitute. In using this approach, we try to determine the benefits and burdens of the proposal and assess what most people would choose in this circumstance. The name given to this standard, "best interests," sounds lofty and noble. However, we must recognize that it is the lowest standard we use.

Limitation of Treatment (Including Do-Not-Resuscitate Orders)

Between two-thirds and three-fourths of discussions in clinical ethics are about limitation of treatment. In the not too distant past, professionals and laypersons alike believed that if a treatment was available, it should be used. Beginning in the mid-1970s, it became evident that many treatments could postpone death but some were only "partial cures." Often patients were saved from death but left in a condition from which they could not recover, dependent on some type of technology for continued life (ventilator, dialysis, feeding tube, etc.). In addition, some patients chose not to use burdensome treatments (e.g., chemotherapy) that offered some percentage chance of postponing death but also reduced the patient's quality of life during that life extension, preferring instead to live for a shorter period with a better quality of life.

The Karen Quinlan case was the first publicly aired discussion about limitation of treatment.[6] She was permanently unresponsive (in a **persistent vegetative state**) and was thought to be dependent on a ventilator. Her family wanted to stop the ventilator, but her doctors were unwilling to do so, fearing she would die and they would be culpable for causing her death. After years of court battles the Supreme Court of New Jersey determined in 1976 that it was permissible to stop her ventilator, even if that meant she would die. In fact, she survived another ten years after her doctors slowly decreased her ventilator settings and eventually removed it. But the precedent was established that it is sometimes permissible to stop what appears to be life-prolonging treatment when it is clear that the patient would not want it.

Subsequent legal cases made similar determinations about **cardiopulmonary resuscitation**, dialysis, intravenous fluids, feeding tubes, etc. These court cases are often referred to as "right to die" cases. This is misleading. There is no global right to die. There is a right to refuse treatment, a right to be left alone. This is referred to in philosophical circles as a negative right. But that does not mean there is a corresponding positive right to be made dead; that is, there is no such entitlement to death. If there were such a positive right to die, then it would logically follow that others would have a duty to help a person die. This is clearly not the case.

When a decision has been made by a physician and a patient about limitation of treatment, it is important that other individuals involved in the care of the patient are aware of this. The most commonly encountered situation is when a decision has been made to not use cardiopulmonary resuscitation. This information is most often documented by a **do-not-resuscitate order** (DNR order). This DNR order may be written in the patient's chart in the hospital or nursing home, or inscribed on a bracelet worn by the patient. Other limitation of treatment orders include: do-not-intubate (DNI, indicating a decision to not use ventilatory assistance to

---

6. In the matter of Karen Quinlan, see 70 N.J. 10, 335 A. 2d 647 (1976).

help a person breathe) and do-not-transfer, that is, don't move the patient to a higher level of care, say, from nursing home to hospital, or from the hospital ward to the ICU.

Palliative Care and Hospice

As these value-based decisions became clearer, a new medical specialty arose. The hospice movement focused on whole-person care for patients confronting death, including not only the many physical symptoms[7] but also psychological issues (depression, anxiety), social issues (loneliness, unfinished business), and spiritual concerns (guilt, doubt, need for forgiveness). This movement began in the 1970s in Great Britain under the direction of the founder, Dame Cecily Saunders, then moved to Canada and eventually to the United States.

The earliest hospices began as a parallel group to the medical profession, and occasionally faced resistance. Gradually their great benefits to patients, families, and professionals became evident, and the field expanded into the more formal medical specialty of **palliative care**. Palliative care services are a bit different from the original hospice movement in that the latter is clearly focused on patients at the end of life (generally less than six months prognosis) who are no longer receiving potentially curative treatment, whereas palliative care includes offering services to patients with incurable chronic conditions who may live for some time and/or to patients who are terminally ill but still receiving curative treatments.

Uncertainty

Part of the dilemma, of course, is that we often do not know and cannot tell in advance whether a treatment will work or not. We can get some statistical guidance from evidence-based medicine, but statistics will not tell us what will happen in a particular case. Thus decisions often must be made under the cloud of uncertainty, both clinical and moral uncertainty.

7. Though pain and shortness of breath are the symptoms of greatest concern for patients and families, a host of other symptoms should be addressed in a person with chronic or fatal illness, including nausea, vomiting, constipation, diarrhea, hiccups, cough, dry mouth, urinary difficulties, weakness, fatigue, insomnia, and agitation.

Here we must follow the admonition of theologian Lewis Smedes: "When you can't be certain, be responsible."[8] We must make the best decision we can, given the information we have.

Patients I refer to as "hospice alumni" provide a striking example of clinical uncertainty. The entry criterion for hospice services is generally a prognosis of six months or less to live. And it is generally possible to renew the eligibility of those who outlive this estimate. In addition, many physicians drag their feet and are reluctant to refer patients to hospice until they are in their very last days of life. In spite of this, about 13 percent of patients referred to hospice in the United States each year are discharged because they didn't die.[9]

Another part of the uncertainty dilemma focuses on what it means when we say a treatment "works" or "doesn't work." This leads us into the discussion of **futility**.

Futility

It has become a truism in medicine that there is no obligation for a physician to provide futile treatment. However, the concept of futility is difficult and imprecise. I use the term in its original sense: it will not work, period; that is, it will not have a physiological effect. Some interpret "will not work" to mean will not have a beneficial effect, and they may mean the ventilator or dialysis machine might postpone death, but since the patient is severely cognitively impaired, it will not benefit him or her. In using "futility" in this way, the person has introduced a value judgment, almost always using his or her own values. Still others interpret the term in a quantitative way. They may mean a treatment is futile if there is a 99 percent chance it will not work. Others might set the definition at 95 percent or 90 percent or even lower. Thus, even this quantitative interpretation of futility implies use of personal values. The term "futility" is difficult and somewhat nebulous because it is used differently by different individuals, and it often includes a judgment of value.

My primary concern in the use of futility is that it sometimes becomes

8. L. Smedes, *Choices: Making Right Decisions in a Complex World* (New York: HarperCollins, 1991).

9. A humorous personal experience is documented in Art Buchwald's book, *Too Soon to Say Goodbye* (New York: Random House, 2006).

the physician's trump card. He or she can say, "That treatment is futile, therefore I don't have to provide it." This ends the discussion. Don't get me wrong. I believe there are treatments that are futile, and I believe a physician must have the prerogative to say, "I will not provide futile treatment." However, I think we need to guard against the situation where the physician (or nurse, or other clinician) says "it's futile" when in fact he or she means "I don't think it's a good idea."

Withholding versus Withdrawing Treatment

A generation ago physicians were taught that it was better to withhold a treatment than to withdraw it. The thinking was that if a patient was being maintained on a treatment, it must be continued. If the physician decided to withdraw the treatment and the patient died as a result, the physician bore some responsibility for the death. Thus physicians were often reluctant to begin a treatment if there was very little likelihood that it would work. But as more technologies were developed that had the potential to postpone death but leave the patient "half-cured," this concept has been refined.

The Quinlan decision, as well as being the first public discussion of the issue of limitation of treatment, set a precedent that some treatments that could sustain life became optional in some circumstances.

Further discussion among theologians, philosophers, and clinicians helped solidify the concept that there is no difference in these two actions. In fact, it is now understood that it is ethically better to try a treatment that has a very high chance of not working and then to withdraw it when it is completely clear that it will not work. Withholding it in the first place would have missed those few patients in whom it might have worked.

Conflict

Given the complexity of decisions to be made and the vagaries of capacity and surrogacy, differences of opinion are inevitable. There may be differences of opinion between patient and physician, between patient and family, between two or more family members, between physician and nurse, between primary physician and specialist, and the list goes on. Most often these differences of opinion can be worked out through direct discussion, sometimes by soliciting another opinion from another specialist, sometimes by mediation. Rarely, it is necessary to go to court for guidance about who has the final authority to make decisions.

When there is conflict regarding a treatment decision, it is tempting to think that someone is right and everyone else is wrong. In a few cases the ethical issue is between right and wrong. It is wrong to take an action that has the intention of ending a patient's life, for example (see Case 11.01). However, in the vast majority of cases presenting for ethics consultation, the conflict is between right and right; that is, two (or more) options are available, neither is clearly wrong of and by itself, and the decision-makers have to decide which option is better in this particular case. One of the aims of the ethics consultant is to draw some boundaries, indicating that options A, B, and C are "ethically permissible" but options D and E are outside the boundaries of acceptable medical practice, that is, they are "wrong."

In many of these cases of right versus right, it is possible to determine that "in this case" a certain action may be impermissible when, in another situation, it might be permissible. For example, not using a feeding tube in Case 6.03 was felt to be impermissible because it would be contrary to our understanding of the patient's values. But in Case 6.04 it was felt to be permissible to forgo a feeding tube because that was consistent with the patient's wishes and values.

In some circumstances the decision about permissibility versus impermissibility may be based on the intention, rather than on the action. For example, in Case 8.02 it was determined to be impermissible to limit treatment based on the family's perception that the patient had a poor quality of life, though it would be permissible to limit treatment based on a poor prognosis.

Sometimes conflict seems particularly acute when professionals recommend withdrawal of life-sustaining treatment. They may have been thinking about it for a few days, seeing the patient either not improving or actually deteriorating. But they approach the family at a specific time to recommend stopping the ventilator (or other means of life support), and the family is not prepared. Even if they have been updated on the patient's condition, even if they have heard the words, they may have not let themselves consider the option of changing goals from survival to comfort. It may require some time; it may require setting some short-term intermediate goals for them to be convinced that it is time; it may require significant support from the clinicians, social worker, chaplain, or personal clergy.

Please refer to appendix 2 for a listing of cases in this book that address the following issues raised above: advance directives, patient autonomy, capacity and competence, conflict, futility, informed consent, substituted judgment, surrogacy, uncertainty, withholding and withdrawal of treatment.

Conflicts often arise because of different perspectives, different experiences, different relationships, different emotions, or different loyalties. But the conflicts that seem to generate the most intense discussion are those based on different cultural values or religious beliefs. These conflicts are sufficiently unique and important that we will devote a full chapter to them. Please refer to part III, chapter 9 for discussion and cases that address this critically important issue.

Ethics Committees and Consultants

Differences of opinion sometimes lead the clinicians or the family to request an ethics consultation. This service is relatively new in medicine. Hospitals began to form ethics committees in the late 1970s and early 1980s. Roman Catholic hospitals were in the forefront of this activity, developing Medical Morals Committees.

Ethics committees originally had three functions: education, policy review, and case consultation. Many hospitals found the process of consultation by committee too cumbersome because it was too difficult to gather the fifteen or twenty members in a timely fashion. In addition, clinicians often found the process intimidating, resembling a court proceeding, and were thus reluctant to seek help from such a committee.[10] As a result, a large number of hospitals chose to provide case consultation using a subcommittee format. Using this method, two, three, or four committee members, usually from different disciplines, go to the patient unit, review the chart and speak with relevant individuals, and render an opinion.

The next step in the development of ethics consultation was that some hospitals, particularly larger hospitals, hired individuals to teach ethics and provide ethics consultations. Some were clinicians with additional

10. Before my arrival at Loma Linda University Medical Center in 1990 to establish an ethics consultation service, such consultations were done by the entire ethics committee, and they provided from two to four consultations per year. Within a few months of a changed format to consultations by an individual ethics consultant, we provided an average of two consultations per week.

training in ethics; others were individuals whose primary training was in philosophy or theology who had developed an interest in the medical arena. Because of the diversity in training and preparation for ethics consultants, no credentialing process has yet been established. However, the American Society for Bioethics and Humanities has developed a forty-page booklet[11] to help hospitals as they search for qualified and competent clinical ethicists.

Hospital Environment

Individuals who only infrequently enter the hospital setting may find things confusing, primarily because of the many professionals involved in caring for patients with complex problems. In some settings, especially smaller hospitals, the patient's primary physician is in charge of the patient's care, which is provided with the help of consultants, nurses, social workers, chaplains, and patient representatives.

Many hospitals are moving to a "hospitalist" system in which some physicians work only in the hospital and care for a larger number of patients who have been referred by their primary physician. This offers a number of increased efficiencies, but the trade-off is the lack of familiarity with the person and his or her values, and the absence of a longer-term relationship. This hospitalist system may be in place in small or large hospitals.

In teaching hospitals, many of which are fairly large, even more professionals may be involved in patient care. While the patient will always have one physician (called the attending physician) who is responsible for his or her care, most of the bedside work will be done by physicians in training (i.e., residents and interns). Medical students may also be part of the team. And there may be several nurses on different shifts, as well as nursing students. One of the frustrations for families in these settings is knowing with whom to talk. This is exacerbated by the fact that these training teams rotate frequently, sometimes monthly, and in other settings even more often.

Often dilemmas that present as ethics consultations come about merely as the result of lack of sufficient communication between pertinent individuals. And thus the resolution may entail gathering those people to-

11. American Society for Bioethics and Humanities, *Core Competencies for Health Care Ethics Consultation* (Glenview, Ill.: ASBH, 1998). Available for purchase at www.asbh.org.

gether in the same room at the same time to listen to each other. But alas, not all dilemmas can be resolved this simply. In this book we will look at dozens of cases that resulted in clinical ethics consultations. Some merely required better communication; others presented significant dilemmas, the resolution of which required an understanding of the concepts and precedents outlined in this chapter; still others involved differences in religious belief.

Precedents in Clinical Ethics

To the reader unfamiliar with clinical ethics, the information presented in the case discussions may appear confusing or arbitrary. There are, however, some reasonably well established precedents that can give guidance. Some have been outlined in this chapter. Some will be further elucidated in case discussions.

My colleague, Dr. Robert Macauley, has developed a flow chart for teaching medical students that includes several such precedents, and he has allowed me to use this chart in this book (see page 21). On first view it appears overwhelmingly confusing, but on closer inspection it is fairly easy to follow. For example, starting at the top of the chart, if the patient and the treating physician (or team) agree, and the patient has decision-making capacity (DMC), there is no ethical dilemma, and treatment may proceed. If they disagree, or even if they agree but it is not clear if the patient has DMC, there is a series of steps to follow that involves an assessment of the patient's capacity, the use of an advance directive, the recognition of the authority of a surrogate, and possibly even overriding the patient. This is not presented as a way to arrive at "the answer," but as a tool to help follow the reasoning presented in specific case discussions.

*   *   *

References on the Ethical Foundation of Medicine

American Medical Association's Council on Ethical and Judicial Affairs. *Code of Medical Ethics, 2004-2005: Current Opinions with Annotations.* Chicago: American Medical Association, 2005.

Beauchamp, T., and J. Childress. *Principles of Biomedical Ethics.* 5th ed. Oxford: Oxford University Press, 2001.

Campbell, A., G. Gillett, and G. Jones. *Medical Ethics*. 3rd ed. Oxford: Oxford University Press, 2001.

Engelhardt, H. T. *The Foundations of Bioethics*. 2nd ed. New York: Oxford University Press, 1996.

Gert, B. *Bioethics*. 2nd ed. Oxford: Oxford University Press, 2006.

Jonsen, A. R., M. Siegler, and W. J. Winslade. *Clinical Ethics*. 6th ed. New York: McGraw-Hill, 2006.

Lo, B. *Resolving Ethical Dilemmas: A Guide for Clinicians*. 3rd ed. Philadelphia: Lippincott Williams and Wilkins, 2005.

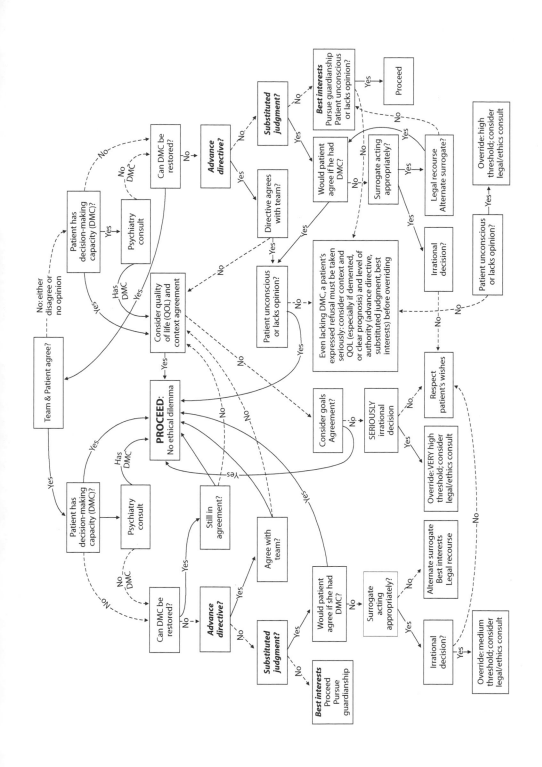

CHAPTER 2

A Theological Foundation

Writing this chapter seems like an exercise in hubris — a nontheologian trying to demonstrate to readers, many of whom may have far more theological training and expertise than he, that contemporary clinical ethics has a unifying theological foundation. Certainly there are many books on this topic already, some of which are listed at the end of this chapter. I would encourage you, the reader, to explore those that come from your own theological tradition.

But I am going to try to do more than that. I hope to show that the three monotheistic faith traditions — Judaism, Christianity, and Islam — share some basic theological beliefs that are foundational for our thinking about these clinical issues. This should help to focus our understanding of how this basic theological approach differs from the nontheistic worldview that is so common in contemporary clinical ethics. This is perhaps an example of extreme hubris.

I got the idea and the courage to undertake this daunting task while speaking at a conference at West Virginia University in Morgantown in 1994. The title of the conference was "The Spiritual Dimension of Illness, Suffering, and Dying." Leaders in medical ethics from these three monotheistic faith traditions were invited to share their perspectives on issues at the end of life. I left the conference exhilarated because I came to realize that more foundational elements unite us than divide us. What a breath of fresh air!

I suspect that my own Christian tradition will be visible between the lines here, but my intent is not to be a Christian apologist or an evangelist. Rather, I hope to show that in spite of significant differences in our understanding of our relationship with and obligations to the Divine, we share some fundamental beliefs about who we are and how we should care for each other.

I have patterned the outline for this chapter and borrowed some of the content for it from the small book that came out of a 2004 Lausanne Forum in Thailand, *Bioethics: Obstacle or Opportunity for the Gospel?*[1] While this small treatise comes from a Christian perspective, the points I have chosen to underline here are generally consistent with my understanding of Judaism and Islam in many regards.

What Does It Mean to Be Human?

People of faith believe that a divine Being — Yahweh, God, or Allah — created the heavens and the earth, and specifically that he created humankind in his own image, the ***imago Dei***. We may differ on our understanding of that concept, and I don't pretend to know exactly what it means. But it does seem clear that God views created humans as different from the rest of creation. We have been given stewardship over the rest of his creation, and we are able to be in relationship with him.

A secular worldview does not, of course, consider the *imago Dei*, but rather focuses on personhood. Proposed criteria for personhood have varied over the past few decades, from the fourteen characteristics of neocortical function proposed by Joseph Fletcher[2] to the single concept of self-awareness espoused by Michael Tooley.[3] This leads to the difficulty of defining which humans are persons and which are not, which deserve protection and care and which do not. It may even allow some nonhumans to be considered persons.

The Sanctity of Human Life

The *imago Dei* present in each human is a gift from a loving divine Creator. He considers human life to be set apart from the remainder of creation, to be sacred. And because of this, he has enjoined us not to shed the blood of

---

1. *Bioethics: Obstacle or Opportunity for the Gospel?* ed. R. Chia et al., Lausanne Occasional Paper no. 58, Lausanne Committee for World Evangelism (2005).

2. Joseph Fletcher, *Humanhood: Essays in Biomedical Ethics* (New York: Prometheus Books, 1979).

3. Michael Tooley, *Abortion and Infanticide* (Oxford: Clarendon, 1983).

innocent human beings. Further, his love is extended especially to the weak and vulnerable, implying that we, too, as bearers of his image, should offer protection and care to the sick, the disabled, the very young, and the aged.

It is interesting and noteworthy that the concept of the sanctity of human life is not absent from a secular worldview. The term is often used in a nontheistic context to indicate the value of human life. In my way of thinking, it is difficult to explain the genesis of this understanding without invoking the creation narrative. In fact, some discussants of medical ethics from an atheistic perspective recognize this difficulty. For example, Peter Singer calls the unwavering protection of human life "speciesism," and he asserts that "progress" will not be made in the public policy arena (e.g., on issues like euthanasia) until the notion of the sanctity of human life is eliminated.[4]

The Fall, Suffering, and Death

For centuries, philosophers and theologians have struggled to explain the presence of evil, suffering, and death in a world created by a loving and merciful God. My simple understanding is that it was not intended, but was permitted by God.

God created humans in his own image, placed them in an idyllic setting, and gave them dominion over his creation. But the prospect of being like God proved to be too tantalizing; temptation gave way to sin. Adam and Eve disobeyed God. This resulted in punishment from God — the necessity to work by the sweat of one's brow, the pain of childbirth, and the prospect of sickness, suffering, and death. Thus the theistic worldview includes not only the sanctity of human life but also the finitude of human life.

Suffering is allowed by God. It is not without purpose, however. Even though some suffer in vain, that is not God's purpose. Occasionally suffering is corrective, that is, as C. S. Lewis says, pain is God's megaphone, a way to get our attention. Suffering may be developmental, to help us grow toward maturity, to make us more like Christ, or to draw us closer to him. He may allow suffering to bring glory to himself. People of faith may be able to intellectually accept these statements of purpose in suffering, but let's face it, no one likes to suffer.

4. Peter Singer, "The Sanctity of Life," *Foreign Policy,* September-October 2005; available at http:www.utilitarian.net/singer/by/200509 — .htm.

In contrast, the secular worldview almost always sees suffering as bad — and it is. Though some may see some benefit in suffering ("no pain, no gain"), the majority of secularists seek to eliminate all suffering. I believe the relief of suffering is noble, and in fact is part of the calling of the ministry of healing. At the same time, we must recognize that sometimes our efforts will be inadequate. Most people of faith believe there is a limit here. In the process of relieving suffering, we are not allowed to destroy human life.

The Quality of Life

The concept of the sanctity of human life is inviolable from a theistic perspective. But what's all this talk about quality of life? Many people of faith get hives whenever the phrase is mentioned. But because the fall of humankind brought suffering and death into the world, we must admit that individual human lives have varying quality. Some have limited functional or intellectual capacities. Some have chronic pain or suffering. In spite of this, each individual human life is of inestimable worth because each bears the image of God.

It is very appropriate to be wary of discussions about quality of life. Secular ethicists often use quality of life as the yardstick to determine whether an individual's life should be preserved. They may espouse that someone who is severely demented, or is severely developmentally delayed, or has sustained severe brain damage, has such a poor quality of life that society has no obligation to protect or even preserve that life.

One thing I think we can all agree on, however, is that an individual's quality of life is a subjective determination that only he or she can make. Repeated studies have shown that both professional and personal caregivers underestimate the quality of life perceived by the patient.

For some theists, sanctity of life always trumps quality of life. This leads to what is called a vitalist stance — if it is possible to preserve life, it must be done, regardless of its quality. However, we must first recognize that human life is finite. In addition, human lives have varying quality. One of the pressing questions before us as we contemplate dilemmas in clinical ethics is to try to determine when the quality of life is so low that there is no moral obligation to preserve that finite life. I suspect we will not all agree on where that line should be drawn, but let us at least accept that we must try to draw the line.

The Ministry of Health Care and the Hope of Eternity

Divine love, mercy, and compassion dictate that we, the bearers of God's image, should reach out to care for those who are ill and suffering. We should try to prevent and alleviate the ills of the fallen world. At the same time, we must realize the limits of our current situation. We will not be able to eliminate suffering and death. We still have to deal with terminal illness and death, and do it as compassionately as we can. But almost all theistic faith traditions believe in an eternity with the Divine, free from suffering and death. The pathway and requirements vary, but the faithful can joyously look forward to paradise.

Many people in health care and clinical ethics, even those who do not personally hold a theistic worldview, respect these beliefs when expressed by patients or families. Not infrequently, however, differences of belief system will lead to conflicts, often dealing with moral obligations or with hoped-for supernatural intervention in natural events.

Miracles

All three of the monotheistic faith traditions support a belief in divine supernatural intervention in the course of human lives. Specific instances of miracles are recorded in their respective sacred scriptures. But do miracles still occur today? Some say yes, and some say no.

Unfortunately, the words "miracle" and "miraculous" are often trivialized so that phenomenal recovery from a serious illness or injury or the use of a powerful new drug is often incorrectly made to sound like a supernatural intervention. Such occurrences may be the wonderful application of medical knowledge, brought about by the diligent use of human intelligence, and allowed by providential grace, but they do not qualify as miraculous unless they truly defy human logic. Even this qualifier is suspect since human logic is admittedly limited and imperfect.

How does the health-care professional respond when a patient, or more often a family member, requests that treatment be continued — treatment felt to be inappropriate by the professional — because the family is praying for and expecting a miracle? Should the response be different if the professional is also a person of faith?

A belief in miracles need not cripple the practice of medicine, nor even have a major impact on our decisions. A colleague once said to me,

"God is not ventilator-dependent." The implication is that the patient's life may be dependent on the use of external support, but God's omnipotence and sovereignty are greater than that. If he decides that an individual should go on living, in spite of life-threatening illness and dependence on human technology, then he is able to intervene in a supernatural way — without our help. This line of reasoning may or may not give some solace to family members. It does not, however, satisfy those few who believe that God will not perform a miracle unless that praying individual has sufficient faith to continue human efforts awaiting God's intervention.

God Is Sovereign, but Humans Have Dominion and Are Stewards

Most individuals coming from a theistic worldview believe that God is omniscient and omnipotent. Translated into the realm of clinical ethics, this would mean that he ultimately determines whether an individual lives or dies. Different traditions vary on the human component here. This raises the issues of dominion and stewardship.

The fact that God gave dominion to humankind implies his sanction of the scientific enterprise including medical care, research, and the development of medical technology. But the balancing tenet of stewardship implies that we are responsible and accountable for how we use our knowledge and technology. We have liberty, but only within the moral boundaries established by the Divine.

Even those in medical ethics who do not seek the will of God recognize boundaries. They often say, "The ability to act does not justify the action." And they seek other guidance to determine where those boundaries are or should be, for example, the accepted principles of beneficence (doing good), nonmaleficence (doing no harm), and justice (treating people without discrimination). But far and away the dominant principle in secular medical ethics today is autonomy, the patient's right to self-determination. Deferring to the will of the individual rather than to the will of God allows the acceptance of some decisions/procedures that are disallowed by consideration of the other theological concepts and precepts outlined above. For example, relying on parental autonomy might be seen by some to justify termination of a pregnancy because it has been discovered that the developing fetus has **Down syndrome**, whereas relying on the theological concept of the *imago Dei* would be seen by most to preclude such a decision.

Justice

Justice is a complicated issue with many perspectives and nuances. But for the sake of this discussion, let us define justice as getting what we deserve. Many faith traditions include a concept of deserved punishment for those who do not seek God's will or follow his commands. In the Christian tradition, we look beyond justice to God's mercy (not getting what we deserve) and his grace (getting what we do not deserve) for those who have sought and found personal redemption.

From a secular worldview, justice means treating equals equally, without discrimination. This is certainly consistent with theistic teaching. But this view of justice often goes on to focus on the protection of personal autonomy, and as we have discussed above, the predominance of autonomy is antithetical to a theistic worldview.

With these fundamental theistic precepts in mind, let's begin the walk through muddy water. Let's look at some ethical dilemmas encountered by patients, families, and health-care professionals, and try to apply some of the foundational principles of clinical ethics and theology.

*　　*　　*

References on the Theological Foundation of Medical/Clinical Ethics

Ashley, B. M., J. deBlois, and K. D. O'Rourke. *Healthcare Ethics: A Catholic Theological Analysis.* 5th ed. St. Louis: Catholic Health Association, 2006.

Brockopp, Jonathan E., ed. *Islamic Ethics of Life: Abortion, War, and Euthanasia.* Columbia: University of South Carolina Press, 2003.

Cahill, L. S. *Theological Bioethics.* Washington, D.C.: Georgetown University Press, 2005.

Davis, J. J. *Evangelical Ethics: Issues Facing the Church Today.* 3rd ed. Phillipsburg, N.J.: Presbyterian and Reformed, 2004.

Dorff, E. N. *Matters of Life and Death: A Jewish Approach to Modern Medical Ethics.* Philadelphia: Jewish Publication Society, 2004.

Feldman, D. M. *Health and Medicine in the Jewish Tradition.* New York: Crossroad, 1986.

Harakas, S. S. *Health and Medicine in the Eastern Orthodox Tradition.* New York: Crossroad, 1990.

Hathout, Hassan. "Medical Ethics: An Islamic Point of View." Available at http://ww.islamonline.net.

Jakobovits, I. *Jewish Medical Ethics: A Comparative and Historical Study of the Jewish Religious Attitude to Medicine and Its Practice.* New York: Bloch, 1975.

Kilner, J. F. *Life on the Line: Ethics, Aging, Ending Patients' Lives, and Allocating Vital Resources.* Grand Rapids: Eerdmans, 1992.

Lammers, S. E., and A. Verhey, eds. *On Moral Medicine: Theological Perspectives in Medical Ethics.* 2nd ed. Grand Rapids: Eerdmans, 1998.

Meier, L. *Jewish Values in Health and Medicine.* New York: University Press of America, 1991.

Meileander, G. *Bioethics: A Primer for Christians.* 2nd ed. Grand Rapids: Eerdmans, 2005.

Organization for Islamic Learning. "Encyclopedia of Bioethics: Islam." Available at http://www.islamiclearning.org. See other articles on this Web site.

O'Rourke, K. D., and P. Boyle. *Medical Ethics: Sources of Catholic Teachings.* Washington, D.C.: Georgetown University Press, 1999.

Rahman, F. *Health and Medicine in the Islamic Tradition: Change and Identity.* New York: Crossroad, 1987.

Steinberg, A., and F. Rosner. *Encyclopedia of Jewish Medical Ethics.* Jerusalem: Feldheim Publishers, 2003.

PART II

CHAPTER 3

Ethical Issues in Heart Failure

Not that long ago, a person died when his or her heart stopped. But in the middle of the twentieth century, researchers realized that this was merely "pump failure," commonly called a cardiac arrest.[1] Sometimes the pump failed because the heart muscle's intrinsic electrical stimulus stopped, and the heart stopped its rhythmic contracting. This is called **asystole** (systole is the name for contraction of the heart muscle). At other times, however, the pump suddenly failed to produce effective cardiac output because the muscle was overstimulated by erratic and uncoordinated electrical activity. This is called **ventricular fibrillation**. In either case, there is no cardiac output, no circulation of blood to the brain or other organs, and in just a few minutes the organs and tissues begin to experience death from lack of oxygen.

Closed-chest **cardiopulmonary resuscitation** (CPR) was introduced in 1960 as a method that could sustain the circulation for a time. This mechanical pumping was merely a temporary measure to be used while it was determined whether anything could be done to restore the heart's intrinsic contractions, for example, by applying an electrical shock to try to disrupt the uncoordinated ventricular fibrillation or by giving drugs to correct other causes of loss of function.

CPR was used initially only for cardiology patients (e.g., those being monitored after a heart attack) or for cardiac surgery patients. Soon it was recognized that cardiac arrest was merely a sign of some underlying prob-

---

1. Cardiac arrest needs to be distinguished from congestive heart failure, sometimes called "heart failure." Cardiac arrest is sudden. Congestive heart failure is chronic and may go on for years. In this chronic heart failure, the heart muscle is weak; it continues to pump, but at a reduced capacity, resulting in weakness, shortness of breath, and swelling of the ankles.

lem, whether of cardiac or noncardiac origin (e.g., lack of oxygen, **sepsis**, electrolyte imbalance). With this recognition, "crash carts" began to appear throughout hospitals so doctors and nurses would have all the equipment and medications at hand, and "code 99's" were called rather regularly when a patient had a cardiac arrest.

At that time in history, there was a heavy burden on bedside health-care professionals, nurses in particular, to make a snap judgment whenever they found a patient who had "arrested." Should they call a code or not? It was recognized early on that delayed CPR was automatically failed CPR — if not used in the first few minutes, it will not work, or worse by most assessments, it will restore circulation, allowing survival, but with residual brain damage from lack of oxygen. There is not time to think about whether it should be used or not; no time for discussion, collaboration, or consultation. Frequently, nurses and house staff (physicians in training) developed a system of anticipating this question and documenting (or more often not documenting) a decision that some patients would not receive CPR.

This dilemma of uncertainty began to be resolved in the United States in the late 1970s when many hospitals adopted policies stating "Call a code for every patient found in cardiac arrest unless there is a **do-not-resuscitate order** (DNR order) written in the chart." This shift received judicial support in 1982 when a court sanctioned a hospital in Queens, New York, for using purple adhesive dots on the nursing chart to signify a covert DNR decision by the professionals. The default for in-hospital CPR quickly spread nationwide, and in 1988 the Joint Commission on Accreditation of Healthcare Organizations[2] required a DNR policy for hospital accreditation.

At about the same time, CPR began moving outside the hospital so that paramedics and, later, laypersons were trained in the technique. Though successful CPR in the out-of-hospital setting was quite uncommon, the few dramatic successes encouraged wider usage. The American Heart Association (AHA) developed protocols for training and for providing CPR. Soon the AHA also adopted a policy of always using CPR, except in very narrowly defined circumstances (e.g., decapitation, rigor mortis). DNR orders for patients living at home (often called "prehospital DNR orders") began to appear in the late 1980s, and are used for some terminally

---

2. The Joint Commission on Accreditation of Healthcare Organizations (JCAHO) is a national assessment and accreditation organization for hospitals and other medical organizations. It focuses on patient safety and quality of care. JCAHO accreditation is required for a hospital to receive a payment from Medicare.

ill patients once a decision is made by the patient (or family) and physician. This allows these families to call 911 for assistance in crisis but tells the paramedics to use comfort measures but not CPR. Currently, over thirty-five states have laws or regulations authorizing prehospital DNR orders.

CPR is unique in that it is an aggressive, invasive treatment that, because of its emergent nature, is given without patient consent. In fact, as per the above history, our society has established a presumption for CPR. This is understandable but somewhat surprising since this unconsented treatment has many possible bad side effects in 20-25 percent of "successful" cases, including broken ribs, punctured lungs, **aspiration** of stomach contents, ruptured abdominal organs, electrical burns, and perhaps worst of all, survival with brain damage from lack of oxygen during the period of arrest (see Cases 7.06, 7.07).

Not only that, but the "success" may be temporary. Though nearly 40 percent of patients currently survive CPR when provided in the hospital, fewer than 30 percent of the total survive the next twenty-four hours, and about 15 percent of the total survive to leave the hospital, some with irreversible brain damage. (This stands in stark contrast to the 75 percent survival rate seen by Americans on TV shows like *ER, Chicago Hope,* and *Rescue 911.*)[3]

This societal presumption for CPR underscores the importance of prethinking the decision, and the burden on health-care professionals to compassionately recommend to patients, or more often to families, when it is time to shift goals from survival to comfort care. This recommendation is frequently resisted by family members who hold out hope for an unexpected, or even miraculous, reversal of what seems to the professionals like a certain downward spiral. Enter . . . potential for conflict.

A significant number of requests for ethics consultation come from this scenario: the patient or the family wants CPR, and the professionals caring for the patient do not want to use it, believing this is an unwarranted assault on a person at the very end of his or her life (see Case 3.05). Occasionally the reverse is the case: the patient or family declines CPR, but the professionals believe the patient has a significant chance to survive the current crisis if CPR were available for use in treating this temporary situation (see Case 3.04). In other instances, family members disagree on whether to use CPR or not (see Case 3.01).

---

3. S. J. Diem, J. D. Lantos, and J. A. Tulsky, "Cardiopulmonary Resuscitation on Television: Miracles and Misinformation," *New England Journal of Medicine* 13, no. 334 (1996): 1578-82.

The options to resolve the first (and far more common) type of conflict include: (a) time, education, and persuasion; (b) (reluctant) provision of treatment that is perceived by professionals to be inappropriate; (c) overriding of family wishes by writing a unilateral DNR order; or (d) subterfuge in the guise of a **slow code**. The last is the name used when the professional caregivers agree, often covertly, to leave the patient officially under **full code status** but when arrest occurs to walk slowly to the bedside, or to intentionally use ineffective efforts, so that their efforts are doomed to fail. This is an immoral deception.

There is quite uniform (and deserved) condemnation of slow codes in the literature of medicine and ethics. In talking with physicians in training about this temptation, I propose as an alternative a fifth option — what I call a "fast code." When the family is unwilling to consent to a DNR order, and the professionals are unwilling to write a unilateral DNR order (as is most often the case), and also reluctant to assault the dying patient, I believe it is appropriate to leave the patient's status "full code," and if arrest occurs, to do full-bore CPR for as long as it takes to be certain it will not work. If that conclusion can be reached in two minutes or five minutes, there is no moral obligation to continue CPR efforts for forty-five minutes or two hours just because the family wants it.

One other issue arises in relation to hospital (or departmental) policy: DNR in the operating room (OR). In some hospitals it is written policy (or unwritten practice) that DNR orders are automatically suspended in the OR or during some invasive procedures where the patient is placed at some increased risk of iatrogenic[4] cardiac arrest (e.g., injection of contrast material for imaging studies). Not many patients with a DNR order are scheduled for surgery, but occasionally a person with incurable cancer may have made a decision to forgo CPR but is still willing to have palliative surgery to alleviate symptoms. In these situations, I agree with an opinion in the *Journal of the American Medical Association* that instead of an automatic use of CPR (i.e., an automatic suspension of the DNR order), there should be an automatic rediscussion of whether to leave the DNR order in place or to suspend it.[5] I personally believe that 90 percent of the time it is appropriate to suspend the order, and thus to allow the anesthesiologist to vigorously treat an adverse cardiac event. Indeed, the intact survival statis-

---

4. Iatrogenic means caused by the treatment; literally "caused by the physician."

5. R. M. Walker, "DNR in the OR: Resuscitation as an Operative Risk," *Journal of the American Medical Association* 266 (1991): 2407-12.

tics from CPR in the operating room are considerably better than in other situations. However, there are some situations where the patient or family may feel that death during a procedure would be acceptable for someone who is in the last days or weeks of life and has merely consented to the procedure as part of vigorous **palliative care**.

Now let's look at some cases where cardiac failure has led to a request for ethics consultation.

Case 3.01

QUESTION

Is it permissible to write a do-not-resuscitate order for this patient when her five children are not in agreement?

STORY

Mildred is seventy years old and has a history of diabetes and hypertension. She was admitted to the hospital with a heart attack nearly two months ago and had coronary artery bypass surgery four days after admission. She has been in the intensive care unit (ICU) since surgery because of multiple complications, mostly involving her lungs. At one time she was off the **ventilator** for a few days, but it had to be resumed. Her pulmonary status has recently worsened in spite of continued full treatment. Her ICU and consulting physicians are convinced she will not be able to **wean** from the ventilator and are recommending a **do-not-resuscitate order** (DNR order) with consideration of withdrawal of support soon.

The patient has no written **advance directive**, and her ability to communicate during her prolonged ICU stay has fluctuated. Her daughter, Betsy, reports that on admission she said she wanted full treatment "temporarily," without elaboration about what that meant. After discussing the issues, the ICU team and her five adult children have concluded that she probably would not want long-term ventilator support, but there is lack of consensus on a DNR order, with two of them adamantly believing she should have "one more chance." Ethics consultation was requested by her social worker to try to resolve this conflict.

The patient has been a housewife all her adult life and has been widowed for sixteen years. Her husband was a telephone lineman. She lives alone, next door to Betsy. She has been active and social, quilting and playing cards, a Methodist who has not recently been active in church. The social worker reports that there has been some significant family stress during the past eighteen months, apparently involving property, finances, and responsibilities.

Her nurse reports that since surgery Mildred has been unable to engage in meaningful conversation most days, but she is more alert today than she has been recently. I spoke with her, in the presence of Betsy and her nurse. I explained my understanding of her condition and prognosis. She agreed that if she should deteriorate with continued treatment, she would not want to be resuscitated. She seemed to newly understand the choice between long-term ventilator support and withdrawal of life support, but she was not ready to make a decision to limit or withdraw the ventilator support.

DISCUSSION

Patients with **decision-making capacity** should be encouraged to make an informed choice for or against specific treatments, based on their wishes and values. When treatment decisions must be made for a patient without decision-making capacity who has not left a written advance directive, we use **substituted judgment**, asking those who know the patient best to make the decision the patient would make based on their understanding of the patient's values and wishes.

For patients with borderline or fluctuating capacity, the goal should be to optimize their cognition and have a discussion with them. If they seem to understand and are able to express their wishes, these should almost always be followed, especially if their choice is consistent with previously expressed wishes. This is true even if their **surrogates** are uncertain of what they would choose or what might be in their **best interests**, or even if surrogates disagree with them.

In this case, the patient now seems to understand her poor prognosis. She has agreed with a recommendation for no resuscitation but is not yet ready to make a choice about long-term ventilator support. Her expressed wish is of greater importance than the opinion of some of her children that "she should have one more chance."

RECOMMENDATIONS

1. It is appropriate to write a DNR order for this patient based on both the very small likelihood of success and her agreement to this recommendation. If any of her adult children object, ask an ethics counselor to meet with them along with someone from her care team.
2. It would also be appropriate for her ICU caregivers to talk with her again about the use of the ventilator when she is cognitively clear, preferably with some family present. This should not be repeated so frequently as to be perceived as harassment.

FOLLOW-UP

Four days after the consultation, the patient told her physician that she wanted to continue on the ventilator and did not want life support withdrawn. Plans were initiated for transfer to a long-term ventilator facility, but a bed would not be available for a few weeks. Some of her children became frustrated with her unwillingness to withdraw support and asked if her cardiac medications could be stopped. They were told that since she had been unwilling or unable to switch goals from survival to comfort care, it would not be ethically permissible to do so surreptitiously unless her death were inevitable and imminent. Over the next two weeks she gradually deteriorated with decreased responsiveness and increased swelling, and she developed overwhelming **sepsis**. She died on the ventilator, with her family present.

COMMENT

Family conflict about nonmedical issues often surfaces in the ICU when important treatment decisions have to be made for a loved one. Lines are drawn, heels dug in, voices raised. Sometimes these tensions can be relieved by a frank discussion in which participants are asked to set aside differences that cannot at that time be resolved and to agree on seeking the patient's wishes or best interests. Sometimes the clinical dilemma can be resolved by further conversation with the patient, when that is possible, preferably with family present to observe the patient's responses.

It seems sad that this patient died in the ICU, unable to communicate easily with her family. Could something more have been done to relieve her reluctance to meet death? Could she have benefited from spiritual counsel, from a better understanding of **palliative care**, from some sense that her children were cooperating? Was there some point where the inevitability of her death was sufficiently certain that it might have been justified to withdraw support over her objection? Even in retrospect, questions remain.

Case 3.02

QUESTION

How should we make decisions about resuscitation status for this confused woman with no designated surrogate?

STORY

Nellie, a ninety-seven-year-old woman living alone in her own home, was admitted to hospital four days ago with weakness, decreased mobility, and confusion. She was found to have pneumonia and **sepsis, renal insufficiency**, and dry gangrene of one toe. She has responded surprisingly well to treatment but remains frail, somewhat confused, and at risk of further complications. Dr. Roberts, who has not previously known the patient, has attempted conversation with her about her wishes regarding resuscitation and **intubation**, but she has given inconsistent responses. He believes that **cardiopulmonary resuscitation** (CPR) with chest compressions is unlikely to work if Nellie's heart should stop because of her very frail ribs, but he can't be absolutely certain.

The patient has generally avoided medical care. She was hospitalized for a few days eight years ago with dehydration and then transferred to a nursing home. Her nurse says Nellie remembers vividly the nursing home stay and says it was terrible.

Nellie was an elementary school teacher, retiring about thirty years ago. She has been widowed for many years, has no children, and has no living relatives. She has no guardian and no written **advance directive**. She lives in her own home and mostly takes care of herself, but she has daily help with cooking and cleaning from a woman named Bernadette who has known her only in this capacity, and only for about two years. She has an attorney whom she has known for twenty years who is in charge of her financial affairs. He is reportedly not available today, but a progress note written by Dr. Roberts says the attorney believes the patient would not want heroic measures.

Nellie has no designated **surrogate**. I spoke with her. She was chipper and reasonably clear in her responses, but occasionally incomprehensible. I introduced myself as "Dr. Orr from the Ethics Committee." She seemed to have some level of understanding, saying with a smile, "Then you better do the right thing," but she repeatedly called me "Father." She said she was an active Roman Catholic all her life, but has been unable to go to church for many years. When I asked her if she would want to go to the intensive care unit (ICU) and have machines or tubes if she should worsen, she said, "Well I guess so — if it would help." I then suggested that if some treatments were not working, it might be appropriate to stop them, and she also agreed. She said she had no close friends, and when I asked if we should talk with Bernadette or her attorney if we had questions about treatment, she seemed uncertain.

DISCUSSION

When treatment decisions must be made for patients who are unable to participate in the discussion, we try to use **substituted judgment**, that is, we try to make the decision they would make, based on their written instructions, previously spoken wishes, or an understanding of their values. When this is not possible, we drop to the lower decision-making standard of doing what is in their **best interests.**

Some patients choose to defer to a physician for decision making. Older patients in particular often "trust the doctor" to do "what is best" with little thought about self-determination. This may be especially true for a patient who has had little contact with the medical profession in recent years when patient autonomy has become dominant.

This patient does not currently seem capable of or interested in detailed discussion about her treatment wishes. When led in conversation, she has somewhat vaguely spoken of wanting effective treatment but not ineffective treatment. She seems to trust the medical professionals to make such decisions rather than her caregiver or attorney.

RECOMMENDATIONS

1. Continuing current treatment aimed at survival and hospital discharge is appropriate for this patient.
2. If there are treatment modalities that two physicians agree have a very low chance of working or would involve a disproportionate burden for the patient, it would be permissible to write orders to withhold them. Absent this, it would be appropriate to use any treatment that has a reasonable chance of achieving the patient's goal of survival; for example, if her care team believe that CPR for cardiac arrest would not be effective, a **do-not-resuscitate order** could be written. If, however, it is not clear, it would be ethically preferable to begin CPR and then use clinical judgment at the time about how long to continue.
3. If difficult decisions must be made about life-prolonging treatment that may or may not be effective, or that entails significant burden, it would be appropriate to discuss this with her, if possible, or with her caregiver and attorney, recalling her Catholic heritage. But if that input does not give clarity, it may be necessary to pursue legal guardianship.

FOLLOW-UP

Dr. Roberts had another conversation with Nellie about resuscitation and ICU care. It is not certain how clearly she expressed her wishes, but orders were subsequently written for no resuscitation or intubation. Several days later she agreed to transfer to a nursing home for convalescence with the plan to return home when she was able.

COMMENT

Making treatment decisions for socially isolated patients can be very challenging when they are not able to fully engage in the needed discussions. Efforts can be made to improve their **decision-making capacity** or to search out individuals who may know something about their values or wishes. When neither of these avenues is productive, we are forced to drop to the lower standard of doing what is in the patient's best interests. Sometimes it is relatively easy to use this standard, for example, when aggressive treatment has virtually no chance of being beneficial. But when outcomes are less certain, this is not an easy calculation since individuals have such varying thoughts and values. In general, we tend to err on the side of doing more rather than less in these situations. And we sometimes engage in leading conversations with patients who have borderline decision-making capacity.

When trying to make a treatment decision for a patient using the best-interests standard, one should still recall what is known of that patient's past behavior (e.g., avoiding medical care) and values (e.g., Roman Catholic heritage). Knowing this small amount about the patient's values may help us lean one way or the other in an ambiguous situation.

Case 3.03

QUESTION

Is it ethically permissible to keep this cognitively impaired patient who is deteriorating at the rehabilitation hospital under "full code" status (versus transfer to an acute care hospital's intensive care unit)?

STORY

Rudy is a fifty-five-year-old man recently paralyzed from a spinal cord injury who has been experiencing pulmonary deterioration for forty-eight hours. He has been severely developmentally delayed since birth. He lived in a state institution for developmentally disabled individuals for over forty-five years. Since that institution closed nine years ago, he has lived with and been cared for by Jerry, a man who had been on the institution's staff and had known him for two or three years before it closed. Until recently he was quite functional; he could walk, choose his food and clothing, shop with supervision, and socialize (parties, annual trip to the beach). He is nonverbal but able to communicate. For the past two years he has had intermittent neurological symptoms (weakness, falls) that were found to be from spinal stenosis, a narrowing of the bony vertebral canal causing pressure on his spinal cord. Surgical correction was scheduled, but before it took place he fell again and sustained a spinal cord injury in his neck that has left him nearly quadriplegic.[6] He had surgical fusion to stabi-

---

6. Paralysis of all four extremities.

lize the fracture site three months ago, but of course this did nothing to restore movement to his limbs. He **weaned** from the **ventilator** about three weeks after surgery and was then transferred to the rehab hospital with a goal of returning to Jerry's home for continued chronic care in this more debilitated condition.

Rudy has had problems with recurrent pulmonary emboli, blood clots that form in veins and migrate to his lungs, a rather common problem in patients immobilized from paralysis. To prevent recurrence he was first **anticoagulated**, and later a filter was inserted in the large vein in his abdomen to catch emboli (clots on the move). In spite of this, for the past two days he has had progressive respiratory symptoms felt to be from pulmonary emboli, perhaps from his upper extremities. He has not had invasive testing since he is already anticoagulated, and confirmation of a diagnosis would not lead to any additional therapy.

He remains in **full code status**, though both his rehab physician and his pulmonary consultant recognize that resuscitation would not likely work if he should have another sizable embolus. The rehab nurses are uncomfortable keeping him at the rehab hospital since cardiopulmonary resuscitation (CPR), **intubation**, and ventilator support are not readily available at that facility twenty-four hours per day.

Rudy's father is deceased; his mother is elderly and unable to participate in decisions; two siblings have little involvement. He has a state-appointed guardian, Juanita, who has known him for eight years. Both Jerry and Juanita understand that his prognosis is guarded, but they are still hopeful that he will pull through this pulmonary setback. They recognize that coordinated care at the rehab hospital is preferable to several days at the acute hospital where he would likely lose ground in his rehabilitation without the coordinated team care. Thus they would prefer to not transfer him now unless there is a reasonable chance that more intensive investigation or treatment would increase his chance for survival. They understand his chance of survival of a major cardiopulmonary crisis is practically nonexistent, whether attempted here at the rehab hospital or at the acute care hospital three miles away.

DISCUSSION

Treatment decisions for an adult who has never had **decision-making capacity** should be made jointly by professional caregivers and surrogates based on what would be in the patient's **best interests**. This best-interests calculation is never easy, and is even more difficult when site of care and availability of needed services require trade-offs.

In this case, the patient has progressed through rehabilitation, his caregiver has been trained in his new needs, and he is nearly ready for discharge. However, new complications now threaten his life. What might be construed as maximal therapy (full treatment, including transfer to acute care) could compromise his rehabilitation and his outcome should he survive the complication. On the other hand, the prognosis for this complication is still uncertain, though it would probably not be much different in either setting. It is quite clear that a sudden cardiopulmonary crisis (e.g., from a large pulmonary embolus) will not be reversible and will end his life regardless of where he is receiving care. His prognosis is less clear if he should experience gradually progressive deterioration (e.g., from multiple small emboli, or even from pneumonia).

RECOMMENDATIONS

After prolonged discussion with his professional caregivers and his two **surrogates**, there was agreement on the following plan:

1. The patient will remain at the rehab hospital to continue his coordinated care.
2. A **do-not-resuscitate order** (DNR order) will be written for no CPR in the event of sudden or rapid pulmonary deterioration.
3. If deterioration is more gradual, however, he will be transferred to the acute care hospital for further investigation and treatment.
4. These decisions will be reassessed as appropriate in light of his clinical situation.

FOLLOW-UP

The DNR order was left in place until his condition stabilized three days later. It was then rescinded in case he should experience some other reversible condition. His rehabilitation continued for two more weeks and he was discharged to Jerry's home.

COMMENT

Specific treatment decisions often involve trade-offs. For example, a man who is found to have recurrent cancer that is not curable may have to decide between accepting chemotherapy that has a small chance of slowing the growth of the tumor but has a high incidence of side effects, versus declining the chemotherapy and thus the potential for some therapeutic benefit, in order to avoid the side effects that can diminish the quality of his remaining life. It is often difficult for a person to apply this type of trade-off decision to himself or herself. It is even more difficult to make such a decision for another, especially one who has never been able to express his or her values.

Case 3.04

QUESTION

Is it ethically permissible to write a do-not-resuscitate order at the parental request of this somewhat impaired young man whose acute illness is still potentially reversible?

STORY

Chris is a thirty-two-year-old man who was admitted to the hospital nearly two weeks ago with pneumonia and pleural effusion (fluid accumulation in the chest, between the lung and the chest wall). No bacteria could be isolated from fluid removed from his chest, so the microorganism causing this serious infection remains unknown. He was treated with antibiotics, but his condition worsened so that he was transferred to the intensive care unit (ICU) with respiratory failure one week after admission. He has been **intubated**, treated with a **ventilator** and chest drainage tubes, and is now beginning to show slight improvement from this life-threatening infection. He is sedated but opens his eyes and interacts with family and staff. His parents have requested a **do-not-resuscitate order** (DNR order). Dr. Jenkins and Chris's nurses are uncomfortable with this request since there is now a reasonable chance that he will survive.

The patient has **Down syndrome** and has a very high level of function. He is an optimist, writes poetry, and is an expert on World War II, especially about the role of soldiers from Michigan. He is also very articulate and does public speaking as an advocate for people living with disabilities. He lives with his mother and helps with household chores. His parents are divorced, but his father remains involved in his life and his care. Chris has signed an **advance directive** naming his mother as his **agent** and indicating his preference for **limitation of treatment** if his condition is irreversible. He has an understanding of death and grief, having lost two close friends in separate motor vehicle accidents. He has been followed by Dr. Jenkins for four or five years and has no known cardiac disease, a common physical manifestation of Down syndrome.

His parents and physicians share the goal of treating his infection so that he can return to his previous condition. His parents report that their request for a DNR order is based on their understanding of his reduced life expectancy, and a concern that incomplete resuscitation could possibly lead to survival with further cognitive impairment.

DISCUSSION

In a patient with a serious illness who is unable to participate in treatment decisions, it is important for the family and caregivers to agree upon goals of therapy and on the use or nonuse of specific therapeutic modalities. When the patient's condition is potentially life-threatening, it is particularly appropriate to agree upon what measures will or will not be used if a crisis should arise. An understanding of the patient's wishes and values is the primary guide to making such decisions.

When a patient at baseline has diminished cognition, decisions about goals of treatment should also consider the patient's **best interests**. Discussions about the use or nonuse of treatment should try to estimate the balance of benefits and burdens for the patient, and should not be based on benefits or burdens to others.

In this case, the patient's caring family has a good understanding of his wishes and are striving to make decisions consistent with those wishes and with his best interests. With his healthy heart, a cardiac arrest would almost certainly be the result of major progression of his acute illness. Thus a decision to not resuscitate him from an arrest is not inconsistent with his wishes or best interests.

RECOMMENDATIONS

1. Though many would assert that full treatment for this patient, including **cardiopulmonary resuscitation**, would be the ethically preferable option, it is not ethically impermissible to write a DNR order for him based on his parents' understanding of his wishes.

2. If his condition should worsen or fail to improve after an adequate trial of therapy, it would be appropriate for his caregivers to rediscuss goals of therapy with his parents. An ethics counselor should be asked to participate in such a discussion if it becomes necessary and is desired by the parents.

FOLLOW-UP

Chris continued to improve slowly, was **extubated** five days later, and was transferred out of the ICU. His parents were delighted with his progress. He was discharged home ten days after the consultation.

COMMENT

Both health-care professionals and family are expected to advocate for sick patients, especially for those with preexisting vulnerability, for example, from developmental disability. It is thus not surprising that Dr. Jenkins and Chris's nurses were uncomfortable with his parents' request for a DNR order. They might have presumed that the parents were weary of caring for him; or more altruistically, that the parents were concerned about what would happen to him if they should die first. Further discussion, however, showed that everyone involved had the same goal — survival and return home. The parents sought to avoid his suffering through a prolonged dying process if he was not going to survive, and also the possibility of a lower quality of life if he should require resuscitation but only be "half-cured." When their motivation became clear, the professional caregivers might have tried to dissuade them from their request. But understanding their degree of caring, and understanding that a cardiac arrest in Chris would indeed be a sign of major deterioration, they felt it not unreasonable to accede to the parents' request.

Case 3.05 ───────────────────────────────────

QUESTION

Is it ethically/legally permissible to write a do-not-resuscitate order for this dying man who says he wants "everything" done?

STORY

Reginald is a thirty-nine-year-old prisoner with a long history of alcohol and other chemical abuse, plus liver disease from hepatatis C, complicated by recurrent liver failure with **encephalopathy** and life-threatening hemorrhages from dilated veins in his esophagus. He also is reported to have a history of schizophrenia, though this is not well documented in his hospital chart. He has been in prison for several months. He was sent to the hospital yesterday after progressive lethargy for twenty-four to forty-eight hours. He has been found to have recurrent liver failure with effusions of fluid in his chest and abdomen. Though awake on admission, he has deteriorated quickly and is now barely arousable.

On admission here he said, "I'm not ready to die," and he indicated he wanted "everything done" in spite of being informed of his prognosis. He indicated that he would like a liver transplant, the only treatment that could possibly reverse his rapidly progressive decline; however, he is not a candidate. He has had considerable fluid removed from his chest and abdomen and is receiving medication to try to reverse his encephalopathy. His care team and critical care consultant agree that he is irreversibly dying, and they recommend comfort measures. However, Dr. Newton, his attending physician, requested ethics consultation about the permissibility of writing **limitation of treatment** orders in light of the patient's request for "everything."

DISCUSSION

Decisions about treatment goals and about the use or nonuse of specific treatment modalities should generally be made jointly by a competent patient and his or her professional caregivers. If a patient loses the ability to participate in such discussions, decisions should be based on our best understanding of the patient's wishes. Physicians should follow those wishes whenever it is feasible to do so, even if the physician strongly recommends a different course. However, there is no moral obligation to use a treatment that is physiologically futile, i.e., one that cannot reasonably be expected to achieve the effect of its intended use.

Physicians sometimes inappropriately claim **futility** when they really mean, "I don't think it's a good idea," "it's not medically indicated," or "it's not worth it." However, the term "futility" should be reserved for those uncommon situations where the treatment in question clearly will not work.

This patient has rapidly progressive irreversible multiple organ failure. Aggressive measures like cardiopulmonary resuscitation, drugs to sustain his blood pressure, and **ventilator** support might postpone his death by a few hours or days, but cannot reverse his underlying condition and will not improve his encephalopathy.

The fact that this man is a prisoner or that he has a past history of schizophrenia might lead some to consider him less worthy of fully aggressive treatment. This would violate the principle of justice. He should be given the same consideration as all other patients.

RECOMMENDATIONS

1. If there is professional agreement that aggressive life-sustaining measures will only temporarily postpone his death without improving his encephalopathy, there is no obligation to provide them. Orders to withhold such measures may ethically be written, and comfort measures should be instituted.
2. Measures that could possibly allow him to return to awareness, even temporarily, should be used while efforts are made to summon his family.

FOLLOW-UP

Reginald was treated with antibiotics and laxatives in an effort to reverse his encephalopathy. A **do-not-resuscitate order** was written. He remained unresponsive and died peacefully about eighteen hours later.

COMMENT

This patient's goal was to receive a liver transplant in order to survive, but this goal was not feasible. Failing that, we still had an obligation to try to help him recover from his liver failure and encephalopathy. When this, too, became impossible, there was no obligation to postpone death by a few hours by using means that could not restore his awareness.

Case 3.06

QUESTION

Is it ethically permissible to write a futility-based do-not-resuscitate order for this critically ill woman over the objection of her family?

STORY

Lois is a seventy-one-year-old woman with diabetes who requires dialysis. She had major surgery several months ago for removal of her bladder and both kidneys because of bladder cancer. She developed numerous infectious complications after surgery, including an abscess in her spinal cord and serious infection in her bones. She has been treated vigorously, and was continuing treatment as an outpatient, but was readmitted over a month ago with recurrent **sepsis** and has continued to receive intensive treatment aimed at survival. She continues to have positive blood cultures in spite of antibiotic treatment, a poor prognostic sign. The source of her infection is not clear.

During this hospitalization she has had several episodes of sepsis with a drop in blood pressure and slowing of her pulse requiring **cardiopulmonary resuscitation** (CPR) and transfer to the intensive care unit (ICU) each time. Though she has responded to treatment each time, her physicians are increasingly convinced that her condition is not survivable, and her nurses are concerned that the aggressive treatment is causing her increased suffering with very little benefit. They would like to limit treatment, at least to withhold another use of CPR. The patient is arousable but unable to communicate. She is receiving dialysis, antibiotics, and supplemental oxygen; she is currently not **intubated** or on medication to stabilize her blood pressure.

The patient has no written **advance directive**. Dr. Griswold, her **nephrologist**, who has cared for her for about five years, was able to communicate with her at the time of admission. She said then, as she has always said, that she wanted full treatment. The ICU team report that when the patient has been unable to communicate, her attentive daughter, Bea, has also always requested full treatment, based in part on the observation that "she always pulls through these crises." In addition, her daughter, along with other family, is now requesting that the patient be given less pain medication, fearing that the resulting additional sedation further compromises her ability to get better.

DISCUSSION

When a patient and family agree on treatment goals and on the use or nonuse of specific treatment modalities, those wishes should almost always be followed. The two possible exceptions are true medical **futility** and disproportionate suffering, i.e., when the requested treatment would cause the patient considerable suffering that cannot be relieved but would offer very little in the way of benefit.

There is no moral obligation to provide treatment that will not work. Unfortunately, it is often very difficult to predict if a specific treatment will work without trying it. Physicians sometimes invoke "futility" when they believe the treatment has only a very small chance of working or when, in their clinical judgment, it is not medically recommended in a given situation. However, this recommendation is often based on their assessment that the treatment is "inappropriate," not that the treatment is "futile." Families are often reluctant to accept such a recommendation, especially for a patient who has survived unexpectedly in the past.

It may be ethically justifiable for professional caregivers to decline requested treatment that they believe is inappropriate and is also causing the patient disproportionate suffering that cannot be relieved. They may then say, "In good conscience, I cannot provide the requested treatment." The obligation to relieve suffering remains, and requests to decrease analgesia should generally be resisted unless requested by a patient with capacity or unless that medication truly does compromise the patient's chosen goal.

In our society, patient autonomy is accorded such prominence that a physician should decline requested treatment, based on futility or conscience, only in these very narrow circumstances. This tenet often leads to frustration and professional discomfort in these situations, which can be resolved only through continued discussion.

RECOMMENDATIONS

1. Continuation of full treatment is appropriate for this patient unless her professional caregivers are convinced that some treatment modalities are truly futile or are causing her disproportionate suffering.
2. If intensive treatments for a crisis are clearly not working, they may be stopped in a timely fashion based on clinical judgment; that is, it is not necessary to continue clearly ineffective CPR for a prolonged period just because it has been requested.

3. It is appropriate for professional caregivers to insist on optimal analgesia unless it is a reasonable contention that this reduces her chance of survival.

4. It may be appropriate to hold another family conference, to include not only her current ICU caregivers but also two or three physicians who have a longer-term relationship with her, and also her sister and mother as well as her daughter. Invite an ethics counselor to the meeting, if you wish.

5. It also might be worth exploring whether there are religious, cultural, or personal beliefs that lead her daughter to pursue aggressive treatment.

FOLLOW-UP

The patient's condition deteriorated the next day such that she again required assisted ventilation. Two weeks later she was **extubated** and transferred out of the ICU, but within forty-eight hours she had another cardiac arrest, was resuscitated, and was returned to the ICU. A new abscess was found in her chest. The patient refused surgical intervention but consented to an attempt at needle drainage. This was unsuccessful. She was resuscitated one more time, but about three weeks after the consultation, her daughter agreed to no further measures when her blood pressure again dropped precipitously. She died in less than an hour. Her daughter expressed great appreciation to the entire ICU staff for all their best efforts.

COMMENT

It was situations like this (professionals ready to limit treatment but patients or **surrogates** insisting on continuation of full treatment) that led to the unethical practice of **slow codes** discussed above. It is more appropriate to continue discussion but to also continue the goal of survival unless either of the conditions mentioned pertains (true futility; unrelievable suffering). In regard to CPR, if physicians are not yet ready to proclaim true futility, it should be instituted at the time of cardiac arrest, but how long to continue is truly a clinical judgment based on the situation at the time.

Case 3.07

QUESTION

Please discuss with this patient's sister the ethically permissible treatment options for this man with Huntington's disease and depression.

STORY

Justin is a forty-year-old man who was diagnosed ten years ago with **Huntington's disease.** The disease has progressed as expected, resulting in major disability. With some assistance and lots of planning, he has continued to live independently in a rural apartment, though his independence has become increasingly marginal. He had a psychiatric admission with suicidal depression just over a year ago. Prior to that admission he had requested that a **do-not-resuscitate order** (DNR order) be registered at his local hospital. He lost his driver's license some time ago, but then bought a four-wheel all-terrain vehicle six months ago. The combination of an antidepressant and semi-independent mobility renewed his will to live.

Twelve days ago he was riding his all-terrain vehicle alone early in the morning when he overturned, pinning his left leg. He remained in this position for several hours before he was found by a man walking his dog. When he was brought to the hospital, conservative treatment was used with the goal of saving his leg. When he heard that hopeful news, he asked that his DNR order be rescinded. He was taken to the operating room five days ago to clean up his leg wound, but at surgery it was determined that a below-the-knee amputation would be needed. Since surgery he has remained dependent on a **ventilator** and he has had kidney failure. Both respiratory and renal failure are expected to be reversible; most likely his lungs will improve before his kidneys.

The patient signed a durable power of attorney for health care eighteen months ago naming his sister, Esther, as his **agent**, without explicit directions about the use or nonuse of treatment modalities. Esther is the only unaffected person in their immediate family. Their mother died of Huntington's disease, as did one brother; another brother has Huntington's disease and has survived a serious suicide attempt. Esther describes the patient as very motivated to be independent, with some financial resources to support that goal. He has said repeatedly and adamantly that he never wants to be in a nursing home. She is concerned that he may "give up" when he learns about the amputation, which will seriously threaten his ability to live independently. She thus wanted to talk about his current level of support, prognosis, and future plans.

DISCUSSION

Treatment decisions should ideally be made by fully informed and competent patients. When patients are unable to participate, we attempt to make a **substituted judgment**, that is, we try to make the decision they would make, if able, based on their written **advance directive**, their previously stated wishes, or an understanding of their values.

When life-or-death decisions must be made by or for a patient who has recently suffered an acute event that changes his or her functional ability or quality of life, it is appropriate to not allow the patient or a **surrogate** to make a hasty, irreversible decision before the prognosis for recovery or optimization of function is clear.

In this case, it is not clear if the patient will be able to continue independent living with his underlying disability and his new amputation, or whether he might require long-term care, an option he has found unacceptable in the past.

RECOMMENDATIONS

1. It is appropriate to continue the current plan of care, that is, recovery from his surgery and double organ failure, rehabilitation, and optimization of function.

2. If he should have new life-threatening complications, it would not be inappropriate to discuss again with his sister the goals of treatment, and even to consider **limitation of treatment** if his prognosis becomes significantly worse.

3. If he recovers his ability to participate in decisions, his wishes should be honored. However, he should be encouraged not to make a hasty, irreversible decision. Since it is anticipated that he will likely **wean** from the ventilator before his renal function improves, he may be able to make a thorough assessment and then decide if he wants to continue short-term dialysis. If that sequence does not happen, he could at some point choose to limit treatment (e.g., to forgo antibiotic treatment for infection, or even to forgo fluids and nutrition and accept only comfort care).

FOLLOW-UP

Justin soon awoke and was weaned successfully from ventilator support. When he came to understand that he had had an amputation, he was distressed and depressed. With encouragement from his sister and professional caregivers, however, he agreed to continue dialysis and accept transfer to a rehabilitation hospital in an attempt to maximize his functional abilities.

COMMENT

The question that led to this consultation was about **cardiopulmonary resuscitation** (CPR) versus no CPR. However, the real dilemma was much broader: it was about goals of therapy in the face of an ultimately fatal disease that was already at a fairly advanced stage. Because of the familial nature of this disease, people suffering with Huntington's disease have almost always watched a parent deteriorate and die. People with this disease have a very high suicide rate.

This patient had support from family and professionals as well as adequate resources, so that he chose to continue to fight against this relentless disease. Many who suffer with Huntington's disease are not so fortunate.

This case brings up an important issue. People who undergo a sudden major loss of function often immediately say they want to decline life-extending treatment and die. The paradigm is the young man who breaks his neck in a diving accident and realizes that he is permanently paralyzed from his neck down and that he requires a machine to breathe for him. Many who awaken to this condition say the quality of life is too low and insist they want to stop the ventilator and die. If we relied purely on the principle of autonomy, we would be obligated to honor their request. However, in light of a sudden life-changing event, I believe it is ethically permissible to postpone honoring their refusal. We should insist on a delay, usually a few months, during which we should exert maximal efforts at rehabilitation, counsel, and support. If, then, the patient continues to insist that his or her life is not worth living, I believe we are obligated to honor the patient's request for limitation or withdrawal of treatment.

Case 3.08 ───────────────────────────────────

QUESTION

Is it permissible to turn off this depressed woman's pacemaker at her request?

STORY

Dorthea is a sixty-nine-year-old woman who was well and active until about five years ago when she developed diabetes. She was admitted to the hospital eighteen months ago with recurrent fainting and was found to have an intermittent transient heart block.[7] She reluctantly consented to insertion of a permanent pacemaker. Three months ago her kidney function was found to be about 10 percent (from the diabetes). It was expected that she would soon require dialysis. However, her kidney function has since improved so that dialysis will not likely be needed for some time. She has since said she would refuse dialysis even if it were needed, and she has refused treatment of her profound anemia. She did consent to a colonoscopy last month to see if she had cancer (malignant change was found in one small area, presumably cured). She is now asking that her pacemaker be turned off so that she can die.

I met with the patient and two of her daughters. Dorthea says she wants to die now because (a) she misses her husband, who died three years ago after forty-five years of marriage; they were very close, did everything together, and she says she can't live without him; (b) she can't stand to live in their home (memories), but refuses to move; and (c) she wants to "set her children free." Her three daughters have encouraged treatment, including grief counseling, and have even offered to allow her to live with them, but she has resisted this. She has guns in her home and knows how to use them, but she says she is unwilling to take her own life. She is an inactive Episcopalian. She says her only pleasure is having her children, grandchildren, and great-grandchildren visit, but she feels her misery is also making them miserable.

The patient says she was told when the pacer was inserted that it could

---

7. Heart block is a dysfunction of the electrical conduction pathway in the heart. It can lead to a slowing of heartbeat, and occasionally to temporary stopping for several seconds. Treatment may require the use of medication or a pacemaker.

be shut off whenever she didn't want it. It is her impression that she will die quickly without it; however, her cardiologist expects this would not be the case. (Though she demonstrates no intrinsic rhythm when the rate of the pacer is turned down to thirty beats per minute on testing, most patients do develop some rhythm after several seconds of not beating at all.) She says she is miserable, is not eating (though her weight is down only five to ten pounds), and cannot care for herself or her home, but she doesn't want treatment for her anemia or her grief. When asked, she said she did not have the colonoscopy last month to protect her life. The only reason she consented to the procedure is that she hoped it would show she had cancer that would end her life.

Her daughters have run out of ideas for helping her, and are now supportive of her request. They believe "she wants quality of life over quantity of life," but they recognize that she is refusing treatment that could enhance her quality. They realize she has not dealt with her grief, but are convinced that she never will.

DISCUSSION

Patients have a right to refuse any treatment, even life-sustaining treatment. It may rarely be ethically permissible to force some treatment on unwilling patients who are a danger to themselves or others. Though a patient may be involuntarily hospitalized to prevent suicide, only rarely is it felt justified to seek court authorization to enforce antidepressant medication. When a patient refuses effective and nonburdensome life-prolonging treatment, it is critical to understand the reason behind the request, and then to try to address that reason before considering acceding to the request.

There is no moral or legal difference between withholding and withdrawing a treatment. Thus it is permissible to stop a **ventilator** or dialysis if it is (a) no longer achieving its purpose, (b) causing intolerable symptoms, or (c) merely sustaining life with an intolerable quality. While it would be permissible for a patient to refuse pacemaker insertion, it is an unresolved question whether it is permissible to shut off a pacemaker that is sustaining life without causing intolerable symptoms. Some would argue that it is permissible because it is artificial technology, comparable to a ventilator. Most would argue that it is not permissible because the pacemaker, once inserted, becomes part of the person, and shutting it off is akin to assisting in a suicide.

In this case, the patient has not allowed her reasons for refusal to be addressed. In addition, her request, if followed, would probably not achieve her goal of being quickly dead and might even cause her greater physical distress for an unknown period of time.

RECOMMENDATIONS

1. It would be ethically troublesome to turn off this patient's pacemaker at this time. At a minimum, she should have adequate treatment for her anemia and her depression before it can be concluded that she has an intolerable quality of life.
2. If she does not respond to an adequate trial of treatment, most physicians would remain unwilling to turn off her pacer either because (a) this would be too close to active participation in the patient's suicide, or (b) it might result in worsening her quality of life without actually ending her life. Others might be willing to honor her request, though they should have clear contingency plans for what would be done if she slips into heart failure or unconsciousness but does not die quickly.

FOLLOW-UP

The patient's primary physician reported that he told her and her family that he couldn't even consider stopping the pacemaker until she had had full treatment for her depression and her anemia. Two weeks later she consented to nursing home admission and beginning an antidepressant. Her appetite and mood improved, and inexplicably, so did her kidney function. She stopped asking about turning off the pacemaker.

COMMENT

People who are seriously depressed often hope they will get a fatal disease that will quickly take their life. In this case, the woman thought she had such a fatal disease and that stopping treatment for it would end her life quickly and painlessly. When she learned that this was not the case, she consented to minimal treatment, and this led to an improved outlook.

Pacemakers are unique among therapeutic interventions because, as mentioned, debate continues about whether they are comparable to external technologies, and thus optional, or have become part of the person, and may thus not be stopped to intentionally lead to death. The next case helps to focus this dilemma.

Case 3.09

QUESTION

Is it ethically permissible to turn off the pacemaker in this patient who is dying?

STORY

Marvin is a fifty-seven-year-old retired fireman with a past history of cardiac disease, diabetes, morbid obesity, and alcoholic cirrhosis. Three months ago he had a cardiac valve replacement, and two weeks later a permanent pacemaker had to be implanted for a serious rhythm disturbance. He was discharged home.

He was readmitted eight days ago because of progressive shortness of breath and a weight gain of thirty or forty pounds from fluid retention. He was found to have **congestive heart failure** with massive swelling, a rapid and irregular pulse, and a large accumulation of fluid around his heart. This fluid was removed with a needle, but he has been found to be in intractable heart failure plus kidney failure, and he has developed a bleeding problem from bone marrow failure. He is thus in **multi-organ system failure** with a very poor prognosis for recovery.

Three days ago his family requested no resuscitation or **intubation** based on his previously stated wishes to avoid life support when it did not look as if he could recover. A **do-not-resuscitate order** was written. He has been treated vigorously, but he continues to worsen. Yesterday his family declined repeat removal of fluid from around his heart because of the risk of bleeding and the small likelihood of long-term benefit, and they went on to request that all life-sustaining therapies be stopped and that he be given comfort care. He is currently comfortable and somnolent. Dr. Michaels, his cardiologist, requested ethics consultation about turning off his pacemaker. It is his opinion that the patient's current survival is dependent on the pacemaker-generated rhythm.

He has a large supportive family consisting of wife, children, and siblings. They have been in constant attendance at his bedside and are struggling to cope with his rapid and unanticipated decline.

DISCUSSION

There is general agreement that when critically or terminally ill patients or their **surrogates** choose to change treatment goals from survival to comfort care, it is ethically permissible to discontinue or not institute any external therapy whose goal is life prolongation. Thus it is permissible to stop a **ventilator**, dialysis, medication to sustain blood pressure, antibiotics, feeding tubes, or intravenous fluids unless continued use will ameliorate otherwise unrelievable symptoms. This is also true for an internal device that was implanted temporarily in an attempt to reverse a disease process (e.g., a left-ventricular assist device or a temporary pacemaker powered from outside the body) if it is subsequently found to not be achieving the hoped-for goal. The issue is less clear if an internal device was implanted at an earlier time with the intention of being permanent, for example, a permanent cardiac pacemaker. There is theoretical debate about whether such a device is now "part of the patient's body" or is still a form of life support that is optional.

The ethically important distinction is the intention of the act of shutting off the pacemaker. If the intention is to stop postponing an inevitable death by stopping treatments that are no longer serving their purpose, this is ethically permissible. If, on the other hand, the intention of the act is to hasten death, this becomes ethically problematic. It could be argued that the permanent pacemaker in the latter case is no longer serving the purpose for which it was implanted, and thus it might seem optional. However, since it is internal and free from external connections, the act of slowing its rate or shutting it off more closely resembles the injection of a medication whose intention is to stop the heart than it does the removal of an external ventilator or even a temporary pacemaker that is powered from outside.

RECOMMENDATIONS

1. While it is not clearly impermissible to shut off this patient's pacemaker, doing so raises sufficient questions of physician intention that it is ethically problematic and should probably not be done if the patient is otherwise comfortable and likely to die within a relatively short time.

2. An ethics consultant should be available to meet with the ICU team or the patient's family to discuss this further if they wish.

FOLLOW-UP

The patient died less than two hours later with the pacemaker still in place and functioning.

COMMENT

Even in this case, where death is inevitable and an appropriate surrogate has decided to no longer try to postpone death, the issue of the pacemaker is cloudy. Though the pacemaker here merely postponed an imminent death, placing a magnet on the dying person's chest and sending signals to the pacemaker to stop the patient's heart feels perilously close to giving a lethal injection. Some ethics consultants might disagree with this interpretation and be willing to grant permission to do this act. Once again, this reveals the cloudiness of this issue.

Case 3.10

QUESTION

Should we proceed with resuscitative surgery in this woman who has said she did not want resuscitation?

STORY

Sister Bernadette is an eighty-four-year-old nun with a history of angina who was admitted to the hospital two weeks ago for elective hip surgery. A pre-op cardiac stress test showed significant coronary artery disease, so her hip surgery was postponed until this could be addressed. She had cardiac catheterization and angioplasty[8] of one coronary artery, and was discharged. She was readmitted to the cardiac catheterization lab today for

---

8. Angioplasty is a nonsurgical procedure to open up the flow of blood through an artery, either by dilation or by cleaning out the obstructing material in the artery.

planned angioplasty of a second coronary artery. She signed the consent form, which included standard wording giving consent for other procedures required due to unexpected findings. It is reported to me verbally that she was told one risk of today's procedure was that she might need emergency surgery, and she said she would consent to that if it were needed to restore her health.

The angioplasty procedure was done about two hours ago. Immediately after the procedure she had a severe drop in blood pressure, was returned to the catheterization lab, was reevaluated, and was found to have a ruptured coronary artery. A balloon pump was placed to sustain her vital circulation, and she was immediately transferred to the operating room for emergency surgery to repair the damage. She is at this moment on the operating table, and the team is ready to begin surgery.

During preparation for surgery she had new-onset generalized seizures, suggesting she has suffered brain damage from lack of oxygen. Though survival of such emergency cardiac surgery is quite common, intact survival in an elderly patient who is exhibiting signs suggestive of brain damage from inadequate oxygen is quite unlikely; that is, there is a reasonable chance that she could survive the crisis, but it is likely that she will be left with some degree, probably severe, of neurological deficit.

When Dr. Beckett was discussing the emergency surgery and grave prognosis with her mother superior, he learned that the patient had said in the past that she did not want to be resuscitated or to survive if she should become neurologically incapacitated. The mother superior confirmed this by telephoning another nun who also knows the patient well.

DISCUSSION

Emergency treatment decisions for a patient who cannot participate should be made using **substituted judgment**, i.e., by trying to make the decision that the patient would make if the patient were able. This may be based on the patient's written **advance directive**, on a report of the patient's previously expressed wishes, or on an understanding of his or her values.

In this case the patient consented to hip surgery, to angioplasty, and even to emergency chest surgery if needed, suggesting that her goal was survival. However, given her current grave prognosis for intact survival, her clear statement to two intimates that she did not want resuscitation or survival in an incapacitated condition would seem to outweigh these consents for procedures that were aimed at intact survival.

RECOMMENDATIONS

1. If this patient's physicians are convinced that she has suffered permanent brain damage that will leave her severely incapacitated, it is ethically permissible to honor her previously expressed wishes to avoid resuscitation and impaired survival by stopping current resuscitative efforts (e.g., the balloon pump, **ventilator** support) and to switch goals to end-of-life comfort care.
2. If this is done, she may be cared for in whatever setting will allow appropriate **palliative care** to be administered; that is, she does not need ICU (intensive care unit) care unless it is needed to ensure her comfort.

FOLLOW-UP

Sister Bernadette was transferred to the ICU for intensive comfort measures. She remained unresponsive. The balloon pump was discontinued a few hours later, and she died about twenty-four hours after that with her religious community present.

COMMENT

This was an urgent dilemma requiring a very rapid decision — to do life-saving surgery or not. It almost seems intuitive that this surgery should be done since the patient had specifically consented to surgery for complications of her catheterization procedure. However, analysis of her pattern of consent showed that she wanted to get better to continue her former level of activity. She had said to at least two individuals that she did not want to be kept alive by technology if she were to become disabled. The generalized seizures she had during this crisis portended a grim prognosis for her brain. It might have been possible to save her life, but not to restore her to the level of function she desired. Thus it was ethically permissible to honor her prior request to limit treatment.

Case 3.11 ——————————————————————————————

QUESTION

Is it ethically permissible to ignore this patient's requested do-not-resuscitate order after his suicide attempt?

STORY

Gerald is an eighty-six-year-old man with a history of chronic anemia for which he receives periodic transfusions. He came to the emergency department two days ago with chest pain and was admitted to the intensive care unit (ICU) with a heart attack. On admission he requested a **do-not-resuscitate order** (DNR order), and this was written into his chart. This morning he was found to be unresponsive, and twenty-eight capsules of a barbiturate sedative were found in his bed. His daughter reports that he always carries an envelope with fifty such capsules. This afternoon his respirations were sufficiently depressed, most likely from the barbiturate, that he was **intubated** and is now on a **ventilator**. If he took twenty-two capsules, this is considered a serious overdose but is probably not lethal. The psychiatric consultant recommended an ethics consultation. On examination he appears younger than his stated age and has a fresh haircut.

His daughter, Becky, brought in a medical directive[9] in which he rejected all twelve therapeutic options in all four clinical scenarios presented. In addition, she is named as the patient's health-care proxy. The patient is divorced and has no other children.

Becky reports that her father was a happy, vibrant, and vain person until a serious auto accident eight years ago in which he sustained several fractures and facial lacerations. Since that time he has been depressed, very unhappy with his appearance, and wishing to die. He has maintained that something happened inside his head at the time of the accident. He made a serious suicide attempt about two years ago (overdose) and was angry that he recovered. He has had two prolonged psychiatric admissions and multiple attempts at outpatient therapy with antidepressants and counseling without apparent improvement. Two years ago he fell and broke his right

9. A medical directive is a specific form of advance directive with considerable detail. In it, the principal is asked his or her wishes for or against twelve different treatment options in each of four different clinical scenarios.

arm and has since had difficulty combing his hair, another blow to his concern about his appearance. He has been giving away or designating recipients for all his possessions for several months and recently declared that the task was completed. On his calendar for this week he had written "transfusion" on Tuesday, "haircut" on Wednesday, and "Riverside Cemetery" on Sunday, suggesting that he had planned to take his suicidal overdose of pills imminently.

DISCUSSION

Limitation of treatment requests by competent patients should almost always be honored. A medical directive rejecting all life-sustaining treatment is not an uncommon request from someone eighty-six years old. Occasionally, overriding a limitation of treatment request from a seemingly competent patient may be justified if the care team believes the request to be seriously irrational.

Most clinicians and ethicists believe that depression and suicidal action render a patient not competent to make such limitation of treatment decisions. "Rational suicide" is a designation used by some to denote suicide that seems to make sense, for example, in the face of terminal illness and unrelievable pain, but many believe that suicide is always irrational.

This patient's do-not-resuscitate request on admission with a potentially life-threatening cardiac problem would seem to be rational even with his long history of depression. Lack of a terminal diagnosis makes his suicide attempt irrational and renders his request for nontreatment invalid in regard to the overdose.

RECOMMENDATIONS

1. It is justifiable to ignore this patient's do-not-resuscitate request in order to treat the results of his suicide attempt, that is, intubation and ventilation.
2. It would still be ethically permissible to honor the do-not-resuscitate request if he should have a life-threatening situation that is readily discernible to not be related to his overdose, for example, if he should have an extension of the heart attack with consequent instability of blood pressure.

FOLLOW-UP

Six days after the ethics consultation, the patient's respiratory depression from the suicidal overdose had cleared and his cardiac condition was stable. However, as attempts were made to discontinue his ventilator, he did not awaken. It soon became evident that he had suffered a large stroke sometime after admission that was now causing swelling of his brain. This was felt to be life-threatening and not easily reversible. It was thus felt to be ethically permissible to reinstate a DNR order, to discontinue his ventilator support, and to provide comfort measures. The patient died three hours later.

COMMENT

It is important in progressing through this consultation to keep in mind both intention and prognosis. It was felt to be ethically impermissible to not treat an easily reversible condition brought about by the patient's suicide attempt. At the same time, it was ethically permissible to honor this elderly man's wish to not have aggressive treatment if he were faced with an irreversible condition. This is not splitting hairs but, I believe, a valid moral distinction.

*   *   *

Other Cases Where Heart Failure/CPR Is an Issue

Cases 4.02, 4.13, 5.01, 5.07, 6.08, 8.11, 9.01, 9.02, 9.05, 9.12, 9.13, 10.12, 11.02, 13.05, 14.04, 14.05, 14.08, 14.09

References on Cardiac Disease and/or CPR

Brody, Baruch. *Life and Death Decision Making.* Oxford: Oxford University Press, 1988.

Kilner, J. F., A. B. Miller, and E. D. Pellegrino, eds. *Dignity and Dying: A Christian Appraisal.* Grand Rapids: Eerdmans, 1996.

New York State Task Force on Life and the Law. *Do Not Resuscitate Orders.* 2nd ed. New York: New York Task Force on Life and the Law, 1988.

Randall, F., and R. S. Downie. *Palliative Care Ethics.* 2nd ed. Oxford: Oxford University Press, 1999.

CHAPTER 4

Ethical Issues in Lung Failure

Next to cardiac arrest, the most common way for a person to die quickly is to stop breathing or to stop breathing effectively. This results in a lack of oxygen and a buildup of carbon dioxide, either of which may cause serious organ dysfunction or damage.

Respiratory arrest may occur rapidly, leading to sudden death, but more commonly it happens over a period of hours or days. Respiratory failure occurs when the work of breathing exceeds the capacity of the lungs to do effective exchange of oxygen and carbon dioxide, so that the level of oxygen falls and the level of carbon dioxide rises in the bloodstream. The good news is that several types of "breathing machines" (called respirators or **ventilators**) have been developed that can assist the breathing process by reducing the work expended in breathing. Use of such assistance requires that the patient be **intubated**, that is, have a plastic **endotracheal tube** (ETT) inserted into the airway, most commonly through the mouth but occasionally through the nose. While receiving ventilatory assistance, the patient is almost always sedated since having a tube in one's trachea is very uncomfortable.

Assisted ventilation can often prevent a respiratory death, allowing time for the body to repair the underlying problem, for example, pneumonia or chest trauma. When the underlying problem is resolved, the patient is **weaned** from the ventilator by slowly decreasing the pressure used by the machine or reducing the concentration of oxygen. This weaning may occasionally be done quickly (over a matter of hours), but more commonly it requires a few days.

Sometimes, however, the underlying problem is chronic and progressive such that the ventilator prevents or postpones death but the patient fails to wean. To complicate matters, while the patient's breathing is being assisted by a machine, the muscles the patient ordinarily uses to breathe lose strength from lack of use. Thus the weaning, especially if assisted ventilation has gone on for some time, may involve a period of gradual strengthening of those muscles. This may take several weeks, and in some instances it may not work, so the options are long-term use of the ventilator or discontinuation of the machine, with death almost inevitable (see Case 4.03).

Along with **cardiopulmonary resuscitation**/do-not-resuscitate dilemmas, questions about the use or nonuse of ventilators probably generate more dilemmas (and more ethics consultations) than any other treatment modality. It is not uncommon for patients or families to say "no breathing machines" or for professionals to write do-not-intubate (DNI) orders, that is, do not insert an ETT into the airway, when a decision has been made against use of this treatment modality. Unfortunately, very often when patients or family members say "no breathing machines," they actually mean the patient would not want to be attached to assisted ventilation long-term or permanently, even though the patient might be willing to accept it for a few days. When this misstatement is clarified, the dilemma expands to include the difficult task of predicting whether the patient will ever be able to breathe without assistance (see Case 4.01).

Intubation and assisted ventilation are most commonly needed because of pulmonary (lung) problems (see Case 4.08), but sometimes they are used for problems in the brain or spinal cord that result in the chest not being stimulated to move, called a lack of respiratory drive (see Case 4.14).

Ventilator support is usually started as a short-term measure to give the underlying lung or brain problem time to heal, and this trial of therapy is often anticipated to last a few days. But very commonly the outcome of this trial is uncertain, and thus the "trial" may slowly transition into longer-term use, often without discussion or even a conscious decision. This transition comes into focus two or three weeks after initial intubation because the intensive care physician will want to get the ETT out so it will not erode the tracheal lining. If assisted ventilation is to be continued, the physician will then request consent for a **tracheostomy** (often called a "trach" and pronounced with a long *a*). In this operation a small hole is made in the front of the neck so that a plastic or metal tube can be inserted into the trachea, and the ventilator tubing can be attached directly; this eliminates the need for the ETT to go through the mouth. Such a request often triggers questions of "how long should we continue?" or "what are the chances of weaning?" and not infrequently questions for an ethics consultant or clergy support person (see Case 4.05).

The standard ethics questions of capacity and surrogacy clearly apply in discussion of ventilator use (see Case 4.08). However, these are complicated by the sedation that is almost always used for the patient on ventilator support. Sometimes it is possible to decrease or stop the amount of sedation in order to have a discussion with the patient or to switch from a long-acting sedative to one that is rapidly cleared (see Case 4.12). The issue of sedation also factors into the question of prognosis in several ways. Sedation obscures cognitive function, and families (and clinicians) usually want to know about cognition at the present and in the future before making a decision to stop a ventilator. If it is determined that the patient has suffered severe brain damage from lack of oxygen during the medical crisis, this may change the goals of treatment. In addition, the physician usually wants to diminish sedation during weaning so the patient will be able to participate as fully and clearly as possible in the process. Sometimes, without sedation the patient becomes agitated and families may want to forsake the weaning attempt to prevent patient suffering.

Decreasing sedation to allow communication sounds good on paper, and it sometimes actually works. But even when it is possible to eliminate sedation altogether, the process of communication is challenging. Patients awakening from a period of sedation may be confused or disoriented, for short or long periods. Even if they are awake and alert, they are unable to make any sound because of the mechanical disruption to their airway. They often try to mouth words, but this is usually frustrating to both them and clinicians. Some patients are able to nod or shake their heads, so you can play "20 Questions" with them. In doing this, it is important that each question is clear and can be answered yes or no. Double questions must be avoided ("Would you like us to stop the ventilator and keep you comfortable?"). Some patients can write on a clipboard or use a letter board to form words by pointing sequentially. At other times it is possible to develop communication codes using eye blinks or hand squeezes. Requesting consultation with a speech-language pathologist may sometimes improve communication in these situations.

Predicting weanability is an art form and subject to considerable error. Most ICU (intensive care unit) professionals use measurements called weaning parameters to see how ready the patient is to come off the ventilator, but they are merely educated guesses. Generally, the longer the patient is on the vent, the less likely he or she will wean successfully, because of muscle weakness and because the underlying illness is just too severe to allow independent respiration.

Decisions to stop ventilator support are difficult for families and clinicians, and both may need reassurance and support. When such a decision is made, clinicians often do a "terminal wean." I dislike the term, but the better descriptor is quite cumbersome: discontinuation of assisted ventilation with the expectation that the patient will not survive. The former suggests that the patient will surely die, and we know that this is not always the case — 4 to 10 percent of patients who undergo "terminal weans" actually survive to get out of the ICU or even leave the hospital (see Cases 4.01 and 4.08). Thus, it is important for families to understand that the goal is to stop assisting ventilation to see if the patient can survive. Sometimes we can be very certain; at other times less so. Sometimes the patient dies in a few minutes; sometimes the patient dies in a few hours; sometimes the patient continues to breathe for a few days; and rarely, the patient survives. So we are not guaranteeing death, even though that is usually our best guess. And this brings up the question of paralytic agents.

When it is difficult to ventilate a patient due to resistance (whether from stiffness of the lung tissue or muscular resistance by the patient), a paralyzing drug may be used to eliminate any muscle resistance. If a decision is made to discontinue efforts at assisted ventilation with the expectation that the patient will not survive, the ethics consultant is often asked if the paralytic agent must be stopped first. The concern is that recovery of muscular effort may cause visible struggling during the dying process, and this may be upsetting to the family though it may or may not represent increased suffering for the patient. This has been debated in the literature, and almost all agree that the paralytic agent should be stopped first. If it is continued, there is no longer any question of unexpected survival because we would be guaranteeing death since the paralysis would prevent any effort to breathe by the patient. In addition, when the patient is paralyzed, caregivers have no way of observing signs of physical suffering. Some ethicists and physicians have tried to make a case for not discontinuing the paralytic agent in some unusual cases; they make a strong case[1] but have not yet totally convinced me.

Families often are reluctant to consent to ventilator withdrawal. This

1. R. M. Perkin and D. B. Resnik, "The Agony of Agonal Respiration: Is the Last Gasp Necessary?" *Journal of Medical Ethics* 28 (2002): 164-69.

may be because they think they (or we) would then be "killing the patient" (see Case 4.07). It is important for them to understand that it is the underlying disease that is taking the patient's life. We have been trying to avoid that by using intensive treatment, but when it is clear that the treatment is not going to achieve the desired goal, it is ethically and legally permissible to change treatment goals from survival to comfort care; to stop current efforts and accept the inevitability of the patient's death. Some families want to discuss this question with their clergy support, and this should be encouraged, preferably with the ethics consultant or someone from the ICU team present.

At other times families are reluctant to consent to ventilator withdrawal because they fear the patient will suffocate. Good symptom control is possible, using appropriate steps in withdrawal and well-timed drugs, so patient discomfort can be avoided. The steps taken to ensure patient comfort should be outlined in detail for the family and for the patient if he or she is aware, preferably by someone from the **palliative care** team or an ICU professional who is experienced in and comfortable with ventilator withdrawal.

If a patient cannot be weaned from the ventilator, another option is long-term ventilator support. This is generally recommended for younger patients with neurologic reasons for being unable to breathe (e.g., spinal cord injuries), and less often for older patients or those with intrinsic lung disease (see Case 4.14). However, facilities with beds for long-term ventilator support are few and far between, so a decision for this may involve a major geographic move. A (very) few hospitals have home ventilator programs in which family members are taught how to manage the ventilator and provide several hours per day of personal oversight, with paid support professionals to cover remaining hours.

Let's now look at some clinical dilemmas raised by the use or nonuse of ventilatory support.

Case 4.01

QUESTION

Is it permissible to continue the ventilator on this patient who has said she didn't want to be intubated?

STORY

Linda is a forty-three-year-old woman who had a kidney/pancreas transplant for advanced diabetes three years ago. Three months ago she developed chronic rejection of her transplanted organs and she is back on insulin, though she does not yet need dialysis.

She developed severe back pain after a fall ten days ago and was admitted to the hospital seven days ago for evaluation and treatment. On admission, she consented to treatment, except she specifically declined **intubation** of her airway. Five days ago she developed respiratory failure of uncertain cause and was transferred to the intensive care unit (ICU) where this was initially treated with respiratory assistance via a tightly fitting mask since she didn't want to be intubated. An **MRI** of her back was felt to be necessary to rule out progressive hemorrhage or abscess as the cause of her back pain because these could be treated; without treatment they might lead to permanent paralysis. However, an MRI could not be done while she was using this type of breathing machine. Her sister was able to persuade her to accept short-term intubation for the MRI in order to avoid paralysis from a correctable cause. The MRI was done four days ago. It did show a hemorrhage near her spine, but it was small enough that unassisted reabsorption was expected, so surgical drainage was not required. Unfortunately, the ICU team has thus far been unable to **wean** her from the **ventilator**. Her prognosis is uncertain, but the doctors would like to try for a few more days to reverse any correctable problems. Because of her resistance to intubation, however, they have asked the above question. The patient is moderately sedated and able to respond somewhat to her sister.

The patient and her husband had a son eleven years ago. He has multiple handicaps. He spent his first eighteen months in the neonatal ICU and was on ventilator support at home for several more months. The patient's husband died six months before her transplant, and she has been unable to care for their son; he is now in foster care. Linda's parents are deceased, and she has been dependent on her only sister, Jane, whom she has named as her durable power of attorney for health care.

Jane says the patient has had a long-standing aversion to anything near her face or in her mouth. This worsened after her son spent so many months on a ventilator. The patient has told her sister on many occasions that she didn't want intubation, but she has displayed full trust in Jane's judgment. When this issue was rediscussed recently, Jane told the patient she would probably authorize intubation for a few days for a reversible problem, and Linda reluctantly agreed.

DISCUSSION

When patients are unable to participate in treatment decisions, we attempt to make those decisions using **substituted judgment**, that is, we try to make the decision they would make if they were able, based on their written statements or an understanding of their values and wishes.

This patient has said that she didn't want intubation, but when pressed, clarified this to mean no long-term intubation. She has made several decisions that indicate she wants to survive if possible: she consented to transplantation in recent years; she agreed to admission for this illness and consented to full treatment except for intubation; she later was persuaded to accept short-term intubation in an effort to reverse her current condition. She made these decisions in spite of her unexplained and perhaps irrational fear of having mechanical devices in her mouth or on her face, suggesting that she wanted to survive if possible, but she clearly did not want long-term ventilator support.

In most situations of this sort, it is appropriate to reduce a patient's sedation in an effort to determine the patient's current wishes. In this case, however, the patient's complete trust in her **agent**, coupled with her inordinate fear of intubation, makes this an undesirable option, though this places a heavier burden on her agent.

RECOMMENDATIONS

1. It is ethically permissible to continue intubation and ventilator support for this patient for a short time as long as there is a reasonable chance of her survival when taken off the ventilator.
2. If her agent feels that the benefits of further treatment are outweighed by the patient's stated wishes, it would be ethically permissible to withdraw ventilator support even if this leads to her death, and even if prolonged ventilator support had some chance of allowing survival in another patient.

FOLLOW-UP

Two days later the patient was able to be **extubated**, but her respiratory status remained marginal. She requested orders for no resuscitation and no repeat intubation. She was transferred out of the ICU to receive comfort care, with the expectation that she would not survive. However, she continued to breathe adequately, and several days later she was smiling and accepting of transfer to a rehabilitation facility.

COMMENT

Sometimes it is necessary to look beyond the patient's specific consent or refusal in an attempt to understand the patient's goal and values. In this case, it appeared that the patient's goal was to survive if possible, but she had made some decisions about **limitation of treatment**: (a) no long-term intubation, and (b) toleration of short-term intubation only if she had a reasonable chance of recovery. Determining the tipping point, the point of diminishing returns, is never easy. It is easiest if the patient can participate in this calculation, but when that is not possible, a decision from a trusted **surrogate** is the next best option.

Case 4.02

QUESTION

Is it ethically permissible to accept a refusal of a potentially life-extending tracheostomy from this man with mental illness?

STORY

Bernie is a fifty-two-year-old man who has had cardiac disease for several years. Five years ago he had a two-vessel coronary artery bypass graft with a prolonged stay in the intensive care unit (ICU), which included a **tracheostomy**, and was told he had a poor prognosis for survival. Against the odds, he survived and did well for some time, but his condition has slowly worsened over the past eighteen months. He was admitted two weeks ago with worsening shortness of breath, was found to have an acute heart attack, and was again evaluated for consideration of coronary bypass grafting. This surgical procedure was not possible, but an alternative stenting procedure[2] was done. He is not a candidate for heart transplantation because of severe obesity.

2. Stenting of an artery involves dilation of a narrowed segment of an artery to improve

Since the stenting procedure, he has had a difficult time with **intubation** and **ventilator** support for **congestive heart failure** most of that time. He has been **extubated** twice and has required reintubation both times within minutes or hours. A repeat echocardiogram today shows that his low ejection fraction[3] of 10 percent has not improved (normal is 45-65 percent). No cardiology procedures remain as options. He has now been intubated for about ten days, so personnel are considering performing a tracheostomy to avoid complications from prolonged intubation (erosion and hemorrhage of the lining of the trachea). However, he has said on several occasions to several individuals that he does not want another tracheostomy. He mentioned this to his case worker in a conversation about two months ago; he said it to his ICU caregivers and to the cardiology consultant.

Bernie has a long history of bipolar disorder with several episodes of psychosis leading to difficulties with the law as a young adult. He has done quite well on medication for the past ten years and has consistently made his own treatment decisions, been in charge of his checkbook, etc. He has never married. He lives in a group home for individuals with mental illness and has been known to his case worker (also operator of the home) for more than ten years. He has worked part-time doing auto parts inventory until this admission. He has been aware of his deteriorating condition and made burial arrangements about two months ago. The patient is deeply religious (Christian) and has told his case worker that he does not fear death.

I found him very sleepy, but rousable. He appeared to be aware of my presence and my questions. He again shook his head indicating no tracheostomy, even if that means he will not survive. He chose to continue current efforts to postpone death and get off the ventilator rather than have extubation now with a high chance of death.

DISCUSSION

A patient with decisional capacity is free to decline any and all recommendations for treatment, even if refusal has a high likelihood of leading to

---

blood flow and insertion of a small expandable device intended to keep the artery from renarrowing. This is done in the catheterization laboratory under X-ray observation, and does not involve an operation on the heart or opening the chest.

3. Ejection fraction is a calculation to assess the strength of the heart muscle. It is done by echocardiography, using an ultrasound technique to visualize heart structure and measure heart muscle strength. This measurement is often done in patients with congestive heart failure.

death. This is especially true if the patient is very familiar with the procedure, and is consistent in refusing. When a patient refuses a particular treatment option, it is important to ascertain if all alternative treatment options have been considered.

This patient is dying of irreversible heart disease. He has consistently refused a tracheostomy recommended to assist with **weaning** and to prevent tracheal erosion. He has had a tracheostomy in the past.

RECOMMENDATIONS

1. It is ethically permissible to not perform a tracheostomy in this patient.
2. Apart from a tracheostomy, the patient currently says he would like to survive and get off the ventilator if this is possible. Thus it is appropriate to continue his current therapies, including efforts to maximize his function to enable weaning. Even if prolonged intubation increases his risk of tracheal complications, this may be an acceptable risk if there is a concomitant potential benefit.
3. Given his overall poor prognosis, if his ICU caregivers believe that **cardiopulmonary resuscitation** (CPR) would offer no chance of significant benefit, a **do-not-resuscitate order** (DNR order) may be written.

FOLLOW-UP

There was no change in the patient's clinical condition over the next several days. He remained on **full code status** because there was some uncertainty whether CPR could restore circulation in the event of a cardiac arrest. The patient requested a DNR order of his case manager six days later, and this order was written. About one week later, after the patient had been miserable for several days, and when he showed no sign of being able to wean, his case manager and physician chose to discontinue his ventilator. He was given comfort care and died in two hours.

COMMENT

The issue of surrogacy is important in this case. It is traditional for a spouse or other relatives to act in this capacity. In this case, though there were no involved relatives, a caring person had looked after the patient's welfare for several years, and knew the patient, his values, and his goals. Thus his case manager was an appropriate proxy with significant moral authority.

The final decision in this case was made by his case manager, based on the understanding that the patient's goal of survival without a tracheostomy was no longer achievable, and his apparent unrelievable discomfort.

Case 4.03

QUESTION

Is it ethically permissible to continue aggressive therapy for this dying patient when his primary physician believes it would not be in his best interests and that he probably would not want it?

STORY

Tom is a fifty-nine-year-old man who had surgery six years ago for a slow-growing brain tumor. It later recurred and he had noncurative surgery, irradiation, and placement of a shunt in his brain to prevent pressure buildup. He has been cared for at home by his family, with considerable assistance from visiting nurses and his primary physician, Dr. Alexander, during his long course of gradual deterioration.

He was admitted to the hospital with progressive sleepiness two and a half weeks ago, and a few days later was transferred to the intensive care unit with respiratory failure and **sepsis**. He has now been on a **ventilator** for about two weeks and has had a tracheostomy. Testing has shown increased pressure in his brain such that he will not awaken. He previously had some muscle tone, but now is flaccid.

At a family meeting six days ago, his wife and son agreed to a **do-not-resuscitate order** but were unwilling to consent to the recommended withdrawal of ventilator support or withholding of any measures to treat new crises. A goal was established for home ventilator therapy after family training. They based this goal on their understanding of his previously stated wishes. His wife reported that the patient indicated his desire for full therapy by refusing to complete a living will. A representative from his visiting nurse association was present at the meeting and confirmed that Tom had always said he wanted to survive as long as possible, regardless of his quality of life.

However, Dr. Alexander, who has known him since before his brain tumor, believes Tom would not desire intensive measures when there is no prospect of regaining awareness. In addition, he fears that Tom's condition could slowly progress to total brain death, which his family might not detect if he is at home when it happens. He feels it would be unseemly to continue ventilator support for a corpse. (See the discussion of death by neurologic criteria in chapter 7.)

DISCUSSION

When a patient is no longer able to participate in treatment decisions, we try to use **substituted judgment**, that is, we try to do as the patient would wish. This may sometimes be assessed by the wording of a written **advance directive**; absent that it is best approached through conversation with those who know the patient best, usually family and professional caregivers.

When a family establishes a goal of therapy for a patient based on an understanding of the patient's wishes, the professionals involved in his or her care almost always honor those wishes. Occasionally a professional may decline to provide the services to meet that goal: (a) if the therapy is futile; (b) if it would cause the patient unrelievable suffering; or (c) if there is credible evidence that the chosen goal is not what the patient would choose. In addition, health-care professionals may decline to provide services that make them professionally uncomfortable by transferring care to another professional.

In this case, the family is caring and united in their understanding of the patient's wishes, and this is corroborated by his visiting nurses. However, the patient's long-standing physician believes he has a different understanding of the **best interests** of the patient as well as the patient's wishes and values.

RECOMMENDATIONS

1. It is ethically permissible to continue current measures, which are not physiologically futile and are not causing the patient unrelievable suffering.
2. It would be good for Dr. Alexander to talk again with the family, to explain the basis for his different understanding of the patient's wishes, and his recommendations for further management.

3. If the family remains steadfast in its current goals, the primary physician may continue to provide care, instituting extra measures to address his professional concerns, such as frequent home visits to assess the patient's neurologic condition. Alternatively, he may choose to decline further care by transferring responsibility to another physician.

COMMENT

Patient autonomy is foundational in contemporary Western medical ethics. Families have the responsibility to honor the known wishes or values of the patient. Physicians are generally bound to honor those wishes and values as well. However, that does not mean that physicians are mere technicians who automatically do as they are told. They have the responsibility to educate patients and families, and when they disagree with patient or **surrogate** choices, they may attempt to persuade them. However, physicians should not place undue pressure on decision-makers, nor use manipulation (biased disclosure of facts) or coercion (threats) to get decision-makers to change their minds. If a decision-maker remains steadfast in a choice with which the physician is not comfortable, the physician may choose from the options mentioned above.

Case 4.04

QUESTION

Please help discuss treatment options when the patient's spoken wishes are not consistent with his written advance directive.

STORY

Harry, an eighty-year-old man, was admitted to the hospital three weeks ago with a recurrent small bowel obstruction. Surgical intervention was postponed for a few hours because of his poor pulmonary function, but was undertaken when the symptoms of obstruction worsened. At surgery he was found to have multiple adhesions[4] that required removal of a short

4. An adhesion is a band or sheet of scar tissue that may develop between two or more

piece of small bowel. Post-op he has had multiple complications including persistent respiratory failure (requiring continuous use of a **ventilator**), air leaks from both lungs (requiring drainage tubes in his chest), pneumonia caused by a microorganism that is difficult to treat because of its resistance to most antibiotics, and development of a leak of bowel contents through his abdominal wall. While his overall prognosis is very poor indeed, none of his current problems is felt to be insurmountable. His pulmonary situation is probably the most tenuous.

The patient has a past history of severe chronic lung disease (he was on continuous supplemental oxygen at home) and chronic alcoholism. He has had small bowel obstruction twice in the past. One episode about two years ago required surgery and three months in the hospital (of which one month was in the intensive care unit [ICU], three weeks on a ventilator), during which his physicians declared a very poor prognosis for survival. The other episode, three months ago, was successfully treated with conservative measures and did not require surgery.

The patient's only daughter, Cynthia, reports that Harry completed an **advance directive** (no copy on chart) several months ago in which he named her as his **agent** and checked the option from the standard wording that he didn't want to survive on life support. However, when she asked him if he understood that this meant he would not be put through another extended ICU stay, he said the experience was not bad since he didn't remember most of it. Also, the admitting surgeon told him that this admission would likely be as difficult as the one two years ago, or perhaps more so, and he indicated that he wanted full treatment to proceed.

Harry's daughter describes him as a blunt, stubborn, independent person who bucks the trends. He operated a small newsstand for many years until his respiratory problems forced him to give it up. She reports that his quality of life was objectively not great (congregate living, limited mobility, mostly self-care), but that he seemed to cope with it well. His only pleasures in life are drinking and seeing his family, though he doesn't get along well with a few of them. Cynthia says the patient is nonreligious and does not appear to be spiritual. She knows the patient fears death and may have some unfinished interpersonal business that he has been unwilling to confront.

---

surfaces as an aftermath of a surgical procedure, most commonly seen in the abdomen. This abnormal tissue may cause compression or obstruction of function of intra-abdominal organs.

DISCUSSION

When a patient has lost **decision-making capacity**, we try to make difficult treatment decisions using **substituted judgment**, that is, we try to make the decision the patient would make if the patient were able. This may be based on the patient's written advance directive, previously spoken wishes, or an understanding of his or her values. A written advance directive often requires some interpretation by those who know the patient best and know the circumstances in which the patient composed the document.

In this case the patient has named his daughter to be his **surrogate**, indicating that he trusts her to make treatment decisions and believes she knows his values and wishes. Though he wrote in the advance directive document that he didn't want long-term life support, he has indicated to both his daughter and his ICU physicians that he wanted to survive if at all possible, and he didn't mind a prolonged ICU course if that was needed.

RECOMMENDATIONS

1. It seems ethically appropriate at this time to continue treatment aimed at survival.
2. If the patient develops further complications that suggest an even more dismal chance of survival, it would then be appropriate to rediscuss with his daughter goals and possible **limitation of treatment**.
3. If the patient continues in a stable situation without improvement, at some (difficult to determine) point it would be appropriate to (a) try to awaken him to discuss the option of long-term vent support with him, or (b) rediscuss with his daughter the prognosis and treatment options.
4. If the patient improves, it might be wise to have a chaplain or social worker talk with him about his fear of death and unresolved issues with other people.

FOLLOW-UP

For the next two weeks the patient's condition waxed and waned, but his poor mental function made it impossible to talk with him about his wishes or other issues. He subsequently developed another episode of **sepsis** and was treated vigorously, but he died in the ICU on full support.

COMMENT

It is tempting to look back on this case and wish that the health-care professionals had been able to persuade the patient or his daughter to accept some limitation of treatment so that he could have received compassionate **palliative care** rather than dying on full treatment in the ICU. The problem, of course, was uncertainty. There was no way to be sure of the outcome without trying. In addition, all involved in his care were trying to honor their understanding of his wishes and values.

Case 4.05

QUESTION

Should we continue ventilator support and do a tracheostomy in this patient who has poor prospects for weaning from the ventilator and has said in the past she didn't want long-term support?

STORY

Rita is a seventy-two-year-old woman whose aortic valve has been narrowing for a few years and who has had symptoms of shortness of breath and occasional chest pain for about three years. Earlier evaluation had suggested that she was not a good surgical candidate because of obesity, chronic lung disease, immobility, and diabetes. Three weeks ago she had a more severe episode of chest pain and was admitted to the hospital. From a cardiac standpoint she was felt to have strong indications for valve replacement, but this was felt to be "very high risk" for the above reasons. She consented to risky surgery and short-term **intubation**, and the surgery was done twelve days ago. She initially did well and was **extubated** three days after surgery. However, just two days later she was transferred back to the intensive care unit in respiratory failure and again she agreed to short-term intubation. One week later she is now stable, but is not **weaning** from the **ventilator**, and it is felt that she will require a long, slow weaning process, necessitating **tracheostomy** and surgical insertion of a feeding tube soon. There is a **do-not-resuscitate order** (DNR order) written in her chart, but the physician who wrote it did not write the customary accompanying note explaining the justification for the decision.

The patient signed a living will just a few days before admission in which she requested withdrawal of support if she had an irreversible mental or physical condition with no reasonable expectation of recovery. An accompanying durable power of attorney for health care names Ronald Williams as her **agent**.

The patient is alert, able to nod yes and no, and able to write on a clipboard. I explained her current situation and the above questions. When asked if we should continue her current treatment, she initially wrote "Call Rena" (her only daughter) and then "Call Ronald Williams," and she also correctly wrote their phone numbers. I said I would do that but suggested that she tell us whether to continue, and she nodded yes when asked twice.

Rena reports that her mother has been in gradually declining health for many years; she has given up bingo and quilting, which she formerly found enjoyable. She is pleased that her mother indicates she wants to continue treatment, but understands that new complications or failure to wean may lead to a decision to withdraw support and give comfort care.

DISCUSSION

Treatment decisions should ideally be made jointly by the patient who has **decision-making capacity** and his or her professional caregivers. Only when the patient is not able to participate do we use **substituted judgment** to make decisions, using the patient's previously written or spoken wishes as a guide.

This patient has a poor prognosis, which might be interpreted to fit the "no reasonable expectation of recovery" clause in her living will. However, her written **advance directive** need not be invoked or interpreted as long as she retains the capacity to participate in decisions including the naming of her **surrogate**. We also do not need to seek consent from her named surrogate as long as she is able to make her own decisions.

RECOMMENDATIONS

1. It is appropriate to honor this patient's request to continue her current level of treatment.
2. If she remains stable but fails to wean so that a decision must be made about a tracheostomy and feeding tube in another week or two, this

should be discussed with her, along with the best possible guess at her prognosis for eventual weaning.

3. If a new crisis intervenes, the question of limiting treatment should be discussed with her, if she is able, or with her named surrogates (Ronald Williams, named in writing, and daughter Rena, named verbally).

4. The DNR order now in place may be justified if (a) her professional caregivers believe there is no reasonable chance she could survive a cardiac arrest, or (b) she has indicated to them that she does not want **cardiopulmonary resuscitation**.

FOLLOW-UP

Two days later the patient's surgical chest wound opened spontaneously. This made the prospect of weaning even more unlikely. The wound was covered with a sterile dressing and her surgeon recommended wound closure in the next few days if her condition was stable. Over the next three days she developed new infection and became unresponsive. Her surrogate and her daughter agreed that she would not want to continue vigorous treatment at this point. Her support was withdrawn and she died quickly.

COMMENT

Sometimes health-care professionals quickly jump to surrogate decision-making when the patient is still able to participate. If this patient is able, she should be encouraged to do so. However, some patients may feel overwhelmed and have full confidence in their chosen agent to do what is best for them. It is permissible for the patient to defer to a designated agent.

Some people of faith worry that giving the patient such decision-making authority in life-and-death situations is an inappropriate use of autonomy, feeling that God is in charge of such ultimate matters. Certainly a belief in the sovereignty of God would suggest that he is able to make the ultimate decisions in spite of human efforts. At the same time, a belief in human dominion and stewardship would suggest that individuals have been given the ability to exert some authority in such matters. Decisions on the use or nonuse of ventilator support are not completely different from those on the use or nonuse of antibiotics. The difficulty, of course, is that some individuals, whether devout in their faith or not, may choose to continue death-postponing therapies beyond a point that seems reasonable to others. I believe we must grant some latitude to human reason.

Case 4.06

QUESTION

What should be done for this patient with viral pneumonia and a poor prognosis when the family is not in agreement?

STORY

Gertrude is a seventy-eight-year-old woman with a history of chronic lung disease and chronic pain from a degenerative condition of her spine. She was admitted one month ago with worsening shortness of breath. She was treated vigorously while diagnostic workup was undertaken. Her pulmonary condition slowly worsened and she required **intubation** and **ventilator** support about two weeks ago. Her diagnosis is atypical pneumonia, possibly from a herpes virus (found on **bronchoscopy**), with **adult respiratory distress syndrome**. In general, this condition has a 50 percent survival rate after prolonged ventilator support (from one to six weeks on average, but sometimes months). Since she has shown no improvement so far, it seems likely that she will require a prolonged course of support.

At the time that she was intubated, she appeared to be ambivalent and deferred to a daughter, who made the decision. It is nearing time to consider **tracheostomy** (to prevent complications from prolonged intubation) if prolonged support is to be undertaken. Her history of chronic pain raises the possibility of a more difficult **wean** than average. She has been fully sedated, but this was stopped about twenty-four hours ago. With this condition and prognosis, her professional caregivers believe it would be acceptable either to continue vigorous support or to withdraw support with the expectation that she would not survive.

The patient is a widow who was living independently prior to this illness. She has four adult children. She has been a faithful Methodist all her adult life. She has no written **advance directive**, but one daughter reports that she has said in the past that she "didn't want heroics," though she did not elaborate.

A family conference is convened: one son and two daughters were in the room; one daughter and her husband from out of state were on the conference phone; also present were Gertrude's attending ICU (intensive care unit) physician, her nurse, the ICU social worker, a medical student, and myself from Ethics. Her course, current condition, and prognosis were reviewed. While the son-in-law was inclined to choose tracheostomy and continued efforts at survival, other family members were uncertain.

DISCUSSION

When treatment decisions must be made for a patient who has lost the capacity to participate in discussions, we try to make a **substituted judgment**, that is, the decision the patient would make if able. We try to construct this using a written advance directive, previously spoken statements, or an understanding of the patient's values. When this is not possible, we drop to a lower standard of decision making and try to do what appears to be in the patient's **best interests**.

This patient was ambivalent about starting intensive therapy, and we do not have a clear indication of whether she would choose to continue. Her family is divided between changing goals to comfort care, and tracheostomy and continued vigorous treatment.

RECOMMENDATIONS

1. It would be ethically permissible either to continue intensive therapy or to withdraw support and give comfort care.
2. Her family members are appropriate **surrogates** at this time, and her care team should accept their best estimate of what she would want if her wishes cannot be elicited. It is appropriate to attempt a conversation with her if withdrawal of her sedation does not lead to disproportionate suffering. However, since she deferred to her children about initiation of ventilator support, it would not be surprising if she did the same here. Thus, pursuit of her autonomous choice should not be overly aggressive.

FOLLOW-UP

Her son-in-law convinced the rest of the family to consent to a tracheostomy with continued trial of therapy for a week. The clinicians were doubtful that one more week would make a significant difference, and were thus reluctant to do the proposed surgical procedure if there was a possibility of discontinuing support in a week, so her endotracheal intubation was continued. Her daughter and son-in-law were encouraged to come to her bedside. They arrived from out of state three days later, and after seeing her, agreed with the rest of the family that support should be withdrawn. This was done, and she died in a few hours with her family present.

COMMENT

A picture is worth a thousand words, and a bedside visit often helps a surrogate decision-maker come to a clearer decision. Sometimes the family member from out of state is reluctant to agree to a decision to limit therapy for social reasons — for example, estrangement, guilt about not visiting or being involved. But more often, they cannot fully grasp the situation until they can see for themselves what the patient looks like.

Case 4.07

QUESTION

Should this chronically ill man's ventilator be stopped? Who has the authority to make decisions for him — his wife or his siblings?

STORY

Charles, admitted two weeks ago, is fifty-one years old, has had multiple sclerosis for eight years, and has been disabled for four years from his job in auto tire sales. Until about six weeks prior to this admission he was able to use his legs and get up in parallel bars. However, a recent exacerbation of his disease has caused difficulty speaking and talking, loss of use of his legs, and diminished use of his upper extremities. He was admitted with a staphylococcal pneumonia, and on admission said he wanted full treatment. He quickly progressed to respiratory failure requiring **intubation** and **ventilator** assistance, and to **adult respiratory distress syndrome**. At this point his caregivers in the intensive care unit (ICU) believe it is unlikely he will ever **wean** from the ventilator. He is currently stable, his infectious process is under control, and he is on 40 percent oxygen with relatively low ventilator settings. He responds appropriately to family members. There is a durable power of attorney (not a durable power of attorney for health care) form on the chart signed by the patient eight years ago naming his wife as financial agent.

An ICU management meeting was held four days ago to discuss plans with his wife. She felt that he would choose, in light of his poor prognosis for improvement, to change to comfort care soon. The conclusion of the meeting was that a **do-not-resuscitate order** was written, but the current level of therapy would continue for another week and withdrawal of support would then be reconsidered. When his sister learned the next day that his wife planned to "pull the plug" soon, she became angry and said this would be "murder." In light of the tension between his wife and his sister, his wife said she wanted to resign her role as **surrogate**. I requested a meeting with his wife and two siblings, but his wife was unable to get transportation, so I talked with her on the phone and with his two sisters in person.

His wife reports that Charles was on a ventilator for a short time eight years ago and has said clearly that it would be unacceptable for long-term use. In addition, he said he would not want to be admitted to a nursing home. At this point she believes he would consent to continuation of the ventilator for a few more days, but that he would not want to go longer unless there were a 50 percent or better chance of weaning. His siblings agree that he would not want long-term vent support, but believe it is too soon to quit, especially without an adequate weaning trial, and they would want to continue until there was a 95 percent chance of nonweaning. Both sides verbalize strong antipathy toward the other with accusations about attitudes and motives.

DISCUSSION

When a patient has a poor prognosis for recovery or survival, it is appropriate to discuss ongoing goals and the possibility of **limitation of treatment**. When a previously competent patient loses the ability to make decisions about treatment, we try to make a **substituted judgment**, that is, the decision the patient would make if able. If the patient has left no written **advance directive**, we try to reconstruct the patient's wishes from those who know the patient best.

This patient has a poor prognosis for recovery, and is at a point where many patients would choose to limit therapy. He has made his wife, who has cared for him for eight years, his financial durable power of attorney, but he has no written medical advance directive. She and his sisters agree that he does not want long-term vent support, but disagree regarding how long is an adequate trial and what degree of certainty is appropriate before making an irreversible decision.

RECOMMENDATIONS

1. It is ethically appropriate to continue the current level of therapy. Efforts to clarify and quantify his pulmonary and neurologic prognoses should continue.

2. From an ethics perspective, it would be worthwhile to attempt weaning from the ventilator and from the sedation, if this is medically feasible. If it becomes possible to converse with the patient, his pulmonary and neurologic prognoses should be explained to him, and he may make his own decisions about (a) whether he wants long-term ventilator support, (b) if not, how long he wants to continue vigorous measures before changing to comfort care, and (c) what level of prognostic certainty he would like before making that decision.

3. If it is not possible to converse with him, it would be ideal to seek consensus between his wife and sisters. However, given their level of antipathy, this may not be possible. His wife is the presumptive surrogate, but his siblings could challenge this in court if they strongly object to her decisions.

FOLLOW-UP

One week later another management meeting was held in the ICU with the attending physician, the patient's nurse, the ICU social worker, and his sisters; his wife was unable (or unwilling?) to attend, but the physician spoke with her on the phone. It was emphasized that the patient had been on the ventilator for over three weeks and a decision needed to be made about both a **tracheostomy** for prolonged ventilator support and surgical insertion of a feeding tube. His sedation was weaned last week, and at least two attempts were made to converse with him about his wishes regarding a feeding tube (to which he clearly said no) and a tracheostomy (to which he seemed ambivalent).

Intense rancor and animosity continued between Charles's wife and sisters. At the beginning of the meeting the sisters wanted to withdraw support and they said his wife now wanted "everything done," exactly the opposite positions the two parties had held at the meeting one week earlier. I tried repeatedly to refocus the discussion on what the patient would want, but the parties were unable to relinquish their seeming need to cast the other in a bad light and violently oppose the other's position. His wife reported by phone that she had been told he was improved this morning ("without oxygen for two hours without difficulty"), but after the doctor explained that a two-hour weaning attempt had been made, but failed, she abruptly said, "Well, pull the plug," and went on to put the responsibility for this decision on his siblings.

The conclusion of the meeting was that in light of his failure to improve, his previously stated wishes of not wanting long-term ventilator support or nursing home placement, and his recent apparent confirmation of a wish to avoid long-term support, there was "consensus" that treatment goals should be changed to comfort care. He was **extubated** and given sedation that evening, and he died peacefully in three hours.

COMMENT

Often family disagreement is based on legitimate differences of perspective or differing understandings of the patient's previously expressed wishes or unspoken values. Sometimes, however, the disagreement has to do with an entirely different agenda. It is often necessary to place this apparent source of disagreement on the table by saying, "It is clear that there are differences between you unrelated to our current discussion. We will be unable to resolve those issues here, but I ask that we all try to focus on what the patient would want or, if that is not clear, what would be in the patient's **best interests**." Sometimes that allows family members to set aside old hurts and focus on the issue. Sometimes, as in this case, the animosity is so prominent that the two parties primarily want to disagree. This generates a significant challenge in mediation.

The issue was particularly acute in this case because the patient had signed only a durable power of attorney, a document that gives authority over financial matters, and not a durable power of attorney for health care, which gives authority for treatment decisions. Had he done the latter, his wife would have been legally empowered to make the decision, resolving the conflict. But this might have further inflamed the interpersonal animosity. As it was, his siblings were granted more voice, and the "consensus" that was ultimately reached might reduce future name-calling and blame-casting. Then again, it might not.

Case 4.08

QUESTION

Is it ethically permissible to stop ventilator support at this man's request when he still may be successfully weaned from the machine and may be currently depressed?

STORY

George is a seventy-five-year-old retired railroad engineer who was admitted ten days ago with an exacerbation of chronic lung disease. His condition worsened and he was **intubated** five days ago and attached to a **ventilator**. He has been treated vigorously, but has indicated in the past few days that he wanted to be **extubated** and go home. He understands that this would mean that he would die. The ICU (intensive care unit) team are reluctant to stop so soon, feeling that more can be done to reverse this situation. They believe he might **wean**, though it would likely take a few weeks. They are also concerned that his long-term antidepressant was inadvertently stopped at the time of admission, and they have asked Psychiatry to assess the role of depression in his request.

The patient has been slowly deteriorating from chronic lung disease for several years. He had not been on a ventilator prior to this illness, but he has been on home oxygen (nights and as needed) for two or three years. His activity level has been slowly fading. He has told his wife and only son that he knew he would die soon. He and his wife moved from their home in the country to a mobile home in town several months ago because of his increasing disability. He has still been able to get out of the home, drive his car, and visit friends. He has said in the past that he would not want to live on long-term life support, nor if he were totally disabled and immobile.

The patient has been intermittently depressed since their daughter died of cancer fifteen years ago. He had most recently been on an antidepressant for nearly three years, and his wife believes it was effectively controlling his depression.

There is no **advance directive** in the chart. His wife and I tried to arouse him, but he was sleepy from recently administered sedation and unable to have a meaningful conversation.

DISCUSSION

A patient with **decision-making capacity** is free to accept or decline any treatment. Before accepting from a patient an irreversible decision to decline life-prolonging treatment, it must be clear that the patient fully understands both the implications of the decision and the alternatives. It is also important to ensure that adequate time has elapsed for the patient to give it sufficient thought, and that such issues as a treatable depression are not adversely coloring his or her decision.

In this case, the patient has recognized the terminal nature of his chronic condition and appears to have resigned himself to death in the foreseeable future. He has also given some thought to his end-of-life treatment wishes. Treatment for his chronic depression had apparently been successful, though it is not clear if his recognition of his deterioration has exacerbated the depression or if stopping his antidepressant could be coloring his current request.

RECOMMENDATIONS

1. It is appropriate to maintain his current level of therapy pending at least the following: (a) completion of the psychiatry evaluation, and (b) further discussion with him and his wife about the possibility of weaning over a period of several weeks.
2. If the patient continues to request withdrawal of the ventilator after both above issues are resolved, it would then be ethically permissible, even obligatory, to honor his request.

FOLLOW-UP

Evaluation by a psychiatrist found the patient able to answer questions. He said he did not want to die, but also did not want the **endotracheal tube** to remain in place. The psychiatrist recommended resuming his most recent antidepressant plus a trial of a faster-acting mood stimulator. The patient had a good response to this with improved outlook in just a few days, and he agreed to continue ventilator support. He weaned off the ventilator nine days later and consented to reintubation if needed. He remained bright and cheerful and was transferred to a rehabilitation facility when a bed became available two weeks later.

COMMENT

The role of depression in patient decisions to refuse or discontinue life-sustaining therapy is often difficult to assess. A realistic recognition that one's chronic disease is progressing, and that one's future will likely include incapacity, can be depressing. But it is difficult to justify continuing a patient with a poor prognosis on unwanted life support for the few weeks it may take to see if the depression will lift with medication.

In this case, the patient did have a chronic disease with a poor prognosis, but in addition, he had a chronic depression and his effective treatment had been inadvertently stopped. Fortunately, he responded quickly to the mood stimulator, and continued treatment of his depression allowed his mood to lift, reaffirming his will to live.

Case 4.09

QUESTION

Is it ethically permissible to honor the refusal of relatively low-burden life-saving treatment from this man with schizophrenia when there is a professional difference of opinion about his capacity to make decisions?

STORY

Jeffrey is a sixty-two-year-old man who last evening was found by neighbors to be hallucinating. They called 911, and he was brought to the emergency department (ED). He was evaluated and found to be somnolent, with low oxygen and high carbon dioxide levels in his blood. After treatment with noninvasive pulmonary support (i.e., by tight-fitting mask), his blood gases improved but did not normalize. He awakened and said he would accept medications but refused to continue the mask, and said he did not want ICU (intensive care unit) care, **cardiopulmonary resuscitation**, or other major interventions. When told he would likely die without the mask, he said he understood and still did not want it. His **decision-making capacity** was evaluated by two ED physicians who felt he lacked capacity, and by a psychiatrist and an ICU physician who felt he had capacity. Without the mask-assisted ventilation, he again became somnolent.

Jeffrey has a known history of schizophrenia, low thyroid function, high blood pressure, and chronic lung disease. The psychiatrist who knows him well reports that he has refused treatment on many occasions in the past. During his lucid interval in the ED tonight, he said he stopped all his medication about two months ago, leading to an additional diagnosis of possible myxedema coma (profoundly low thyroid function), which is reversible but has a mortality rate of 30-40 percent. It is recorded in the chart that he has no family or friends and no regular source of medical care.

I was called at home just after 2 A.M., and after discussion with his hospital physician who had not previously had contact with him, I said it was ethically permissible to temporarily treat him over his objection, placing him in restraints if needed, until we had a better understanding of his clinical condition, his prognosis, and his capacity. When I arrived on the ward a short time later, he was unresponsive and had just been placed back on mask-assisted ventilation. He is also being treated with antibiotics and thyroid replacement medication. Initial lab reports suggest he is profoundly hypothyroid but not in the myxedema coma range.

DISCUSSION

A patient with decision-making capacity has the right to refuse treatment, even lifesaving treatment. Assessment of capacity may be difficult, especially in a patient with **encephalopathy** or psychosis. It is ethically permissible to override a patient's refusal of treatment if the patient appears to have some defect in understanding or reasoning, serious harm is likely unless there is intervention, and the probable benefit from intervention (e.g., preservation of life) outweighs the probable harm of intervention (deprivation of freedom). Neither psychosis nor depression automatically indicates lack of capacity, though either may in specific instances.

This patient's current refusal of major interventions is consistent with his past attitude toward treatment. His willingness to accept death to avoid temporary, moderately burdensome treatment raises a question of depression. His refusal of some treatments and acceptance of others might at first raise questions about his capacity — he appears inconsistent about treatment goals. On the other hand, this may merely represent his assessment of benefits and burdens of specific treatments since someone who is incapacitated from depression might be more likely to refuse all treatments.

RECOMMENDATIONS

1. Because there is a difference of opinion among his caregivers about his capacity, it is ethically permissible to temporarily impose life-preserving treatments over his objection.
2. The primary short-term goals of treatment should be to preserve his life and to try to restore his decision-making capacity.
3. When his encephalopathy has been corrected, there should be further conversation with him about (a) his goals of therapy and (b) his reason for refusing ICU care or the mask to help him breathe. If his initial psychiatric evaluation did not include an assessment for depression, this should be done as well.
4. If the patient can articulate adequate reasons for his refusal (such as his assessment of the relative benefits and burdens of various treatments) and he is deemed to be not depressed, then it would be ethically permissible to honor his requested **limitation of treatment**.

FOLLOW-UP

He did not improve with mask-assisted ventilation, and since he had clearly refused **intubation** in the past, it was not felt to be ethically permissible to impose this treatment. Thus, the mask was discontinued and the goals of treatment were shifted to comfort care. However, he awakened again a few hours later and was in florid psychosis, now clearly without decision-making capacity. Since he had refused life-preserving treatment when having capacity, in the view of some professionals, these measures were not added.

The next day he was awake and conversant, and said he was comfortable but hungry. Procedures were begun to pursue guardianship. However, he again slipped into unconsciousness and died.

COMMENT

Determination of decision-making capacity is an art, not a science. To have capacity a person must understand the necessity of a decision, must be aware of the treatment options, must understand the likely outcomes with the various options, and must be able to rationally manipulate the information to make a decision. Occasionally health-care professionals will disagree about whether a specific patient has capacity or not. This makes it difficult when decisions are necessary about the use or nonuse of life-preserving therapy. In the face of such uncertainty, it is better to opt for life-prolonging treatment until more information can be learned about the patient's wishes or values.

Case 4.10

QUESTION

Is it appropriate to limit life-sustaining treatment from this critically ill woman who some believe is indicating that she wants to go to heaven?

STORY

Margaret is an eighty-year-old retired schoolteacher who was admitted six weeks ago for cardiac valve replacement and coronary artery bypass grafting. Since surgery she has been dependent on a **ventilator** (and has had a **tracheostomy**) and is also currently being treated for serious infection. Two days ago she pointed upward and mouthed the word "heaven." Her daughter, Rebecca, who was present, suggested other possible meanings for the gesture, but it quickly became clear that her mother was saying she was ready to die and enter eternity. (She had made this gesture several times in the past, but it was unclear to observers what she was trying to indicate.) Nursing and pastoral care staff are also convinced that she is requesting a shift in goals from full treatment to comfort care. Yesterday an order was written specifying no **cardiopulmonary resuscitation**.

The patient completed a durable power of attorney for health care about three weeks prior to admission, specifying Rebecca as her primary **agent** and her son-in-law as an alternate. I had a long conversation today with both of them. In the midst of their sadness, they are confident that the patient is truly requesting that we let her go. They describe her as a woman of faith, and thus her reference to going to heaven is consistent with her values. They are also very clear that if she had not indicated to them that she wanted to discontinue aggressive treatment, they could never have authorized it. The patient's husband is elderly, often confused, and rarely leaves their home. They also have a son, but he has had little contact with the patient in recent years.

One must consider in this case that the patient is changing goals after battling long and hard, and she was recently started on medication for depression. Obviously she has reason to be sad, given her long stay in the intensive care unit (ICU) and poor prognosis. However, given her limited ability to communicate, one must be sure that her judgment is not being clouded by a mood disorder. To help determine if this was the case, I asked her daughter and son-in-law whether she would have consented to further treatment if she could have known, prior to entering the hospital for surgery, that she would be in the ICU for this length of time and then face prolonged mechanical ventilation and nursing home care. Both, without hesitation, firmly said absolutely no. This offers some reassurance that the patient's current request for **limitation of treatment** is consistent with her values and priorities.

I attempted to speak to the patient herself, but she was not able to follow simple commands nor indicate that she understood what I was saying.

DISCUSSION

There appears to be no significant ethical dilemma at this time. Based on the principle of patient autonomy, patients who possess **decision-making capacity** have the right to refuse any treatment, even that which is life-sustaining. It is quite likely that the patient's decision-making capacity is somewhat compromised — which is to be expected after an extended ICU stay — but the consistency of her expressed wishes is reassuring. The question of depression must also be addressed, but (as mentioned above) her family has no doubt that she would have chosen limitation of treatment if she had been able to foresee this decision point in advance.

If one were to argue that the patient currently lacks decision-making capacity, the onus of decision making would then fall to her agents. Both of the patient's agents support the shift in goals, appropriately applying the **substituted judgment** standard, basing their decisions on what the patient would want, not on what they think is best for the patient (or what they would like to see happen). They very honestly admit that they don't want to see the patient die, but they are able to put their own grief aside to honor her wishes.

RECOMMENDATIONS

1. It is ethically permissible to withhold life-sustaining treatment from this patient and switch goals to comfort care.
2. Before doing so, the patient and her family members (specifically, her husband and son) should have the opportunity to say good-bye. It might be helpful to coordinate their visits with the patient's medication schedule, to maximize the patient's awareness during the visits.
3. The **palliative care** service is always available to utilize their skills and experience in this area to ensure maximal pain- and symptom-control at the end of life.

FOLLOW-UP

The patient's family gathered at her bedside for a final farewell and a time of prayer. She was given some sedation by the ICU team, and her ventilator was turned off. She received two more doses of sedating medication over the next three hours for mild signs of respiratory distress. She died comfortably with her family present.

COMMENT

A patient's spiritual beliefs often enter into his or her decisions at the end of life. In this case, the patient was not only prepared to die but she also fought the good fight, recognized that the outcome was not satisfactory, and made her decision to stop the fight and allow her overwhelming disease process to take her life. Both the fact that she made the decision herself and the fact that it was based on her long-held beliefs gave comfort to her family in the midst of their grief.

Case 4.11

QUESTION

What is the appropriate course of action in the case of an intubated patient who was subsequently found to have orders for no resuscitation or intubation?

STORY

Ethel is a seventy-five-year-old woman with a complex medical history, including oxygen-dependent chronic lung disease, **congestive heart failure**, coronary artery disease, mild **dementia**, and osteoporosis (thinning of bones) leading to recent compression fractures of her spine. She was admitted from her assisted-living facility yesterday in respiratory distress, probably from **aspiration** of stomach contents after choking. After I consulted with her brother (a physician who shares power of attorney with his daughter, though not specifically for health care), it was decided to **intubate** her and give her ventilatory assistance. Subsequently it was discovered that she had a standing **do-not-resuscitate order** at her assisted-living facility, signed by Dr. Hernandez, her primary physician. She was admitted to the intensive care unit, and **limitation of treatment** orders were written (in consultation with the patient's brother) that specified no **cardiopulmonary resuscitation** (CPR) and no other invasive treatments. Antibiotics are being administered, and she is still intubated, having rapidly failed a **weaning** attempt earlier today.

On her last admission two years ago, the patient expressed a wish to not be intubated or subjected to CPR, documented by Dr. Hernandez. He also reports that he had a conversation with the patient in the last few months where she explicitly stated that she did not want any extraordinary measures, by which he felt sure she meant intubation and CPR. He had no doubts about her **decision-making capacity** at that time.

Ethel was a nurse in the armed forces before retiring nearly twenty years ago. She never married, and her only family is her brother and his children. She had long been a zealous volunteer but in recent years had become "very, very, very frail," according to her brother, and she now depends on a wheelchair for mobility. Her family reports that they never had any specific discussions with her about her treatment wishes, but they had a general sense that she "didn't want a whole lot."

Attempts at lightening her sedation led to marked agitation, and she is currently minimally interactive. Radiological studies revealed pneumonia in two lobes of her lungs, and the probability of her weaning off the ventilator soon (i.e., before **tracheostomy** becomes a consideration) is felt to be slim.

DISCUSSION

Autonomy is a foundational principle in medical ethics. The physician, then, must ascertain what the patient's wishes are, either through present conversation (if the patient has decision-making capacity) or by seeking **substituted judgment.**

In this case the patient does not have decision-making capacity, and it is not restorable given the amount of sedation required to prevent agitation. Her previously stated wishes regarding intubation (on her last admission, her assisted-living facility patient record, and recent conversations with her primary physician), however, are clear. Since we know her wishes, there is no need to move on to a lower **best interests** calculation. It is also relevant to note that while she has no assigned **surrogate** decision-maker (in the absence of a durable power of attorney for health care), by convention this role would fall to her closest relative (i.e., her brother). That person's responsibility is to do what the patient herself would want done, which is clear from her prior statements.

It should also be noted that there is no ethical difference between withdrawing and withholding. Thus, the fact that she is currently intubated does not change the fact that she expressed a desire not to be on a **ventilator.**

These matters were discussed in detail with her brother, niece, and nephew. It was decided that the ventilator be continued for another "one or two days" to give family members the opportunity to say good-bye, and to confirm that she is not weanable.

RECOMMENDATIONS

1. It is ethically obligatory, based on the principle of autonomy, to respect the patient's previously stated wishes regarding intubation.
2. That said, it is ethically permissible to temporarily delay **extubation** in order to (a) give her loved ones the chance to say good-bye and be present (if they wish) when she dies, and (b) provide further confirmation that she is not imminently weanable. While a period of twenty-four or even forty-eight hours might be appropriate for this purpose, further prolongation of her intubation (assuming no significant improvement in her condition/prognosis) would run contrary to her expressed desires.
3. If a decision is made to shift to comfort care, all modalities should be brought to bear to maximize the patient's comfort.

FOLLOW-UP

Two days later there was no significant change in the patient's condition. She was extubated with family present, and she died in a few minutes.

COMMENT

A generation ago it was believed that it was morally wrong for a physician to stop a treatment that was postponing death because the physician would then be causally responsible for the death. Consequently, physicians were reluctant to begin a treatment that had only a small chance of success, fearing the patient might become "stuck on" the treatment. Slowly (and painfully) it became established that there is no moral, legal, or professional difference between not starting and stopping a treatment. There still may be a psychological difference; it is emotionally more difficult for a physician to stop a ventilator, or dialysis, or transfusions, or a feeding tube that is sustaining a patient's life, knowing there is a high likelihood that the patient will not survive, than it is to not start the treatment in the first place. It feels "more active." However, one could easily argue that it is on a higher moral plane to start, try, and stop a treatment than to not start it at all. In the former case, an effort was made, and this is different from not trying and wondering if there is a small chance that the treatment would have worked.

Case 4.12

QUESTION

Is it permissible to not institute potentially life-extending chemotherapy and stop ventilator support for this patient at the request of her family?

STORY

Virginia is a sixty-eight-year-old practicing attorney who has been very healthy and has avoided medical care and ignored medical advice until this illness. She was treated two weeks ago by an urgent care physician for a respiratory infection, and she reluctantly agreed to hospital admission nine days ago when it had not responded to oral antibiotics. A chest X-ray showed a large pneumonia. Four days after admission, before her diagnosis was certain, she deteriorated and required transfer to the intensive care unit, **intubation**, and **ventilator** support. It has subsequently been determined that she has an incurable cancer of the lung that has spread to her liver. The malignant tumor is currently obstructing a major airway, and the pneumonia has developed beyond that obstruction. It appears that the cancer has sufficiently compromised her airway that it is unlikely she can be **weaned** from the ventilator without first starting chemotherapy to shrink the tumor.

The oncology consultant says there is a 40 percent chance her tumor will respond to chemotherapy (if it is started immediately) and she could survive for several months. Without chemotherapy, he anticipates she will not be weanable and she will likely succumb within four weeks. Her family has requested no chemotherapy, and her hospital physician, who has not previously known her, is reluctant to comply with this request since she has a reasonable chance of significant improvement.

I met with her physician and her close and caring family, three adult children and their spouses plus two of her own siblings. They report that she has always been an active woman who greatly enjoys her family, loves to eat, cook, and travel. Although not religious, she does believe in God; her beliefs about life after death are not known. She also previously told her family she did not want to be kept alive with machines, and she has commented negatively about several people she knew who had lingering illnesses. The family at first requested that chemotherapy not be done. After further discussion, they agreed that starting chemotherapy with the goal of **extubation** and discharge home was reasonable and in her **best interests**. They further agreed that an effort should be made to involve her in the decision.

I next met with the patient, family, and care team after the patient's sedation had been stopped. She was alert and appeared to understand the explanation of her condition and the treatment options. She indicated that she did not want chemotherapy, but she did want to go home.

DISCUSSION

Patients with **decision-making capacity** should be given the opportunity to make their own treatment choices after being adequately informed of the options and likely outcomes. For those who have lost this capacity, families can usually give the best estimation of patient values and probable treatment choices. They should base their choices on their understanding of the patient's wishes, not on their own preferences. If they decline therapy that the team feels is in the patient's best interests or that they believe most patients would choose, every effort should be made to restore the patient's decision-making capacity since some people may make sweeping statements against therapy when they are well but may feel differently when they are confronted with a life-threatening situation.

This patient has clearly said in the past that she would decline aggressive interventions to prolong her life. She now appears to be making a choice that is consistent with that past expression. However, she also says she wants to go home, and this is not an option in her current condition.

RECOMMENDATIONS

1. Now that her mental status has improved so that she can make decisions, repeat conversations should be held over the next day or two with her care team and her family to make sure she understands the consequences of her choice. It would be ethically permissible to try to persuade her to accept chemotherapy with the short-term goal of extubation and discharge home, but manipulation (e.g., overstating the benefits or understating the risks) is not permissible.

2. If she remains steadfast in her refusal of chemotherapy, all other therapies are also optional. She (or her family, if she loses decision-making capacity) could choose to forgo antibiotics or other acute interventions, or could even choose to stop her ventilator. Since a choice to stop the ventilator would result in significant shortening of her life, that step should probably not be taken immediately upon request. Rather, it should be considered and reflected upon to ensure that it is a clearly understood and confirmed decision.

FOLLOW-UP

After further discussion with the oncology consultant, the patient firmly decided against chemotherapy, realizing this would preclude her going home, and she further indicated she wanted the ventilator stopped immediately. Her family supported her choices. Her physician felt the patient needed at least twenty-four hours to contemplate this irreversible decision. All agreed on a twenty-four-hour wait and repeat discussion. (Her physician confided to me that she was also reluctant for the patient to forgo life-extending treatment without a better understanding of spiritual matters.)

I was asked to facilitate the repeat discussion the following day. The patient was sitting up in bed, wearing fresh makeup, interacting with her family, including writing lighthearted messages on a clipboard. Everyone seemed to have a clear understanding of the situation, the options, and the consequences. The patient reaffirmed her choice against chemotherapy and for immediate extubation. I asked her if there were any conversations she needed to have with others, and she said no. I asked if she was ready to meet God, and she said yes. I reviewed with her that it was not expected she would survive after extubation, but that this outcome was never guaranteed. She wanted to know about the time sequence, the comfort measures that would be used, etc. Her physician went over the steps that would be taken, up to extubation. The patient's daughter said, "And then you will meet Jesus." In an effort to reemphasize that survival was a small possibility, I immediately said, "Or maybe not." The physician gave me a frightful glance, thinking I was commenting on the patient's spiritual future. (Professionals must be careful that their comments are unambiguous.)

Two hours later, the physician gave the patient injections of morphine and sedatives and extubated her. She was given one more small dose of sedation about thirty minutes later, and she died thirty-five minutes after that. An autopsy showed the tumor was even more extensive than had been realized, causing speculation that it would probably not have responded to chemotherapy.

COMMENT

Physicians are often reluctant to agree with family decisions that will shorten a patient's life. Restoring the patient's ability to participate in such decisions will often alleviate this concern because we are more apt to accept such a decision from the patient than from the patient's family. Even then, we must ensure that the patient is not acting on impulse, but has adequate time to reflect on such a momentous decision.

Physicians of deep faith who believe in life after physical death are often reluctant to agree with life-ending decisions made by patients who may not have contemplated their eternal future. The role and level of health-care professionals in such discussions remain a topic of significant discussion.

Case 4.13 ——————————————————————————————————

QUESTION

Must we continue futile support in the intensive care unit for this dying man at the insistence of his daughter?

STORY

Malcolm ("Mac"), age sixty-four, is an architect who was found to have an incurable cancer of the esophagus five months ago. He came to the emergency department thirty-five days ago with shortness of breath, and it was found that his tumor was compressing the large airways going into both lungs. He was emergently **intubated**, admitted to the intensive care unit (ICU), and given ventilatory support, which has now continued for more than a month. Vigorous treatment has failed to shrink the tumor, and the ICU physician and oncologist are both convinced that his condition cannot be improved. Efforts have been made to awaken him to discuss **limitation of treatment**, but he remains too confused to understand or to engage in meaningful conversation. Because of his unawareness and his very poor prognosis, his professional caregivers have said they believe continued ICU care is futile.

Mac has been a widower for several years. His only son, Paul, and his wife, Lindsey, have been very attentive and willing to consent to any therapy that has been suggested so far. When presented a few days ago with information about his terminal condition and imminent death, however, they were unwilling to consider or even discuss any limitation of treatment, insisting that he remain in the ICU, on **ventilator** support, on **full code status**. They stated that their deep religious faith required them to do everything possible to preserve life, and they were counting on God to perform a miracle. They report that the patient was also a man of deep faith who would insist on this approach.

Mac's ICU nurse reports that he remains unresponsive and does not appear to be uncomfortable. She further reports overhearing a conversation between Paul and Lindsey about the need to get the patient's signature on a document that would finalize a real estate venture that he and his son have developed. An attorney came to the ICU to obtain the patient's signature a few days ago, but Mac was unable to understand or sign the document.

DISCUSSION

When it is clear that a patient is dying, is unaware, and cannot improve, it is appropriate to review the patient's treatment and to consider limiting life-extending treatment. Decisions for or against the use of such therapies should be based on the patient's wishes, expressed by the patient verbally or in writing. While it may occasionally be suspected that family members have "another agenda," the presumption should be that they best know the patient's wishes and values, and their decisions should almost always be honored. Exceptions to this generalization include (a) if the treatment is clearly physiologically futile, as determined by at least two physicians, and (b) if the treatment will be unable to restore the patient's awareness and is causing unrelievable suffering.

In this case the patient's professional caregivers are convinced that he is dying and will never again have awareness, and they interpret this to mean that continued treatment is futile. However, his family believes that he would want to continue treatment while they are praying for divine intervention. Since his current ICU care is postponing his death, it is not truly futile.

RECOMMENDATIONS

1. It is appropriate to continue ICU care, using all reasonable attempts to postpone this patient's death.
2. His son and daughter-in-law should periodically be updated on his condition and prognosis, and should occasionally be asked to consider limitation of treatment if he shows no signs of improvement. These requests should not be too frequent or too forceful so as to be perceived as badgering.

FOLLOW-UP

Mac continued to live in the ICU, on full support, for the next thirteen months without recovering awareness. He had several episodes of **sepsis** and was successfully resuscitated from four cardiac arrests. Two more ethics consultations were requested at intervals, in which essentially the same question was asked, with essentially the same recommendations. When he did not survive the final resuscitative attempt, the ICU physician called his daughter-in-law, saying, "We did everything we could, but I'm sorry to report that your father-in-law has died." Her frustration with his lack of improvement came through in her response: "Well, you obviously didn't do enough!"

COMMENT

Mac's professional caregivers were themselves exceedingly frustrated, believing that their heroic efforts had no reasonable expectation of helping the patient. They believed that they were being poor stewards of medical resources. (Mac's care for this hospitalization exceeded $2,000,000.) It is very easy in retrospect to confirm their belief that the extent of treatment applied here was "inappropriate," but it clearly was not futile in the literal sense.

Case 4.14

QUESTION

Is it ethically permissible for this young man to stop his ventilator so that he can die?

STORY

David is a thirty-four-year-old man who has been on a **ventilator** for nine years. He was readmitted to the hospital two weeks ago for treatment of recurrent pneumonia and has improved. He asked yesterday if his ventilator could be stopped.

Nine years ago he sustained a neck fracture in a diving accident that left him quadriplegic and ventilator-dependent. He went to a rehabilitation facility where his family learned to care for his medical needs, and he was discharged home on ventilator care. His pulmonary situation was stable for several years. He was able to be off his ventilator for several hours at a time and go out in his van with friends. However, in the past two years he has had ten hospital admissions for atelectasis[5] or infection. His secretions have increased so that he requires suctioning several times through the night, and

---

5. Atelectasis is the collapse of a portion of the lung, usually caused by obstruction or compression of small airways.

he is no longer able to be off the ventilator for even short periods. He has had vigorous treatment with antibiotics, chest physical therapy, and repeated **bronchoscopies,** and it is the consensus of his care team that his pulmonary situation will not improve and will likely steadily deteriorate.

He has had excellent care from his mother and sister with help from home nursing twelve hours per day. He has a voice-activated computer that facilitates many personal tasks. He has been very involved in his care, and his nurses describe him as thoughtful, intelligent, and self-assured. Prior to his illness he attended college (history major) and enjoyed classical music. He has several supportive friends who visit him regularly.

His parents divorced a few years after his accident. His father and only brother live out of state. The patient states that his sister has "put her life on hold" to assist with his care, and for this he feels grateful but not guilty.

He has been thinking for the past eight months that he wanted to stop supportive treatment so that he could die, but articulated this to his family and care team just yesterday.

On examination he is alert, articulate, and in no apparent respiratory distress. He is able to speak a few words at a time using a speaking valve. He says his life as a "quad" was tolerable until two years ago, but the progressive pulmonary disease has made it intolerable. He would continue treatment for another nine years or more if he could return to his condition prior to the progressive pulmonary deterioration. He is now frightened of suffocating and wants to avoid that. He would take an overdose of a sedative and ask someone to disconnect his ventilator, but he recognizes that this is not permissible and wants to work with his team to find the best comfort care possible as his disease takes his life. He reports that he is not depressed, though he knows what it is like to feel that way, as he was despondent for several weeks after his accident.

I talked with the patient, his mother, best friend, primary hospital nurse, and one of his home care nurses.

DISCUSSION

It is generally felt that there is no moral obligation to continue life that is dependent on technology when the burdens to the patient of that life outweigh the benefits to the patient. It is also the legal and moral consensus that the health-care team should pursue the treatment goals of the competent patient. Thus, even if he were not terminally ill from progressive pulmonary disease, it would be ethically permissible for this patient to choose to discontinue his antibiotics and ventilator if he felt the burdens of continued treatment were disproportionate to the benefits of continued life. His progressive pulmonary disease and terminal prognosis are further reasons that make it reasonable to change treatment goals from life prolongation to comfort care.

It is not acceptable either legally or from a professional ethics standpoint for any member of his care team to assist him with an act of suicide. It is, however, ethically permissible to give him adequate sedation to ease his respiratory distress as long as the intent and the doses are not aimed at hastening death.

RECOMMENDATIONS

1. It is ethically permissible to honor this patient's request to discontinue his ventilator. Before this is done, however, all efforts should be made to ensure that his distress and fears have been addressed and that he then be given the option of continuation of ventilator support.
2. It is also ethically permissible to give him sedation prior to discontinuation of his ventilator as long as the doses used are for sedation only, and are not intended to hasten his death.

FOLLOW-UP

After further discussion with his professional caregivers, he went home on prophylactic[6] antibiotics to prevent recurrent pneumonia. This worked for the next six months during which David felt he had an acceptable quality of life. When at that time he did develop another life-threatening infection, he remained at home. He had a brief celebration of his life with family and friends. His long-standing pulmonary physician went to his home, gave him a small dose of sedation, and removed his ventilator. He died peacefully in about three hours, having received three additional doses of sedation when he showed signs of mild respiratory distress.

COMMENT

In hearing about this case, some express concern that this represents euthanasia. However, the patient died of his inability to breathe without me-

6. Prophylactic antibiotics are used to try to prevent anticipated infection.

chanical assistance. He and his caregivers had successfully treated that inability for nearly ten years, but when the patient found continued efforts inadequate, he chose to discontinue treatment, allowing the disease to take his life. His doctor did not give him anything to cause his death; he stopped therapeutic efforts to prevent death when they were no longer wanted by the patient.

*   *   *

Other Cases Involving Respiratory Failure/Ventilators

Cases 3.07, 5.07, 5.08, 7.03, 7.10, 7.11, 8.06, 9.01, 9.02, 9.05, 9.06, 9.07, 9.10, 9.12, 10.02, 10.03, 10.04, 10.06, 10.07, 10.08, 10.10, 11.01, 11.04, 11.05, 11.06, 11.07, 13.08, 13.12

References on Ethical Dilemmas in Lung Failure

Hastings Center. *Guidelines on the Termination of Life-Sustaining Treatment and the Care of the Dying.* Briarcliff Manor, N.Y.: Hastings Center, 1987.
President's Commission for the Study of Ethical Problems in Medicine and Biomedical Research. *Deciding to Forgo Life-Sustaining Treatment.* Washington, D.C.: U.S. Government Printing Office, 1983.

CHAPTER 5

Ethical Issues in Kidney Failure

We don't often think of the kidneys as "vital organs." This may be because almost everyone has two, and even then, we can get along on one-half function of just one. At first glance it seems that the Creator gave us an oversupply. However, as we age, kidney function slows and may fail. Kidney failure (renal failure) leads to many ethical dilemmas, some that are quite different from those attending the failure of other organs.

Renal failure may be sudden in onset (e.g., from toxins, interruption in blood supply, obstruction of urine outflow) or it may come on slowly and silently. It may be reversible or irreversible. Uncertainty about whether it will reverse or not often leads to ethical dilemmas.

Irreversible kidney failure, also known as end-stage renal disease (ESRD), is somewhat different from other types of organ failure in that two types of long-term therapy for it are effective in postponing death for a considerable period. The first type of therapy, dialysis, substitutes for kidney function with a "kidney machine" that is intermittently attached to the patient's blood vessels (called hemodialysis) or uses a filtration process of instilling and removing fluid from the patient's abdominal cavity (called peritoneal dialysis). Dialysis in the United States is most often done in outpatient dialysis centers, but both hemodialysis and peritoneal dialysis can also be done in the patient's home after training of the patient and caregiver. The second type is kidney transplantation.

Patients with ESRD are most often started on hemodialysis, done for a few hours at a time, three times per week, and placed on the waiting list for transplantation. It is generally agreed that a patient's quality of life is better after transplantation than it is on hemodialysis because the patient does not have the inconvenience of being tethered to a machine for several hours each week, and because he or she does not experience the symptoms of fluctuating azotemia (accumulation of toxic chemicals routinely removed by kidneys).

When first developed in the 1960s, both dialysis and transplantation introduced significant ethical issues. Both had limited access when first introduced, and both were expensive. Some hospitals that offered hemodialysis established selection committees to determine which patients with ESRD would be treated. Some of those committees received significant professional and public criticism for using both medical and nonmedical selection criteria, that is, considering such things as social worth. This ethical dilemma of limited access was significantly diminished with the infusion by industry of major money into the dialysis enterprise so that more dialysis machines were available, but the problem of cost to the patient or insurance company remained.

The first kidney transplant was done in 1954, but early use was very limited because a person's body recognizes a transplanted organ as "foreign" and builds up antibodies to "reject" it. Until the development of effective ways to combat tissue rejection through drugs called immuno-suppressants, only a few living donations between identical twins were done because their identical tissue types avoided the rejection issue. With the introduction of azothioprine in 1963 and especially after cyclosporine was introduced in 1983, kidney transplantation expanded rapidly. Some transplant operations used a living donation procedure similar to the twin donations, but most used kidneys donated from someone who had just died (cadaveric donation). Patients began waiting in line for transplantation while continuing dialysis.

The development of these treatments for ESRD marked the first time the (non)system of U.S. health-care finance confronted an effective but expensive chronic therapy on a large scale. Most insurance companies did not pay for either of these new modalities, and most individuals could not afford them. In 1972, after a congressman brought a relative with ESRD to the floor of the House of Representatives and told his peers that she would die because she couldn't afford dialysis, Congress established the Medicare ESRD Program. Under this program, anyone with ESRD, regardless of age, qualifies for Medicare, so there is guaranteed payment for dialysis and kidney transplantation. Thus the U.S. government singled out kidney failure as the only disease process whereby all citizens have equal access to treatment. But this did not solve all the access problems (see Case 5.03).

Introduction of the Medicare ESRD Program stimulated even greater production of dialysis machines and more dialysis centers. Most viewed Medicare funding for ESRD as a huge societal relief, and some saw it as a lucrative opportunity. Some criticize **nephrologists** for being willing to dialyze anyone, including persons with end-stage **dementia** or those in a permanent vegetative state. Others criticize families for demanding dialysis in these situations because it was available and paid for by someone else. Regardless of the cause, the pendulum swung from underutilization to overutilization. Professional organizations continue to work on criteria for appropriate utilization.

Access to transplantation is not so easily addressed. Factories can't make new kidneys. Because dialysis postpones death in so many people with ESRD, and because transplantation is generally preferred over chronic dialysis, the waiting list for transplantation has grown tremendously and continues to grow each year. In 2009, over 85,000 individuals were waiting for kidney transplantation in the United States, and the average waiting time was two and a half to five years.[1] Efforts have been made to increase donation/retrieval rates for cadaveric kidneys, but the small impact has not been nearly sufficient to meet the still-growing demand. Efforts are now aimed at living donors, and in 2003, for the first time, kidney transplants from living donors exceeded cadaveric donors.

Living donation raises the question of risk to the donor. A healthy person donating a kidney has a mortality risk of 0.03 percent (3 deaths per 10,000 donations), but a significant risk (1-10 percent) of morbidity, that is, nonlethal sickness, usually short term. In living donation, most often the donor gives a kidney to a specific individual, a practice called directed donation. Family members are often asked to consider donating a kidney because they have a higher chance of tissue compatibility. There is always a concern about subtle coercion (rarely spoken) in these requests. The practice of altruistic directed donation between strangers was at first discouraged, but has gained acceptance at most transplant centers as tissue compatibility is now deemed to be of lesser importance.

In addition to retrieval and procurement issues, allocation of available kidneys also raises ethical issues. One of these is the ongoing clinical debate of how much weight to place on tissue typing. Should a person with an uncommon tissue type, or one who developed tissue antibodies from earlier failed transplantation, be delayed or even deprived of a donation because of some increased risk of rejection (see Case 14.07)? What is the

1. Current data available at www.unos.org.

relationship between personal choice of the patient and stewardship of the profession or society?

Another allocation issue involves racial disparity. African Americans represent a disproportionately large amount of ESRD because they have a high incidence of hypertension and diabetes that can lead to kidney failure, but they receive a disproportionately small number of kidney transplants. Some of this disparity is because African Americans also have a low donation rate, and at least some of the tissue-typing factors are related to race.

But probably the largest source of ethics dilemmas, or at least the most common reason for ethics consultation in ESRD, involves the starting or stopping of dialysis in a person with a poor prognosis for recovery or survival. It is not uncommon for a critically ill patient to suffer failure of multiple organs, including the kidneys. This often occurs in a cascade fashion: the heart or lungs fail due to direct disease, and the consequent poor circulation leads to failure of kidneys, liver, and bone marrow. This situation is called **multi-organ system failure** and generally has a very poor prognosis, especially if it continues for more than a few days. Should dialysis be used in such a patient? If so, for how long (see Case 5.01)? Conversely, should dialysis be imposed over the objection of a patient who wants to stop (see Cases 5.11 and 5.12)? What about the use or nonuse of dialysis for a patient who is mentally impaired (see Case 5.05)?

In talking about whether or how to limit therapy that is in use, it is often easier for families to accept the withdrawal of dialysis than the stopping of a **ventilator**. We can give families a pretty high degree of assurance that **palliative care** efforts can adequately address the shortness of breath feared when the ventilator is withdrawn. But we can absolutely guarantee that when a patient dies from kidney failure, the patient will be obtunded[2] from azotemia and thus unaware of any suffering. Health-care professionals often view death from kidney failure as a "good and peaceful death."

Let's look at some dilemmas in clinical ethics that focus on kidney failure.

---

2. "Obtunded" is a term that describes suppressed consciousness, meaning the patient is either minimally responsive or totally unresponsive. This obtundation may be from a number of different causes.

Case 5.01 ————————————————————————————————

QUESTION

Should we start dialysis on this critically ill patient if her two surrogates disagree?

STORY

Margaret is thirty-nine and chronically ill with multiple problems including chronic leukemia and malnutrition. She has now been hospitalized for several months, much of it in the intensive care unit (ICU) on a **ventilator** for recurring episodes of respiratory failure and **sepsis**. She is only intermittently able to participate in treatment decisions. There has been conflict between her husband, Oscar, and her mother, who have countervailing wishes. Her mother has been in nearly constant attendance, has consistently urged full intensive treatment, and has expressed concern that Oscar has not been a good caregiver. He has visited little, seems resigned to her ultimate death, and has been willing to consider **limitation of treatment**. Application for court-appointed guardianship has been considered, but has not been pursued in an effort to avoid escalation of this conflict. Margaret has no written **advance directive**. However, when asked who she wanted to make her decisions, she has said she wanted her husband to be her **surrogate**. In spite of this, she has almost always acceded to her mother's wishes about full treatment when she was able to participate in the discussion.

The patient is again in the ICU on a ventilator with sepsis caused by a bacteria resistant to most antibiotics, and this episode is accompanied by progressive renal failure. She has been treated aggressively, and is somewhat improved with a stable blood pressure, but the nephrology consultant, Dr. Loudon, says her renal failure has progressed to the point of needing dialysis very soon. She remains unresponsive. Today her mother remains undecided about the use of resuscitation, but wants Margaret to have dialysis. Oscar has requested a **do-not-resuscitate order** (DNR order), which has been written, and has said he does not want her to have dialysis. The ICU care team believes her condition is grave but wants advice on who has the authority to make these decisions.

DISCUSSION

When treatment decisions must be made for a patient who has lost the capacity to participate, we try to make a **substituted judgment**, that is, the decision the patient would make if able, based on a written advance directive, previously spoken wishes, or an understanding of the patient's values. Only when it is not possible to make a substituted judgment do we drop to the lower **best interests** standard.

This state, unlike most states, has no statutory hierarchy to automatically name a surrogate medical decision-maker when a patient has lost **decision-making capacity** and has not left a written advance directive. Medical professionals thus rely on tradition to identify an appropriate surrogate, and generally this process is straightforward. Sometimes, however, two or more individuals will claim surrogate authority. This is not problematic if they agree on what treatment should be used, but it becomes quite difficult if they steadfastly disagree. Irresolvable disagreements must often be resolved in court.

In this case, the patient has verbally named her husband as her surrogate but has followed the recommendations of her mother. She is again unable to participate in an urgent decision, and her two potential surrogates disagree.

RECOMMENDATIONS

1. Efforts to establish agreement between the patient's husband and mother should continue. If they continue to disagree on dialysis or other major treatment decisions, emergency guardianship proceedings should be initiated so the court can tell us who is to be her legal guardian.
2. If death-postponing decisions must be made before a guardian can be named, the treatment should probably be started pending the court's decision.
3. Even if this decision-making crisis is resolved at the bedside, it would be prudent to ask the court to appoint a legal guardian in order to help resolve such conflicts in the future.

FOLLOW-UP

Dr. Loudon met with both the patient's husband and her mother and explained her poor prognosis. All agreed to a trial of dialysis, recognizing that it may not change things, and might lead to the need for long-term dialysis if she does survive. Three days later the patient had a cardiac arrest while in the X-ray department, and her mother, who was present, insisted on full **cardiopulmonary resuscitation** in spite of the DNR order. It was successful, but she remained in **multi-organ system failure** and her condition continued to deteriorate over the next fifteen days. At another management meeting with both her husband and mother present, Margaret's primary care physician strongly recommended withdrawal of support since her prognosis was so dismal and rapidly worsening. They reached agreement to withdraw most of her support, so dialysis, medications, fluids, and nutrition were stopped, but her ventilator was continued. Two days later her mother agreed to stop the ventilator, and Margaret died in less than an hour.

COMMENT

It is not uncommon to encounter differences of opinion about whether to start dialysis or not — differences of opinion between patient and family, between family and professionals, or even between family members, as in this case. The good news is that dialysis can be started as a "trial of therapy" to see if it achieves the desired outcome, and it can as easily be stopped. For some reason, it is easier for families to agree to stop dialysis than to stop ventilator support, probably because the therapy is intermittent and the subsequent death is not so temporally tied to the act of stopping.

Case 5.02

QUESTION

Is it permissible to not perform lifesaving dialysis in this man with a stroke on the basis of his family's refusal?

STORY

Herbert is a seventy-five-year-old retired engineer who went to the emergency department two weeks ago with leg pain, shortness of breath, changed mental status, and mild left-sided weakness. Workup on admission showed an oxygen deficit, and a lung scan showed that he had had a pulmonary embolus.[3] Past history shows that he had coronary artery bypass graft surgery three years ago with multiple complications — dialysis for two months, intensive care unit for four months, hospitalization for a total of five months.

On admission two weeks ago he was treated with oxygen and with heparin to prevent further clotting. Two days later his left-sided weakness progressed to full paralysis, and a **CT scan** of his brain showed a large, nonhemorrhagic stroke, presumably from a blood clot in spite of the heparin. He has had no neurologic improvement in the subsequent twelve days. He appears to have minimal awareness most of the time, but has on a few occasions been able to communicate. He has also had deteriorating kidney function and will need dialysis if he is to survive. His family has struggled with decisions and has now requested limitation of therapy — no **cardiopulmonary resuscitation**, no **intubation**, no dialysis — believing this would be consistent with his wishes. Since his neurologic condition is stable, his physicians are somewhat uncomfortable not using dialysis to prevent his death.

His wife, son, and daughter-in-law describe him as optimistic, vigorous, energetic, even "hyperactive." He loves life and is well loved by family and friends. He has made it clear to them on more than one occasion that he does not want to go through another illness like his protracted hospitalization and dialysis three years ago. When his wife was in a convalescent home for a few weeks last year, he again stated that they were to "let me go" if he were to be "stroked out like those patients." His nurse reports that he is intermittently able to interact, and on one occasion he wrote on a clipboard that he wants to die and "Go to God." He is a devout Christian, and his family believes he is spiritually ready to die. His wife says if she were to choose for him, she would request dialysis, full aggressive therapy, and eventual transfer to a rehabilitation facility so that he could live, even if disabled from a stroke. But she recognizes his right to choose limitation of therapy, and she will reluctantly accept that. Her son and daughter-in-law are in agreement that his wishes should be followed.

---

3. A pulmonary embolus is caused when a blood clot forms in a vein, usually deep in the leg, breaks off and travels to the lungs, obstructing small or large vessels and interfering with oxygenation of blood.

DISCUSSION

Patients with **decision-making capacity** should be fully informed of the available therapeutic options and the expected outcomes. They may then choose, and that choice should almost always be honored, even if it will lead to an earlier death. It is occasionally ethically permissible to override patients' choices against life-prolonging treatment if they appear to have some distortion of thought process that might lead them to make an irreversible decision that they might potentially regret.

This patient's family is willing to honor his request to do less than maximal therapy for his condition. Because his current request is consistent with his previous statements, it seems unlikely that his request is prompted by a reversible depression brought on by his illness. In addition, he has had some interaction with patients disabled from strokes, and he himself has experienced dialysis for several weeks.

RECOMMENDATIONS

1. The patient's physician and family should attempt to review the treatment options with him before his kidney function erodes to the point of interfering with his comprehension. In particular, his current wishes about dialysis (short term and chronic) should be elicited. It might or might not be appropriate to discuss antibiotics, transfusions, fluids and nutrition, etc.; decisions on those modalities might be inferable from the tone of his response.
2. If the patient is unable to participate in such a discussion, his family's understanding of his previously stated wishes may be accepted as a valid **substituted judgment**.
3. If the patient chooses to forgo life-prolonging measures, it is ethically permissible to change his treatment goal to comfort care. His care setting and all treatment orders can then be reviewed in light of this.

FOLLOW-UP

Herbert's doctor, wife, and son met with him to discuss treatment options. By way of head nods and finger squeezes, the patient made it clear that he did not want dialysis, even if that meant he would die. He had no objection to other measures (antibiotics, fluids and nutrition, physical therapy). He remained comfortable, but with diminishing function. He died seven days later.

COMMENT

Dialysis is not generally perceived to be uncomfortable, though it is moderately burdensome to patient and family. This patient had experienced it in the past, so was making an informed decision. His wife's position ("I would choose for him to have dialysis if it were up to me, but I know he will not want it, so I must respect his wishes") could have been lifted right out of a textbook on clinical ethics: the patient's informed choice trumps wishes of the **surrogate**.

The family's understanding that the patient was spiritually ready to die brought considerable comfort to them in the midst of their grief.

Case 5.03

QUESTION

Is it ethically permissible to move a patient to the top of the dialysis waiting list if he has extenuating circumstances?

STORY

George is twenty-nine years old and single. A computer programmer, he has known he has incurable cancer of the pancreas for several months. He has just completed a course of chemotherapy that has irreversibly damaged his kidneys, and he is being maintained in hospital with hemodialysis three times per week. His oncologist estimates that his life expectancy is less than six months. He is being discharged from the medical center, which is fifty-two miles from his parents' home where he will be living. He can almost entirely care for himself, but he is unable to drive.

A rural dialysis center is located just eight miles from his home, and the nurse in charge would like to provide requested dialysis for George. The problem is that the center has a waiting list of fourteen patients. New patients are added to the bottom of the list, and are accepted when someone leaves the list (transplant, death, moving away). The list moves very slowly, and it is not anticipated that George will make it to the top for eight to twelve months.

The nurse manager at the dialysis center asks for an ethics opinion about bumping this patient to the top of her list.

DISCUSSION

When I encounter a question about allocation of scarce resources, I often refer to an excellent book entitled *Who Lives? Who Dies? Ethical Dilemmas in Patient Selection.*[4] The author lists several possible criteria for patient selection that have been used over the years and devotes a chapter to each, concluding that some have greater ethical justification than others. He lists and groups the potential criteria as follows:

- Social Criteria: (1) social value; (2) favored group; (3) resources required; (4) special responsibilities
- Socio-medical Criteria: (5) age; (6) psychological ability; (7) supportive environment
- Medical Criteria: (8) medical benefit; (9) imminent death; (10) likelihood of benefit; (11) quality of benefit
- Personal Criteria: (12) willingness; (13) ability to pay; (14) random selection

This case pits patient A, who has been on the waiting list for some time and has a longer life expectancy, against patient Z, who is new on the list and doesn't have long to live. The starting presumption is that each person on the list has an alternative location where he or she is receiving dialysis, though less conveniently. In addition, it is assumed that a fair procedure is in place for adding new patients, so the dialysis center would have to find an extenuating circumstance to justify altering the procedure. Of Kilner's listed criteria, the only one that seems to apply to our case is quality of benefit. (While you might be tempted to invoke imminent death, that doesn't really apply here because the issue is not *whether* the two patients will get dialysis or die of kidney failure, but *where* they will get dialysis.)

So the question becomes: Does saving from four to six hours of driving time per week for patient Z justify postponing the acceptance of patient A for dialysis at the rural facility for another several weeks? Part of the consideration might be whether patient Z can drive himself, or whether someone else will have to drive him 16 miles or 104 miles three times per week.

4. John Kilner, *Who Lives? Who Dies? Ethical Dilemmas in Patient Selection* (New Haven: Yale University Press, 1990).

RECOMMENDATIONS

1. The benevolent offer of dialysis at the rural facility is tempting and has strong emotional appeal. However, the length of drive doesn't appear to me to rise to the level of moral importance to trump the fair procedure already in place.

2. The rural dialysis center could propose an option of asking patient A (and perhaps B and C?) if he or she would voluntarily allow patient Z to jump queue, but I would not recommend that because the emotional appeal of the case borders on being coercive.

FOLLOW-UP

No follow-up information is available.

COMMENT

Allocation of resources is a major issue in health policy, but it is not often encountered in clinical ethics where we are focused on what is best for one patient. This case is the exception that makes the rule.

Case 5.04

QUESTION

Is it permissible to let this child go home without dialysis if he and his mother are refusing it?

STORY

Jose is twelve years, nine months old and was born with spina bifida, a developmental problem with incomplete closure of the spinal column, and variable neurologic disabilities. He is paralyzed in his legs and unable to empty his bladder; the resulting urinary pressure led to kidney failure three or four years ago. He also has had a shunt for hydrocephalus (increased fluid in and surrounding the brain) surgically placed, and is reported to be mildly developmentally delayed. He was admitted to the hospital two weeks ago with fever.

His kidney failure has been treated with hemodialysis for nearly four years. His most recent vascular access catheter had been in place for ten months but had to be removed last week because of localized and systemic infection that was found to be the source of his fever. After diligent attempts (four hours in the operating room under general anesthesia), it has proven impossible to place another catheter, so hemodialysis is no longer an option. Kidney transplantation has been discussed in the past, but the patient and his mother have rejected that possibility because of the extensive preparatory surgery that would be required and the prolonged wait for an available kidney (currently sixteen months). The only other option is peritoneal dialysis. While this would likely be temporarily successful, it is not generally recommended for a patient who had the type of bladder surgery he had because it would place him at higher than average risk for peritonitis, a painful, life-threatening infection in the abdominal cavity. It is very unlikely that peritoneal dialysis could be maintained for sixteen months while he waited for a kidney for transplantation.

Jose's mother has requested that he be allowed to go home to die without further interventions. She says, "He has suffered enough." Jose also wants to die at home, not in the hospital.

Jose has been cared for by his widowed mother with considerable support from other family members. They were all prepared for him to die ten months ago when there was a major problem finding a site for catheter access, and they look upon this unexpected time as a gift. He has done quite well during this time. He enjoys TV and video games and visits with cousins. He loves being at home where he is the center of attention.

Jose's mom is a dedicated mother and caregiver who loves him and has his **best interests** at heart. She is a religious person (Christian) but does not go to church. She does not have a good understanding of peritoneal dialysis. She is very apprehensive about the possibility of peritonitis; she fears this would cause him great suffering and mean he would probably die in the hospital.

Jose is alert and conversant and appears to understand his situation well. He recognizes that he will die if peritoneal dialysis is not done. He understands that death is permanent, and he expects to go to heaven where he will be healthy and will no longer need a wheelchair. In addition, he says he would be able to meet his father, who died about ten years ago. He says he would be willing to accept a catheter in his chest (his request) in order to continue treatment, but he refuses a catheter in the abdomen. He could not give a reason for this apparent discrepancy, even on repeated questioning. It probably has to do with his concept of peritonitis.

DISCUSSION

There is no moral obligation to pursue technological intervention to prolong life if the patient feels the burdens outweigh the benefits. Patients with **decision-making capacity** may decline life-prolonging therapy, and **surrogates** who are acting in the patient's best interests may do the same. Such decisions should be made by a patient or surrogate only after receiving adequate information about all possibilities and the consequences of each option.

Parents are generally appropriate surrogates for their children, but adolescents should participate in treatment decisions to the level of their understanding. Minors who have been forced to mature because of chronic illness are often able to participate in treatment decisions at an age when others might not have adequate understanding. Children with developmental disabilities generally need additional protection by a surrogate, but should be encouraged to express their values and wishes if they adequately understand the options and the consequences of their decisions.

In this case, Jose's mom had been a good surrogate and advocate for him. She is now ready for him to participate more fully in difficult treatment decisions. His developmental disability does not appear to preclude this, and his coping with chronic illness has prepared him to do so.

RECOMMENDATIONS

1. Jose and his mother should be given more information about peritoneal dialysis and encouraged to accept a trial of therapy. In addition to talking with the **nephrologist**, it might be worthwhile for them to talk with patients (or family) who are using this treatment. Is there a video description of peritoneal dialysis available?
2. After thorough discussion, if Jose continues to be willing to accept a chest catheter but not an abdominal one, it might be good to have someone else (perhaps a child psychologist) talk with him to try to elicit his reasoning and to assure us that he is making an informed choice.
3. After thorough discussion, if Jose and his mother are in agreement in declining peritoneal dialysis, that decision should be honored. They should then be given assistance with hospice home care.

FOLLOW-UP

After watching a video of the procedure and talking with patients receiving peritoneal dialysis, Jose and his mother (reluctantly) consented to insertion of the peritoneal catheter and a trial of this form of dialysis. Jose subsequently became sullen and withdrawn. He was discharged home on peritoneal dialysis, but he frequently refused the procedure, complaining of abdominal pain, and was unwilling to take even mild oral analgesics. He continued to display ambivalence and hostility. After two weeks the peritoneal dialysis was discontinued. He received hospice care until he died at home about a week later.

COMMENT

It is unusual to allow a twelve-year-old to take the lead in life-and-death decisions, especially one who is felt to be mildly developmentally delayed. However, Jose had matured beyond his years due to his chronic illness. In addition, he and his mother basically agreed about how to sort out his poor choices. However, it was important for both to understand the options well before making an irreversible decision. Even though their ultimate choice (to stop dialysis with the anticipation of death) was the same as their initial choice, I believe it was worthwhile for them to receive additional information and to give the proposed therapy a trial. Without this, there might have been uncertainty, especially on the part of the surviving mom, about whether the best decision had been made.

Case 5.05 ———————————————————————————————

QUESTION

Is it appropriate to continue chronic high-tech support for this cognitively impaired woman with poor quality of life? Who is her appropriate surrogate?

STORY

Patricia is a fifty-one-year-old woman with preexisting disability (mild developmental delay, dependent personality, diabetes with resulting failing vision and poor kidney function, seriously impaired motility of her gastrointestinal tract) who was admitted five months ago with a life-threatening urinary infection. She had a protracted stay in the intensive care unit and was unresponsive for the first two months. She has been on hemodialysis since a few days after admission. She has had several surgical procedures (for placement of a **tracheostomy**, feeding tube, and several dialysis catheters). She was **weaned** from the **ventilator** after about six weeks. She is now more stable but will require permanent dialysis and may need permanent **total parenteral nutrition** (TPN) for her gastrointestinal dysmotility. She has become fairly alert and answers simple questions, but she has been unable to participate in physical therapy and unable to learn how to use a speaking valve in her tracheostomy. Her renal social worker reports that she understands (by mouthing words) that she is on dialysis ("to take poisons out of my blood") and that without it she would die, but she does not find dialysis uncomfortable.

She has been married for twelve years to Robert, who is also mentally disabled with recurring schizophrenia. When she was admitted, he was distressed and deferred treatment decisions to her father (nearly eighty years old), who has consistently requested full therapy. Her parents have been living some distance away for five years, and her mother, disabled from a hip fracture and a stroke, is cared for at home by her husband. Robert now seems somewhat better able to cope, and yesterday he agreed to **limitation of treatment** orders (no resuscitation and no reattachment to the ventilator) because he felt she would not want those aggressive therapies if she should worsen. Uncertainty remains about the continued use of her high-tech support (dialysis, TPN) and what to do for other complications such as recurrent serious infection.

Georgina, this patient's advocate through the Department of Mental Health, has known her for thirteen years and contacts her every one to three weeks. She reports that the patient has been well networked but is very dependent for personal care on Robert. She has particularly enjoyed eating and talking, the two activities that may now be permanently impossible. It is her opinion, however, that the patient would not mind a dependent existence as long as she was comfortable and aware of her surroundings. Patricia's primary physician reports that the patient had previously been terrified at the prospect of dialysis, but that she easily accommodates to new challenges.

DISCUSSION

When making treatment decisions for previously competent patients, we try to use a **substituted judgment** standard, that is, we try to make the decisions that the patient would make if able. These can be learned from a written **advance directive**, previously spoken wishes, or an understanding of the patient's values. If none of these is available, then we drop to a lower **best interests** standard.

Choosing a **surrogate** for a no-longer-competent patient may be easy or difficult. By tradition we consult with family members and other individuals who have intimate knowledge of the patient's wishes and values. Generally a spouse is felt to have the most moral authority in these situations, but if the spouse's ability is compromised, because of either baseline mental health difficulties or coping difficulties, it is often appropriate to share such responsibilities with others who know and care for the patient.

In this case the patient has some ability to communicate but limited ability to discuss treatment goals or modalities. Several individuals have long-standing relationships with her and some understanding of her values, but she has offered no direct written or verbal statement. The consensus of those with whom I spoke was that she would probably accept high-tech interventions and total dependence as long as she was comfortable.

RECOMMENDATIONS

1. In light of her protracted hospital course and fragile condition, the current limitation of treatment orders do not seem inappropriate.
2. It is also appropriate to continue her current level of support with a goal of survival as long as she is comfortable, at least until a surrogate is identified.
3. It would be good to have a conference that included at least her husband, father (by phone), hospital attending physician, outpatient primary physician, social worker, and Georgina, her Department of Mental Health advocate, to discuss her current condition, goals of further therapy, and the use or nonuse of additional modalities. Her attending physician may want to include others (**nephrologist**, gastroenterologist, nutritionist). It is not clear to me whether the patient should attend. Her caregivers should decide this based on whether they believe the discussion might enhance her participation or cause her greater distress. An ethics consultant could facilitate this discussion. If

the group agrees about goals and treatments, and on who should be consulted for specific decisions, there may be no need to seek appointment of a guardian. If this cannot be achieved, appointment of a legal guardian would be very helpful.

FOLLOW-UP

A management conference was held as suggested, and there was consensus that (a) Patricia is not suffering in her present state, (b) she would very likely choose to continue this level of technology as long as it maintained her condition, (c) new conditions or complications that have a reasonable chance of being reversed should be treated, (d) the limitation of treatment orders currently in place is appropriate, and (e) if she has further significant deterioration that is unlikely to be reversed, it would be in her best interests to give comfort care rather than burdensome treatment that almost certainly will not work. There was considerable discussion about surrogacy, and both Robert and her father indicated a trust in Georgina, the Department of Mental Health advocate. She agreed to be available but will contact Robert and Dad before making any major changes in therapy.

Patricia's condition remained stable for six weeks, at which time she again became critically ill with **sepsis**. This was treated aggressively for another two weeks, but when she remained minimally responsive and appeared to be uncomfortable, all agreed it was appropriate to change goals to comfort care. Her dialysis was stopped, and she died in another thirty hours.

COMMENT

This case is an example of developing and exercising a community of individuals who know and care for a patient to assist with major decisions when the patient is unable. It is generally preferable to rely on this type of community rather than on the court system or governmental agencies. The latter are necessary and do a good job in advocating for socially isolated individuals or in situations where there is unresolvable conflict in this social community. However, they are not a satisfactory substitute for the caring and understanding of an intimate community.

Many individuals would find the confinement and limitations of pleasures (talking, eating) experienced by Patricia to be intolerable. Many of those would thus choose to discontinue dialysis. However, those who knew this patient well felt that she would accept dependence and limitations as long as she had awareness and was not uncomfortable.

Case 5.06

QUESTION

Is it ethically permissible to write futility-based limitation of treatment orders for this dying homeless and friendless patient who wants "everything" done?

STORY

Hank is a forty-one-year-old homeless man who has had AIDS and dialysis-dependent kidney disease for a few years. He has been under the intermittent care of local health-care professionals since he was released from prison about four years ago. He has been a difficult patient in that he has frequently skipped dialysis appointments, stopped HIV medications for weeks at a time, etc. His caregivers have been resigned to his "call the shots" attitude, but have continued to provide appropriate treatment when he has been willing to accept it. His caregivers report that his body configuration has changed from essentially normal to extreme wasting in the past two months.

He was admitted one month ago with abdominal pain and liver dysfunction, but extensive workup failed to find a specific diagnosis. He left **AMA** (against medical advice) two weeks later without waiting for prescriptions for his symptoms. The next day he was brought back to the emergency department by two individuals (identity unknown) because of persistent vomiting, diarrhea, and weakness. Since readmission, he has most often refused to talk and has frequently declined nursing assistance. His one point of consistency is that he has always said he "wants everything done," and as recently as yesterday he repeated this to Dr. Ainsworth, his attending physician, while quite mentally clear. However, Dr. Ainsworth believes the patient is now irreversibly and imminently dying of malnutrition and metabolic imbalance, such that rescue measures (e.g., **cardiopulmonary resuscitation, intubation**) will not work. He also believes that continuing dialysis will not be possible because of his overwhelming chemical imbalances.

The patient has no **advance directive**, no friends or visitors, and no known family. He has declined a nurse's suggestion that he speak with a hospital chaplain. He identifies an AIDS case worker as his next of kin, but this person cannot be located.

DISCUSSION

Treatment decisions are ideally made jointly by patient and physician. When they disagree about the use or nonuse of a specific modality, generally the patient's wish for a treatment should be honored, as long as there is even a small chance the requested modality will be effective. However, a long-standing medical truism says, "there is no moral obligation to provide futile treatment." This has been incorporated into professional practice guidelines and hospital policy. The ongoing difficulty is in deciding at what time in a specific case modalities become futile. Sometimes a second (or third) opinion will help to confirm such an assessment or even de-escalate conflict that is not uncommonly generated on this issue. When there is any doubt, the benefit of that doubt should be given to the patient.

In this case, the patient is dying of an irreversible metabolic derangement. Aggressive cardiopulmonary measures will not reverse this inexorable process, nor will further dialysis.

RECOMMENDATIONS

1. It is ethically permissible to write **limitation of treatment** orders to withhold measures that are truly futile for this patient. Prior to doing so, however, the assessment of **futility** should be confirmed in writing by at least one other physician besides Dr. Ainsworth.
2. Since the patient has consistently requested "everything," any temporizing measures that can reasonably be expected to postpone his death should be continued.
3. If, however, continued efforts to forestall death (such as limiting his dose of analgesics because they cause a drop in blood pressure) will cause him additional suffering, it is ethically permissible to set aside his goal of death postponement for the sake of relief of suffering unless he has specifically stated his preference to endure suffering for temporary postponement of death.

FOLLOW-UP

Consultation confirmed Dr. Ainsworth's assessment of futility. Dialysis was stopped, limitation of treatment orders were written, and a **palliative care** consultant advised on end-of-life measures. The patient died peacefully forty-eight hours later.

COMMENT

Health-care professionals and patients generally work together in developing treatment goals and making decisions about which specific treatments to use or not use. In some cases, however, the patient establishes unachievable goals. In many cases the professionals are willing to pursue those goals as far as is medically possible, but there comes a point when further treatments just plain no longer work. Determining when the point of futility is reached is not easy. Some physicians are tempted to use "the futility card" more quickly than may be justified because they see the inappropriateness of the patient's choice. However, it is ethically mandatory to set aside that bias and to continue treatment, which may indeed seem pointless, until it is clear to at least two physicians that continued treatment will not have any physiological effect. Then the physician is justified in declining to provide continued treatment, even over the objection of the patient or family.

Case 5.07

QUESTION

Is it appropriate to continue full treatment (including ventilator and dialysis) for this patient with a history of avoiding medical care?

STORY

Catherine is a seventy-nine-year-old woman with a history of coronary artery disease (for which she had surgery twelve years ago), diabetes, and end-stage renal disease. She has been on dialysis for four years. She was admitted two and a half weeks ago with worsening pneumonia after several days of outpatient treatment. On the day after admission she had a cardiac arrest and was resuscitated, but has remained unresponsive and on **ventilator** support in the intensive care unit (ICU). She has received full treatment, including treatment for gastrointestinal bleeding. Her pneumonia has now cleared on X-ray, and she has stabilized, but she has failed to **wean** from the ventilator and is still on dialysis three times per week. She has been minimally responsive off sedation for several days. She does not follow simple commands. It is not yet known if she has suffered brain injury from lack of oxygen that could compromise recovery of cognition.

It is anticipated that weaning will take several weeks, and she may require long-term nursing-home care with continued dialysis or, alternatively, considerable family assistance at home. Though the patient has said in the past that she would never want to live in a nursing home, her son continues to request full treatment in spite of the prediction of nursing home placement, saying, "We'll cross that bridge when we come to it."

Her ICU nurse has learned that Catherine refused admission or outpatient investigation for an earlier upper gastrointestinal hemorrhage, and she has repeatedly resisted hospital care, requiring family to sit with her to keep her from signing out **AMA** (against medical advice) during previous admissions. Thus her nurses are concerned that we are currently providing treatment that the patient might well have refused, and they requested ethics consultation.

The patient has been widowed for many years and lives with her only son. She also has two brothers, one sister, and many nieces and nephews. Prior to admission she had enjoyed going shopping on nondialysis days. She found dialysis fatiguing. She has no written **advance directive**. Her son says she is feisty and has always said, "Do everything," when questions of level of treatment arose.

Her longtime dialysis nurse and social worker both report that Catherine has always consented to dialysis, even to changing access sites when needed. They believe that what is perceived as resistance to treatment emanates from fear or lack of understanding, not from a desire to discontinue treatment or lack of a will to live.

DISCUSSION

When a previously healthy patient loses capacity to make treatment decisions, we use **substituted judgment,** that is, we try to make the decisions the patient would make if able. To do this we rely on a written advance directive or we look to those who know the patient best to articulate his or her wishes or values.

In this case, several caring family members report that the patient has a strong will to live and a (reluctant) willingness to undergo burdensome treatments to maintain her previously somewhat compromised condition. This is confirmed by health-care professionals who have known the patient for a long time.

RECOMMENDATIONS

1. It is ethically permissible to continue full treatment for this patient with a goal of weaning her from the ventilator and allowing her to return home.
2. Rediscussion of treatment goals, and the use or nonuse of specific modalities, should be undertaken if it becomes clear that: she has suffered significant cognitive impairment; she will be unable to wean from the ventilator; or her family would be unable to care for her at home.
3. If there is future discussion of changing treatment goals, it might be beneficial to include in the discussion other family members as well as health-care professionals who have known her for some time.

FOLLOW-UP

When she had shown no clinical improvement and no signs of awakening one week later, her son consented to a **do-not-resuscitate order**, though he remained optimistic about weaning her from the ventilator and taking her home. A few days later, venous access could not be achieved in her arms, so dialysis had to be done through a catheter in her groin. Since the son's goal (and presumably the patient's) had been to return home and go shopping, and this would now be precluded by the groin catheter, her son agreed to withdrawal of support, including no more dialysis. She died two days later.

COMMENT

This case demonstrates how well-meaning health-care professionals may misinterpret a patient's history or actions. Information from those who know the patient best may help to sort out such difficulties.

In addition, it points out that specific goals should be kept clearly in mind. Her son's goal of taking Catherine home and once again going out shopping may have been somewhat unrealistic, but it was clear. Once it became clear that this was not possible, he was willing to change goals to comfort care.

Case 5.08

QUESTION

Please assist the intensive care unit team in determining (a) who is the appropriate surrogate for this patient with chronic schizophrenia and an acute critical illness and (b) what level of therapy is appropriate for him.

STORY

Michael is a fifty-nine-year-old man with a forty-year history of schizophrenia and a five-year history of chronic **renal insufficiency** (not yet requiring dialysis), along with severe hypertension and a stroke three years ago. He was found minimally responsive in his home three days ago, was taken to the emergency department, was **intubated** to protect his airway, and was admitted to the intensive care unit (ICU) critically ill with a large acute myocardial infarction (heart attack), worsened renal failure, and a profound anemia. He has been receiving full therapy, including sedation, daily hemodialysis, and continued **ventilator** support for **congestive heart failure** and pneumonia. There is currently no reason to suspect brain injury from lack of oxygen.

He remains critically ill with **multi-organ system failure**, but none of his problems is clearly lethal. He will need ventilator support for at least a few more days and long-term dialysis, though he has a poor overall prognosis for survival.

Michael has a sister out of state and a brother who lives close by, but neither has had much contact with him in recent years, and it is not clear if either has been named as durable power of attorney for health care or legal guardian. He lives with an eighty-year-old woman and her developmentally delayed son; no contact information is available at this time. His current primary physician, Dr. Fitzgerald, has seen him only twice and reports poor compliance with medications and visits, and frequent refusal of testing. Dr. Fitzgerald believes the patient usually has **decision-making capacity** in spite of his chronic mental illness. He believes the family is disinclined to use long-term dialysis, but he does not know if this has been discussed with the patient.

DISCUSSION

When a patient loses the capacity to make decisions due to illness, our goal is generally to restore the patient's decision-making capacity if possible, and failing that to use **substituted judgment**, that is, try to determine what the patient would choose if able (from a written **advance directive**, from previously spoken wishes, or from an understanding of his or her values). If it is not possible to learn what the patient would want in this manner, we drop to a lower **best interests** standard.

Since there is no reason to suspect that this patient has lost the cerebral capacity to make his own decisions, and since none of his conditions is clearly lethal, it is appropriate to continue standard aggressive therapy with a goal of restoring his capacity to decide about long-term goals. It would be appropriate to continue to search for other sources of substituted judgment (see below).

If decisions must be made before he is able to participate and without additional information about his wishes or values, his aversion to medical treatment in the past might be a statement of values suggesting he would be disinclined to long-term dialysis. However, since he has not declined treatment when confronting a life-and-death situation, this cannot by itself be construed as refusal of dialysis.

RECOMMENDATIONS

1. Continuation of full therapy seems appropriate for this patient at this time. If his condition should deteriorate before he can be talked to about his wishes, and it appears very unlikely he can survive, it would be permissible to write **limitation of treatment** orders based on **futility**.
2. Efforts should continue to contact the woman with whom he has been living to see if she has any additional reliable information about his wishes or values.
3. If it is not possible to restore his decision-making capacity and no further information becomes available about his wishes, decisions about further goals and about the use or nonuse of specific modalities

should be reached by consensus among his professional caregivers, his siblings, and any others who know him reasonably well.

FOLLOW-UP

The son of Michael's caregiver visited. Though reported to have developmental delay, he appeared to the ICU team to be quite capable, if somewhat "slow." He said he didn't think the patient would want long-term dialysis. However, contrary to earlier reports, he felt the patient had been compliant with medical care in the past.

The patient subsequently awoke, was **weaned** from the ventilator, and continued to receive dialysis three times per week. He consented to a **do-not-resuscitate order** if his condition should worsen, but he wanted to continue dialysis. He was discharged one month after admission, and three months later the dialysis service reported that he was doing very well.

COMMENT

With this patient's multisystem disease, poor overall prognosis, chronic mental health condition, and history of poor compliance with past treatment, it might have been tempting to withhold chronic dialysis. However, for the reasons articulated above, it seemed prudent to continue full treatment until his prognosis was clearer or until we had clearer guidance about his wishes.

Case 5.09

QUESTION

Is it ethically permissible to restrain or sedate this patient in order to continue her chronic dialysis?

STORY

Mildred is a seventy-eight-year-old woman who has been on dialysis for four years. In addition, she had some behavioral symptoms, poor memory, and confusion for a few years, which progressed to a formal diagnosis of

dementia three years ago. At that time she was "agitated, aggressive, confused," and was treated initially with a mood stabilizer, with some improvement, and later with a sedative.

Her confusion has worsened and her behavior during dialysis has deteriorated, and she is no longer improved with medication. Questions have been raised by staff in the dialysis unit about her quality of life and her safety. It is reported that she tries to get out of bed, touches sterile catheters, removes dressings, pulls at tubing, curses at staff, etc. — something every minute or two — which mandates one-on-one supervision during dialysis for three hours twice a week. Options considered by the staff in the dialysis unit include having family members as "sitters," increased sedation, and physical restraints to keep her safe during dialysis.

The patient lives in her own home with round-the-clock paid staff. Her son, Rich, and his wife describe her quality of life, except during dialysis six hours per week, as quite acceptable to her and to them. She talks, walks, eats, goes shopping with caregivers, tries to sneak cigarettes, "plans" outings, etc. She strongly resists coming for dialysis every time, recalling it as an uncomfortable place, and does not understand that without it she will die. Her family is convinced that the six hours of misery each week are more than outweighed by the enjoyment of the remainder of her week. They fear that asking her paid staff to sit with her during dialysis could lead to resignations.

DISCUSSION

When a patient is unable to understand the need for unpleasant treatments, it may be ethically justified to restrain the patient against his or her will in order to supply therapeutic benefit, just as we physically restrain a child to give needed immunizations. Sometimes we allow a patient without understanding to refuse an important, but not lifesaving, treatment in order to not infringe on the patient's individual right of freedom. When forgoing treatment is not an option, we generally reserve restraints for those situations that cannot be managed by less intrusive means such as education, persuasion, etc.

In this case, enforcing dialysis over the patient's objection would appear to be ethically justified since her family's perception of her quality of life during nondialysis hours is still very positive. That enforcement should be done in the least intrusive manner that is likely to provide for her safety and the ongoing atmosphere of the dialysis unit.

RECOMMENDATIONS

1. The patient's family should be encouraged to provide someone with a familiar face to sit with her during dialysis.
2. If this is not possible or does not work, it would then be ethically justified to try increasing her sedation or to try a different sedative.
3. Only if (1) and (2) do not prove to be satisfactory should the regular planned application of physical restraints be contemplated.
4. Her family should be encouraged to frequently reassess the balance of burdens and benefits of her treatment on her overall quality of life.

FOLLOW-UP

Rich and his wife took turns staying with Mildred during her dialysis treatments. Her behavior was only slightly better, and it was very stressful for her family, though somewhat less stressful for the dialysis staff. This plan continued for several months, with reports of congenial times at home, before Mildred succumbed to an overwhelming infection.

COMMENT

This case serves as a reminder to health-care professionals that they sometimes see only a patient's worst times — when sick, uncomfortable, confused, etc. They may thus make a judgment that the patient's quality of life is quite poor, when in fact, while that patient is at home, he or she may be more relaxed and appear to enjoy life.

Reflection on this case also allows us to contemplate the place of quality of life in making treatment decisions. If Mildred acted as she did in the dialysis unit all the time, it would still have been appropriate to try all means possible to improve her lot. If, however, all those efforts failed, it would then have been ethically permissible to consider withdrawing dialysis with the expectation that the patient would die. There is no moral obligation to continue life that is dependent on technology if that technology causes greater burden than benefit, or even if continued life is disproportionately burdensome.

Case 5.10

QUESTION

Is it ethically permissible to replace an intravenous line for hemodialysis over the objection of this patient?

STORY

Earl is sixty-three years old and has been on hemodialysis for about one year because of renal failure resulting from his long-standing diabetes. He also has a history of coronary artery disease, stroke, and early **dementia**. He has had several infections in his indwelling dialysis shunts (often called "line infections"), resulting in three admissions to the intensive care unit in the past year with **ventilator** support. He was admitted from his nursing home yesterday with another episode of **sepsis** from a line infection. His shunt was removed and he has been stabilized overnight. He was scheduled to have a temporary dialysis catheter inserted today. Consent had been given by his wife, but the patient said he didn't want it and physically resisted insertion by Dr. Chandler.

His wife reports that Earl was a farmer and cheese maker who has been disabled for twenty-five years from his diabetes and heart disease. He did quite well until about two years ago when he became unable to walk and developed frequent urinary infections. She describes him as a quiet, private person who loved his three children and several grandchildren. Two children are living close by. The other, Jimmy, died of an apparent heart attack while driving four years ago; he was a close pal of the patient.

Both Dr. Chandler and Earl's wife report that he has been ambivalent about dialysis since it started, and since he was admitted to the nursing home four months ago, has frequently said he wanted to stop. He otherwise settled into the nursing home routine better than expected. Dr. Chandler has cared for Earl for some time. He believes that Earl still has **decision-making capacity** in spite of his early dementia.

His wife told Dr. Chandler that Earl told her this morning he wanted to stop dialysis and die unless he could have a kidney transplant, preferably using one of her kidneys. She has hypertension and diabetes and thus is not a candidate for kidney donation. Transplantation was discussed early on, and it was acknowledged that patients report a better quality of life after transplant than while on dialysis. However, it was not felt to be an option for Earl because of his other medical problems.

I spoke with Earl in the presence of his wife, his medical resident, and his nurse. He consistently nodded yes and no to multiple questions and clearly indicated he did not want the line reinserted and didn't want any more dialysis. When asked what would happen without dialysis, he said, "I'll die." He was unwilling to verbalize a reason why he wanted to stop now, but with "20 Questions" said it was not because of pain or other correctable symptoms, but because life on dialysis was not good enough. When his wife asked if it was so he could join Jimmy, he nodded his head, burst into tears, and said to her, "That's mean!"

DISCUSSION

When a patient with decision-making capacity refuses a lifesaving intervention or refuses to continue life-sustaining technology, it is important to determine if (a) there is any correctable aspect of his condition that might persuade him to continue; (b) this choice is consistent with acceptable medical practice; and (c) his decision is consistent with his personality and his values.

This patient appears to his primary physician, his current caregivers, and this examiner to have decision-making capacity. He appears to have reached a rational decision to stop dialysis because of a poor quality of life and a dismal prognosis. His caregivers believe this is not an inappropriate decision. They recognize there may be some element of depression, most likely based on his progressive deterioration. However, protracted grief over the death of his son several years ago may be another factor.

RECOMMENDATIONS

1. If his caregivers believe all efforts at optimizing his quality of life have been exhausted, it would be ethically permissible to honor this man's request to stop dialysis.
2. If there is concern that a treatable depression may be a factor in the timing of his decision, it might be appropriate to try a short course of a rapid-acting mood stimulator. Unless there is a significant likelihood of improving his mood sufficiently to accept continued dialysis, it would be ethically troublesome to impose line reinsertion and dialysis over his objection.

FOLLOW-UP

Earl continued to say he wanted transplantation, though his nephrology consultant feels he is not a good candidate. The transplant surgeon was willing to reconsider his candidacy and said he would pursue an outpatient evaluation. Earl was willing to continue dialysis until a determination about transplantion could be made. He was discharged back to the nursing home.

COMMENT

When any patient declines a treatment recommended by his or her physician, it is important to understand as clearly as possible the patient's reason(s). Sometimes the reason is clear; sometimes it is obscure. It often involves the patient's quality of life, and sometimes that can be improved. But it may also come from depression, or from spiritual or social circumstances. Once the reason is determined as clearly as possible, then the professionals, and perhaps the family, have an obligation to see whether anything can be done to eliminate that reason. If the reason cannot be adequately addressed, then patient autonomy swings the balance toward honoring the request. Only in unusual circumstances is it ethically permissible to ignore a request from a nondepressed patient with decision-making capacity who wants to forgo treatment.

Case 5.11 —————————————————————————————————

QUESTION

Is it ethically permissible to accept this patient's decision to stop dialysis based on intolerable symptoms for which he has refused treatment?

STORY

Melvin is a seventy-year-old man who has a long medical problem list, including diabetes, hypertension, chronic pain, osteoarthritis, back injury, essential tremor,[5] persistent anemia, gastrointestinal bleeding, deep venous

---

5. A chronic tremor, generally of the head and upper extremities. It is not related to another disease process, does not progress, and is resistant to treatment.

thrombosis, and atrial fibrillation. Three months ago he agreed to begin dialysis when his diabetic kidney disease progressed to kidney failure. He did reasonably well with dialysis at first, but in the past month has experienced decreasing quality of life from chronic and acute symptoms. During a recent hospital admission, because of continued chronic pain and uncontrollable tremor, he asked to discontinue dialysis so that he could die. His care was transferred yesterday from the hospital to a local inpatient hospice. The hospice social worker called with the above question.

The patient is a retired railroad worker who was exposed to nerve gas while in the military. The social worker says he talks about recurring war nightmares, including dreams of his own suicidal disembowelment with a samurai sword. He has experienced chronic pain for several years, primarily from osteoarthritis and an old back injury. He has been unable to take mild analgesics (which may cause gastrointestinal bleeding) and has refused opiate analgesics, fearing addiction. The pain has led to sleep deprivation and possible depression. He has also refused psychiatric consultation. Neurology consultation diagnosed his tremor as an essential tremor for which there is no effective treatment. He had told his family doctor prior to his complete renal failure that he never wanted to go on dialysis. His family and professional caregivers were able to convince him to give it a try. Soon after starting, he requested a **do-not-resuscitate order**. Both of the physicians providing care for this patient agree, though sadly, that he is making a rational decision that is consistent with his underlying personality and values.

DISCUSSION

There is no moral obligation to continue technology-dependent life. Patients who are dependent on machines for life may choose to stop treatment if they deem their quality of life to be unacceptable, that is, if the burdens of treatment and of the disease exceed the benefit they perceive from continued existence. When patients express this, it is incumbent on family and professional caregivers to address correctable issues (physical, psychological, social, spiritual) in an effort to optimize their quality of life. However, patients are not obligated to accept those overtures. Only when it is very clear that (a) most people would accept the offered treatment and (b) the benefit of treatment would significantly outweigh the burdens, is it ethically justified to consider imposing treatment over the objections of patients.

In this case, the patient has a long history of declining both invasive and noninvasive treatments. He reluctantly agreed to start dialysis, has tried it for three months, and has now made what appears to be a rational choice to discontinue. Though he has declined other treatments that have the potential to improve his quality of life, he appears to be making an informed choice to forgo those treatments.

RECOMMENDATIONS

1. It is ethically permissible to accept this patient's refusal of dialysis and of other interventions.
2. Good comfort care measures should continue.
3. Reasonable efforts should be made to prevent his suicide, as long as those efforts, in turn, do not greatly infringe on his personal freedom during his remaining days.

FOLLOW-UP

The patient died in the hospice five days later.

COMMENT

When health-care professionals begin providing care to a new patient, they are tempted to think they can provide just what the patient needs. In most cases that is good, and patients may benefit from this perspective. However, if that patient has been chronically ill, and especially if the patient has just undergone a trial of therapy to relieve intolerable symptoms, the newly involved professional must be careful not to push the suggested innovations too hard. It is very appropriate for the professional to review all that has gone on, to offer new insights, and to talk with former professional caregivers to ensure that all reasonable options have been tried. But if reasonable efforts have already been tried, and if the patient has made an informed choice to stop life-extending therapy because his or her quality of life has not been satisfactory, the professional should accept that refusal and continue to provide excellent comfort care measures.

Case 5.12 ───────────────────────────────────

QUESTION

Is it ethically permissible to accept this depressed patient's request to stop dialysis?

STORY

Bernice is an eighty-year-old woman with a history of diabetes, diabetic kidney failure, hypertension, coronary artery disease, and cardiac **arrhythmia**. She has been on hemodialysis for two or three years. She has a past history of depression treated successfully with medication. She fell two weeks ago, sustaining a fracture of her lower left leg that has been repositioned and placed in a cast. At the time of admission, orders were written for no **cardiopulmonary resuscitation**, no **intubation**, and no feeding tube, based on her assessment of her quality of life. Since the fall she has had considerable pain and intermittent **delirium** from analgesics. Her fracture is stable, but because of it she will now require nursing home care. Two days ago she became quite alert; she said she thought she was dying, was miserable, and wanted to stop dialysis. After conversations with her physician, Dr. Rubin, and her children, she decided to continue on for a few days. Today she again refused dialysis, saying she was not getting any better and was ready to die. Her physician and family want to do as she wishes, but Dr. Rubin wants to ensure that she is sufficiently mentally clear to make this life-or-death decision.

The patient has been widowed for many years, living most recently with her daughter. She has just two children, a son and a daughter. They report that she had been in declining health for several months prior to this fall, though they say that her quality of life was still acceptable to her. She has said on several occasions recently that she was preparing to die (sorting things, selecting burial clothes).

I met with the patient and her two children. She is alert and conversant. She says she did have considerable pain in her leg, but this has been controlled with analgesics. She says she cannot stand the nausea and the pain (all over), and she is ready to stop dialysis, understanding that she will die. She agrees that her quality of life prior to her fall was acceptable, and she does not find the prospect of nursing home admission to be unacceptable. When I asked if she would want to go on if her nausea and generalized pain could be better controlled, she thought about it, then said no because she thought she was dying anyway. She is a Roman Catholic and is comfortable with her spiritual condition.

DISCUSSION

Decisions for or against the use of life-sustaining treatment should be made jointly by professionals and an adequately informed patient (or **surrogate**, using **substituted judgment**). It is important that the patient's condition be adequately treated before a decision is made to limit such therapy. This includes adequate assessment and treatment of depression, delirium, and physical symptoms. There is no moral obligation to continue life-sustaining technology if a patient finds the current or projected quality of life to be unacceptable.

This patient had been maintained on chronic dialysis and had found her quality of life to be acceptable. Since her recent fall, however, her ongoing symptoms and her projection for limited improvement have been discouraging. She has had some delirium, which is now improved, and she does not appear to be clinically depressed. She appears today to be capable of making an informed decision. However, it is not clear that she has allowed sufficient time for maximal symptom management.

RECOMMENDATIONS

1. If this patient's professional caregivers believe she has achieved maximal symptom control, or that she has been informed that she might still achieve improved symptom control, but she persists in her request to stop dialysis, then it would be ethically permissible to do so.
2. If she wavers in her request, it would be ethically preferable to plan a time-limited trial (a few days?) for maximizing symptom control. She could still request discontinuation of dialysis at any time.

FOLLOW-UP

After the consultation, the patient changed her mind and wanted to continue dialysis for at least a week, while attempting better symptom control. Three days later her symptoms were better controlled and she agreed to continue dialysis and accept transfer to a nursing home. This was accomplished several days later. The patient was pleased with her decision.

COMMENT

This case highlights the importance of a thorough evaluation of the "whole person" — physical, psychological, social, and spiritual dimensions — before accepting from the patient a refusal of treatment that will lead to death. Chronic symptoms can be overwhelming and may seem never-ending. Excellent symptom management is as important as disease management.

Case 5.13

QUESTION

Should dialysis be continued for this patient when his family is so deeply divided on the question?

STORY

Gerald, a forty-four-year-old man with long-standing diabetes and chronic renal failure, was admitted eight days ago with infection of his dialysis catheter. He is nearly blind from diabetic retinopathy and suffers chronic pain from diabetic neuropathy.[6] According to his family, his mental status has deteriorated during this admission: he is sometimes disoriented, sees things that aren't there, calls them by the wrong names, and insists that he is at home instead of the hospital. He has pulled out several intravenous lines and has intermittently refused medications, making it difficult to administer the proper doses of antibiotics. After extensive testing, the mental status changes have been attributed primarily to **sepsis**. He is still receiving dialysis, but to continue he will need operative replacement of a dialysis catheter and from four to six weeks of antibiotics. His family is deeply divided on whether to continue.

His fiancée, Christie, has been his almost-exclusive caregiver for the last ten years with a little help from the patient's daughter, Jean. Christie's role has been increasingly difficult as Gerald has become less ambulatory

---

6. A neuropathy is failure of function of one or more nerves causing either loss of motor function or (more commonly) a disorder of sensation. The latter may involve either loss of sensation or the presence of abnormal sensations (pain, burning, etc.).

and nearly always bedridden. He has days when he is very confused, depressed, and in pain and says he wants to die. However, both Christie and Jean feel, and the patient confirms, that he desperately wants to go home. If he could go home with the same level of function and continue on dialysis, Christie feels he would be in favor of living. Jean agrees with this plan, but says the decision should be made by her and an uncle (the patient's brother) who is executor of the patient's will. She also has no regard for the opinion of the patient's parents (her grandparents), saying "they don't know" the patient. She prefers not to even include them in the discussion.

The patient's parents, especially his father, and another of his brothers take an entirely different view: they are convinced that the patient doesn't want to live any longer, that he has explicitly told them this several times, and that his medication noncompliance has been reflective of his wish to end his suffering and die. They maintain that Christie and Jean want to prolong his suffering only for self-centered reasons, including financial support they receive on his behalf. Their interactions with Christie and Jean are severely strained and belligerent, including the threat of legal action, and neither side seems eager to consider the other's opinions.

The patient generally gives evasive or contradictory answers when questioned, and although he seems intermittently conversant and coherent, his behavior seems infantile and uncertain. A family conference is scheduled for tomorrow with the entire family, Dr. Nesbitt (Gerald's long-standing primary physician), and the treatment team.

DISCUSSION

When the medical condition of patients precludes their making treatment decisions, efforts should be made to improve their condition so as to restore their capacity. If that is not possible and we do not clearly understand their wishes, treatment decisions should be made using **substituted judgment** by those who know them best. If substituted judgment is not possible, then the **best interests** standard should be used.

First priority should be given to improving this patient's **decision-making capacity** if this is realistically possible (e.g., replacing the catheter and removing a source of sepsis). If this does not restore his capacity sufficiently to clarify his wishes, then the most morally appropriate **surrogate** appears to be Christie, the long-standing caregiver. Her assessment of his best interests should be given the most weight, particularly because of the irreversible life-or-death implications of stopping dialysis.

RECOMMENDATIONS

1. In the family conference, emphasis should be shifted to the patient's welfare rather than the family's conflicting opinions.
2. Before making a final decision, it would be prudent to take all possible steps that might enhance the patient's ability to reason and speak regarding his own wishes.
3. The treatment team should empower Christie to articulate the patient's best interests if they agree that she is the most ethically appropriate surrogate.

FOLLOW-UP

All interested parties were present at the management conference where the treating team outlined Gerald's current condition and treatment options. When I pointed out Christie's moral responsibility, based on her long-standing close involvement, to do as she felt he would want, the opposing family faction became less hostile. There was (reluctant) agreement to reinsert a catheter for dialysis and extend antibiotic treatment.

The catheter was replaced. Gerald continued to have fluctuating levels of consciousness, but consistently agreed to dialysis. He was transferred to a long-term care facility with a plan to return home after the course of antibiotics was continued. This was done, and he died about two weeks after returning home. All family appeared to be at peace with the outcome.

COMMENT

Family conflict can be deep and ugly. It is often based more on other issues — money, relationships, past decisions, etc. — than on what the patient wants or what is in his or her best interests. In states with a statutory definition of who has authority to make decisions, identifying the surrogate becomes easy, but this person may not have the most moral authority. That would have been the case here. While one might wonder about Christie's self-designation as Gerald's fiancée, her ten years of increasing care speak volumes about her dedication to him. Merely laying this out on the table, and refocusing the discussion on what would be in Gerald's best interests rather than on peripheral matters, helped to de-escalate and resolve a very tense discussion.

*   *   *

Other Cases Involving Renal Failure

Cases 3.06, 3.07, 4.01, 9.07, 9.08, 9.11, 11.07, 13.06, 14.02, 14.07

References on Renal Failure

Levinsky, N. G. *Ethics and the Kidney.* Oxford: Oxford University Press, 2001.
Renal Physicians Association and American Society of Nephrology. "Shared Decision-Making in the Appropriate Initiation of and Withdrawal from Dialysis." RPA/ASN Clinical Practice Guideline. Washington, D.C., 2000.

CHAPTER 6

Ethical Issues Involving
Failure of Eating and Drinking

Whether to give nutrition and fluids to patients who are unable to eat or drink has generated a huge amount of news and emotion in recent years. The cases of Nancy Cruzan and Terri Schiavo have been front-page news as they worked their way up to the U.S. Supreme Court in 1990 and 2005, respectively.

Some refer to these matters as "artificial nutrition and hydration," but since the formulas used are similar in content to many processed foods, it is more accurate to refer to this topic as artificially *administered* fluids and nutrition. The way of getting the fluid and nutrition into the patient's body is artificial, and may be of two general sorts. Enteral feedings are put into the gastrointestinal tract (e.g., a feeding tube); parenteral feedings are made directly into the circulatory system (e.g., intravenous fluids).

Artificially administered fluids and nutrition (AAF&N)[1] are not new. Enteral feedings were introduced by John Hunter in 1793, and feeding tubes came into common usage in the early twentieth century. Feeding tubes may be inserted through the mouth (oro-gastric tubes) or nose (nasogastric, or NG, tubes), or through a surgical opening in the abdominal wall (gastric tubes, or G-tubes). In recent years the most common method of insertion through the abdominal wall when intended for long-term use is the **PEG tube**. So simple is the procedure for inserting a PEG tube that this method is sometimes used automatically without much thought. Occasionally it is necessary to position the distal end of the feeding tube not in the stomach itself but beyond the outlet of the stomach, in

---

1. AAF&N is the abbreviation I prefer. Others use AFN (artificial fluids and nutrition) or merely F&N (fluids and nutrition).

the jejunum (the second part of the small intestine). These placements are somewhat more difficult, and the resulting tube is called a **J-tube**.

Parenteral fluids were first used during a cholera epidemic in Scotland in 1831, but intravenous (IV) fluids were not commonly used until after antisepsis was understood in the late nineteenth century. They became more routine in the early twentieth century, thus allowing continued hydration. However, IV fluids alone provide inadequate nutritional support, giving only water, salt, sugar, and perhaps some amino acids. **Total parenteral nutrition** (TPN) was a significant medical advance when introduced in the 1970s, because it allowed the full range of proteins, fats, carbohydrates, and minerals to be administered. The TPN procedure uses balanced mixtures of multiple components, requires highly technical oversight, has significant risks, and is very expensive.

The history of the ethics of AAF&N is a bit different from that of other technologies, precisely because it was not clear when first used that this was technology at all. Many considered long-term AAF&N to be morally equivalent to feeding. In addition, this life-sustaining technology was most often used in patients who were not clearly dying: patients with **dementia**, for example, or after a stroke or traumatic brain injury. Thus, since the patient could survive with AAF&N, and since feeding tubes were considered TLC rather than technology, it was very uncommon to consider withdrawal of feedings prior to 1980.

But the thinking about AAF&N began to change in the early 1980s as the procedures were recognized to be technology and thus optional. The first case contested in court was a 1983 appellate court ruling on IV fluids (*Barber,* California), and the first feeding tube court case was in 1984 (*Conroy,* New Jersey). Both courts said it was permissible in some situations to not use AAF&N; they were optional. But the case of Nancy Cruzan, decided by the U.S. Supreme Court in 1990 (*Cruzan v. Director,* Missouri Department of Health), gave the clearest pronouncement of societal values — AAF&N are medical treatment, not merely sustenance, and thus may be accepted or declined by the patient.

Those who support this perspective, that AAF&N may be used or not used depending on the situation and the wishes of the patient or **surrogate**, maintain that tube feedings are not ordinary care, have both benefits and burdens, and often merely prolong a dying process. When AAF&N are withheld or withdrawn from a person who is unable to swallow, the patient will die in several days from dehydration, not from starvation. Dehydration does not cause the patient to suffer as long as his or her mouth is kept moist; the mouth is the only place in the body where dehydration may be perceived. Those who support this position maintain that a decision to withdraw AAF&N is comparable to decisions to withdraw other treatment modalities such as assisted **ventilation** or dialysis — the therapy would be continued if it were able to accomplish its goal, but when it has been determined that the original goal is not achievable, then the therapy is stopped.

This emerging stream of thought has not been without its critics. Though a consensus has emerged that tube feedings and IV fluids are not appropriate for patients who are imminently dying, some disagreement remains about long-term use in patients who are cognitively impaired. The debate has focused on patients with dementia or those in a **persistent vegetative state**. In particular, conservative/orthodox religious leaders (Roman Catholic, Protestant, and Jewish), along with advocates for people with disabilities and the right-to-life community, have been split on these questions. They have expressed concern that withholding or withdrawing AAF&N is an intentional act that certainly leads to death, and that this practice could be abused.

A North American Catholic consensus developed in the late 1990s that AAF&N were optional in these situations, though there clearly was not unanimity.[2] This consensus became a bit unsettled in March of 2004 when Pope John Paul II issued an allocution saying that feeding tubes are not treatment, and they are morally obligatory in persons who are not terminally ill, specifically in patients in a persistent vegetative state (though he decried the use of that term). Many Roman Catholic moral philosophers look at the question of use or nonuse of feeding tubes in light of proportionality, that is, a balance of the benefits and burdens for a particular patient, rather than assigning an obligatory use because the feeding tube is "ordinary" rather than "extraordinary."

While this moral debate was going on, research data was accumulating that showed, rather surprisingly, that the use of feeding tubes in patients who are cognitively impaired does not on average prolong survival, ensure adequate nutrition, or prevent **aspiration**. Feeding tube usage in patients with dementia varies enormously in the United States, from 9 percent in Maine, New Hampshire, and Vermont to 64 percent in Washington, D.C.

In summary, there is near agreement that AAF&N are generally inappropriate in persons who are terminally ill. There is growing empiric evi-

---

2. J. J. Paris, "Terri Schiavo and the Use of Artificial Nutrition and Fluids: Insights from the Catholic Tradition on End-of-Life Care," *Palliative and Supportive Care* 4 (2006): 117-20.

dence that feeding tubes do not improve outcomes in advanced dementia, leading to a decreasing use pattern in many areas. But significant controversy remains about the use or nonuse of feeding tubes in patients who are permanently awake but unaware (see CASES 6.05 and 7.08).

Above and beyond these policy questions, however, individual ethics consultations will continue to be requested to provide guidance on questions of short-term or long-term usage of AAF&N. And the recommendations may vary in cases that are clinically similar (see CASES 6.03 and 6.04). Those involved in these discussions must be aware of the status of the ongoing debate, and must also be aware of the religious and moral background of the patient and family (see CASE 6.09) and also the beliefs of the professional caregivers (see CASE 6.02).

Let's look at several specific cases where the primary clinical ethics question is about whether to use artificially administered fluids and nutrition.

Case 6.01

QUESTION

Should a feeding tube be used for this man with Parkinson's disease who is now beginning to aspirate oral feedings?

STORY

Mr. Gonzales is an eighty-four-year-old man whose Parkinson's disease[3] has worsened for the last five or six years; a **neurologist** confirmed six months ago that it was in its end stages. He has been treated with several medications but his symptoms have not improved.

After his wife's death a few years ago, Mr. Gonzales lived on his own for a while, but he was admitted to a nursing home two years ago because of falling, poor eating, and confusion in his medications. His condition

---

3. Parkinson's disease is a slowly progressive degenerative disease of a specific part of the brain causing muscle rigidity, tremor, and poor balance. It often progresses to dementia. Its cause is unknown. Progressive neurologic disease of this sort usually leads to death from superimposed infection, often pneumonia.

has progressed so that he is now incontinent and unable to walk or feed himself. His daughter describes him as "pleasantly demented." He usually recognizes family, speaks little, occasionally makes up stories (e.g., recent "travels" to foreign countries), and rarely exhibits the humor that had been so characteristic of his earlier personality. He does not interact with other residents of the nursing home and does not appear to enjoy television. He is on a pureed diet that he seems to enjoy, though he swallows slowly and with difficulty. He recently had his second episode of **aspiration** pneumonia, treated at the nursing home. This has caused the nursing home staff to question whether he should have a feeding tube.

Mr. Gonzales has no written **advance directive** and has been unwilling in the past to engage in any significant discussion with family about his end-of-life wishes, though he has left some funeral and burial instructions. He has three children: a daughter who lives locally and visits frequently, and two sons who live out of state but communicate with him frequently. All agree about not using other aggressive measures (**cardiopulmonary resuscitation**, attaching a **ventilator**, admission to the intensive care unit, etc.) if his condition should worsen acutely.

DISCUSSION

When a patient is terminally ill, all life-extending treatments are optional; the potential benefits and burdens of each treatment in use or under consideration should be weighed in making treatment decisions. When treatment decisions must be made for a patient who has lost the capacity to participate in discussions, we try to make a **substituted judgment** to determine what the patient would choose, based on a written advance directive or his or her spoken wishes. When this is not possible, we must use the lower **best interests** standard, that is, we try to balance the benefits and burdens and make the decision most people would make in this circumstance.

This man is terminally ill from Parkinson's disease. Some types of feeding tubes (e.g., a **J-tube**) might reduce his risk of aspiration and postpone his inevitable death, while others (nasogastric tube, **PEG tube**) would probably offer little or no improvement in his risk of aspiration or life expectancy. The use of a feeding tube could diminish his quality of life by (a) precluding the pleasure he derives from tasting and swallowing and (b) possibly requiring the use of hand restraints.

RECOMMENDATIONS

1. It would be ethically permissible to not use a feeding tube in this patient, while continuing to offer oral feedings and giving good mouth care. If he should aspirate, it would then be ethically permissible to either treat infection (at the nursing home or in the hospital) or continue to give him comfort care without antibiotics.
2. It would also be permissible to use a long-term feeding tube, though most patients/families find that the potential burdens (diminished quality of life from not eating, restraints) outweigh the hoped-for benefit of temporarily postponing death.
3. It would theoretically be permissible to use a short-term trial of a feeding tube, either now or with evidence of recurring aspiration. The goal would be to see how the patient tolerates the tube. Does he require restraints? Does he seem to miss eating? I say theoretically, because the nasogastric or PEG tube may not give sufficient protection from aspiration, and insertion of a J-tube may be a more invasive procedure entailing its own burdens. If a feeding tube trial is chosen, it should be clearly understood by family, physician, and nursing home that it will be discontinued if it becomes clear that it is not serving its intended purpose.

FOLLOW-UP

Mr. Gonzales's family decided against insertion of a feeding tube. He continued to live in the nursing home for another sixteen months, showing signs of continued slow deterioration. He gradually lost interest and ability in eating and was given good **palliative care**, including mouth care. He died in the nursing home with his three children present.

COMMENT

This case represents a very common dilemma. A patient demonstrates signs and symptoms of difficulty swallowing, and family and professionals wonder whether it is appropriate, or even obligatory, to use a feeding tube to assist with feeding and avoid aspiration. Resolution of the dilemma requires an understanding of the clinical situation, including the prognosis; an understanding of the patient's wishes and values; and a calculation of the potential benefits and burdens of the use or nonuse of a feeding tube for the particular patient.

Case 6.02

QUESTION

Is a feeding tube ethically obligatory for this patient with advanced dementia?

STORY

Gertrude ("Gertie") is eighty-three years old and has had **dementia** for about eleven years. She was transferred from the nursing home to the hospital four days ago for the treatment of her third episode of **aspiration** pneumonia in the past four months, and her physician says she can no longer eat anything by mouth and should have a feeding tube (**PEG tube**) inserted. Her only daughter, Anna, is reluctant to give consent for this procedure.

The patient has been a widow for many years. After her husband's death, she continued to live in her apartment, enjoying music, knitting, and going out to her Catholic church just down the street. Anna is close to her and oversaw her care in her apartment for a few years after she was diagnosed with Alzheimer's disease, even hiring live-in help. Four years ago Gertie became incontinent and was unable to get out of bed unless two people lifted her. Anna found a nursing home operated by an order of Catholic nuns who had a reputation for providing excellent care at the end of life. Over the ensuing four years Gertie has slowly deteriorated and now no longer recognizes her favorite nuns or even Anna. She no longer speaks, occasionally smiles, but opens her mouth when food is offered. The nuns have had to feed her with a spoon and eyedropper for the past several months, a process that takes over an hour for each meal.

Gertie has left no written **advance directive**, but early in the course of her dementia she told Anna that she didn't want "a bunch of machines and tubes" when she was dying. It is on this basis that Anna is reluctant to consent to insertion of a PEG tube. On the other hand, Gertie's physician is convinced that continued oral feeding, even as painstakingly done by the nuns, risks recurrent aspiration and perhaps shortens her life expectancy. The nuns are therefore unwilling to take her back without a feeding tube. After the wonderful four years at this nursing home, Anna would prefer not to change to a new facility and new doctor who are willing to care for her without a feeding tube. She would like her mother to die among those who know and love her.

DISCUSSION

Debate continues about the use or nonuse of feeding tubes. Most health-care professionals consider feeding tubes to be medical treatment and optional in any given situation, as is any other treatment. Sometimes they are morally obligatory (e.g., when the patient is unable to eat and has a reversible condition) and sometimes they are not (e.g., when a patient is unable to eat and is imminently dying). In still other situations their use is optional (e.g., when a patient is severely debilitated but not imminently dying, as after a stroke or with advanced dementia). Most professionals are willing to follow patient or **surrogate** wishes in such situations.

Others disagree, believing that feeding by tube is not treatment but an expression of loving care, and as such it is morally obligatory unless the patient is clearly and imminently dying.

This case clearly demonstrates this difference of opinion. The patient's daughter recognizes that her mother has a fatal disease, though a prediction of when she will die is uncertain. She believes that her mother would not want feeding by tube at this advanced stage of her dementia. Her doctor and daily caregivers, however, believe that dementia is not a fatal disease, and they further believe they are obligated to provide optimal nutrition. Her daughter additionally places a high value on her mother's continued care and would prefer that she spend her last weeks with friends.

RECOMMENDATIONS

1. It would be ethically permissible to not use a feeding tube for this patient because of her wish to be free of such encumbrances while dying. She should continue to be offered and given food and fluids by mouth. Should she aspirate and develop a pneumonia, the level of treatment is optional and includes the spectrum of rehospitalization for intravenous antibiotics, oral antibiotics at the nursing home, or comfort care with the expectation that the infection might take her life.
2. The physician and nuns who have provided loving care for this patient should not be required to violate their personal beliefs. Their right of conscience would preclude transfer of the patient back to the same facility without provision of artificially administered fluids and nutrition.
3. Absent an absolute refusal by the patient, her daughter's wish for her to die among friends may outweigh this loosely stated preference, such that it would also be ethically permissible to insert a PEG tube.

FOLLOW-UP

Anna looked at other nursing homes but ultimately consented (reluctantly) to insertion of a PEG tube. Gertie went back to the same nursing home with the understanding that if aspiration should recur, she would receive oral antibiotics at the nursing home but would not be transferred back to the hospital. She died at the nursing home about six weeks after hospital discharge. Anna had mixed feelings about the course of events. She was very pleased that her mother died among friends, but wished she could have honored her mother's wish to avoid tubes at the end of life.

COMMENT

This case illustrates the differences of opinion that may be encountered in dealing with issues of feeding tubes. Sometimes these differences fall along religious lines, but at other times they do not. My understanding from personal discussions and from reading the literature is that the obligation to use feeding tubes is not uniform among those from the Catholic tradition. In this case the physician and nuns took the more conservative stance. It is equally important to recognize their "right of conscience." If this patient's daughter had chosen not to institute tube feeding, the physician and nuns should be supported in their stance and should not feel pressured to accept a patient whose decision (or whose surrogate's decision) violates their personal moral boundaries.

Case 6.03

QUESTION

Is it ethically permissible to place a feeding tube in this patient whose advance directive declines "artificial nutrition and fluids"?

STORY

Evelyn, age seventy-six, has a history of hypertension and atrial fibrillation, a chronic irregularity of heart rhythm. She had a stroke four days ago while visiting her terminally ill daughter. She was brought to the emergency department with weakness of her right side and the total inability to speak. A head **CT scan** done on admission showed no acute hemorrhage, and a repeat scan done yesterday showed a large stroke on the left side,[4] most likely due to a blood clot blocking an artery. She has been given a drug to prevent further clotting and is being fed through a nasogastric (NG) tube. She remains awake, tracks visually,[5] and can follow simple commands such as "please raise your right arm." However, she has had no meaningful neurologic recovery in four days and is unable to swallow or engage in communication. Her caregivers anticipate that she will have little or no neurologic recovery, but they recognize there is some uncertainty about her prognosis because it has been only four days since the event. They have recommended placement of a **PEG tube** if long-term feeding is to be done.

In her chart are both a living will and a durable power of attorney for health care signed and witnessed ten years ago; the latter names one son as her **agent**. She copied from the form this instruction to her agent: "If I suffer a condition for which there is no reasonable prospect of regaining my ability to think and act for myself, I want only care directed to my comfort and dignity, and authorize my agent to decline all treatments (including artificial nutrition and hydration) the primary purpose of which is to prolong my life."

I met with one daughter, two sons, and a daughter-in-law; her other daughter is terminally ill. They report that before this stroke the patient was living alone in senior housing and was fully functional, walking with a cane or walker, driving her car, going to church and bingo. They describe her as a pleasant and quiet woman. Her husband died ten years ago of cancer that spread painfully to his bones. During his terminal illness they signed identical **advance directives** and said they wanted "no machines," but had no further discussion about specific wishes. All family members present agreed that her goal was to avoid prolongation of a painful dying process by the use of machines. They are convinced that she would choose to continue artificially administered feedings until her prognosis was very clear, perhaps for a month, but that she would not want to survive via feeding tube if she could not improve.

---

4. The structure of the brain is such that there is a crossover of pathways, and the left side of the body is controlled by the right side of the brain.

5. Visual tracking means that the patient's eyes follow movement, suggesting the person has some awareness.

DISCUSSION

When treatment decisions must be made for a previously competent patient who has lost the ability to make decisions, we try to make a **substituted judgment**, that is, to make the decision the patient would make. This may be done by reading what the patient has written in an advance directive or talking with those who know the patient's values and wishes.

In this case the patient appointed one of her sons as her agent, and she copied standard wording from a sample document that ruled out use of a feeding tube. Her caring family is convinced that those instructions were written with a different scenario in mind (i.e., one comparable to her husband's terminal illness) and that she would want a trial of artificial feeding until her prognosis, though already quite poor, is more certain.

RECOMMENDATIONS

1. It is ethically permissible to continue to use an NG tube or to insert a PEG tube as a short-term trial to see if she regains the ability to swallow or to engage in conversation about her current treatment wishes.
2. A time limit should be set such that if she has had no significant improvement, artificially administered nutrition and hydration will be stopped to honor her written wishes (her family have suggested a month).
3. If she is transferred to a nursing home, the receiving physician and facility should understand and accept that the PEG is a short-term trial rather than a permanent measure.

FOLLOW-UP

A PEG tube was inserted as a temporary measure, and she was discharged to a nursing home. After about three weeks she began to drink and eat small amounts. This improved so that the feeding tube was removed. Fourteen months later the nursing home staff reported that she had had no further neurologic improvement, she remained unable to speak, but she appeared to be content in her surroundings and was always eager to eat.

COMMENT

It is always troubling to ignore a patient's written instructions about his or her treatment wishes. In this case the exact condition she had written had not yet been met since her long-term outlook was somewhat uncertain only four days after her stroke. In addition, her family felt they understood nuances of her intention that did not come through in the written document.

When a decision is made to undertake a trial of therapy and to transfer a patient from one site of care to another, it is very important that the new health-care professionals are adequately informed about the intent and probable duration of the trial. This is particularly important in relation to artificially administered fluids and nutrition since some professionals and some facilities are very reluctant to withdraw a feeding tube once it has been inserted.

Case 6.04

QUESTION

Is it permissible to not use a feeding tube in this man with an acute stroke who is awake but unable to take sufficient oral nutrition?

STORY

Stephen is almost eighty years old and has a history of vascular disease and hypertension. He fell five days ago and has had severe difficulty speaking. He was admitted, and workup showed that he had suffered a stroke from a large (greater than an inch) **intracerebral hemorrhage** that had extended through the brain tissue into the cavity in the center of the brain. On admission he was found to be awake and alert, but disoriented and speaking unintelligibly. At the request of his family, a **do-not-resuscitate order** (DNR order) was written. Because of inadequate oral intake, intravenous fluids and a nasogastric tube were used; the latter required the use of hand restraints since the patient repeatedly removed it. When his daughter arrived from out of state yesterday, she requested that the feeding tube be removed, and this was done. The patient's prognosis is guarded; he might worsen if bleeding recurs or if he develops hydrocephalus.[6] If this does not happen, he could survive but would likely remain dependent and unable

---

6. Hydrocephalus is an increased pressure of the cerebrospinal fluid inside the skull. There are many causes, one of which is obstruction to outflow of this fluid after a hemorrhagic stroke.

to speak. He remains somewhat awake. Dr. Navarro, the **neurologist** caring for Stephen, has requested consultation because he is uncomfortable not providing tube feedings to this man who is not clearly dying.

On exam, the patient is sleepy but rousable. He tracks with his eyes and tries to talk, but his speech is unintelligible. In the chart is a copy of a "prehospital DNR order" signed by his primary physician and dated three months ago. (I was unable to reach the primary physician by phone as he is out of state for an extended period.) A repeat head **CT scan** taken this morning shows some swelling of the brain but no significant change in the hemorrhage and no sign of increased pressure in the brain.

I met with the patient's oldest son (with whom the patient has lived for the past three years), his daughter from out of state (with whom he lived the five years prior), and his son-in-law. Two other step-siblings are in daily phone contact. His son describes him as a "good-natured old crab" who is stubborn and "never wrong." He divorced many years ago and has lived with several other women over the years. He is Catholic, nonobservant for many years, but he told his children he has "made peace with God" over the past ten years. Until this stroke he was fully functional, though symptomatic from chronic lung disease. They all agree he has said on many occasions, "When my time comes, just let me go. No machines. No tubes." They are certain that he would not want a feeding tube or restraints, even if they were only temporary and even if there were a reasonable chance of survival with some improvement in his functional status.

DISCUSSION

When treatment decisions must be made for a patient who has lost **decision-making capacity**, we try to make a **substituted judgment**, that is, to make the decision the patient would make if the patient were able. This judgment may be based on the patient's written **advance directive**, a report from loved ones of the patient's previously expressed wishes, or an understanding of his or her values, goals, or wishes. Such deliberation assumes that the patient's **surrogate** has the best clinical and prognostic information available and is acting in the patient's **best interests**.

If patients or their surrogates refuse treatment recommended by their physician, it is appropriate to elicit their reasons, and to try to persuade them to accept the recommendation. But if they are firm and rational in their refusal, that should be honored unless the remaining course of therapy clearly falls outside the bounds of acceptable medical practice.

In this case, the patient is currently unable to communicate to us his understanding of his condition or his wishes about treatment. We have no written advance directive, though we do have a prehospital DNR order, apparently written fairly recently by his physician at his request. His caring family is convinced that he would choose to forgo artificially administered fluids and nutrition in this situation, even if some uncertainty remains about his functional recovery. Such refusal is not outside the bounds of acceptable medical practice.

RECOMMENDATIONS

1. It is ethically permissible to accept the substituted judgment of this patient's family that he would not want a feeding tube. If there is a reasonable chance that he will have significant functional recovery, this should be explained to his family so they may reconsider their current request for **limitation of treatment**.
2. Agreement to withhold artificially administered fluids and nutrition does not mean that other treatments should stop. Efforts at prevention of complications and efforts at rehabilitation may proceed with goals of (a) comfort and (b) maximizing recovery within the limits previously set by the patient and articulated by his family.
3. If any of his caregivers are personally uncomfortable with this withholding of therapy they consider to be standard or obligatory, they should be excused from responsibility for his care.

FOLLOW-UP

The day of the consultation Stephen's feeding tube was removed but intravenous fluids were continued. When I pointed out to his physician a few days later that the continuation of fluids without full nutrition would lead to starvation and might also cause fluid overload, the physician (somewhat reluctantly) stopped the intravenous fluids. The next day the patient did develop acute **congestive heart failure** from fluid overload. He was given comfort measures without resuscitation and died in about twenty minutes.

COMMENT

Dr. Navarro's reluctance to discontinue artificially administered fluids and nutrition (AAF&N) is understandable in this case since the patient could probably have survived for some time with adequate fluids and nutrition. However, even when health-care professionals disagree with a patient's choice, it is accepted practice that the patient's wishes in deciding for or against the use of a specific treatment should be honored as long as they remain within the accepted bounds of clinical practice. It seemed fairly clear in this case that the patient would choose to forgo AAF&N in this situation.

Sometimes the question arises whether the person who does not want the feeding tube has an ulterior motive, perhaps relief from the burden of care, perhaps even preservation of financial assets for his or her inheritance. It is almost impossible to rule out such matters, but an attitude of true caring exhibited by the family members helps to alleviate such concerns. It is a truism that anyone close enough to be a surrogate is also close enough to have a potential conflict of interest; this is part of our social and moral fabric.

Health-care professionals also have a "right of conscience," and if a patient's treatment choice, though ethically justifiable, is clearly outside that professional's moral comfort zone, the professional may rightfully be relieved from care of the patient. It is imperative for that professional to ensure that the patient has ongoing care.

Case 6.05

QUESTION

Is it ethically permissible to discontinue feedings for this unaware nursing home patient?

STORY

Judy, a forty-six-year-old woman with a history of untreated seizures, was a pedestrian when struck by a pickup truck nearly six years ago. She was convulsing when paramedics arrived, and her seizures continued for a few days in spite of aggressive treatment. Her family declined professional recommendations for **limitation of treatment** and requested that she receive full treatment. Over the next several weeks she progressed to an "eyes-open coma"[7] and was transferred to the care of Dr. Rupert at Shore

7. "Eyes-open coma" is a term often used to describe the persistent vegetative state.

Acres Nursing Home with a diagnosis of severe brain injury caused by the trauma of the accident and worsened by lack of oxygen during the prolonged period of seizure activity. She has remained stable and has not required rehospitalization. Her nurses report (and her chart indicates) that her eyes are open part of the time but she does not track. She occasionally makes guttural sounds or grimaces when moved, and she withdraws from deep, painful stimulation (e.g., when blood is drawn), but she does not appear to have any awareness of her environment (no smile, no recognition). She is fed via **PEG tube** and still has a **tracheostomy** for suctioning of her airway. A **do-not-resuscitate order** was written soon after admission to the nursing home, and a recent progress note indicates she is not to be given antibiotics or to be transferred to hospital without consulting Dr. Rupert. She has received excellent nursing care and grooming from dedicated staff.

Dr. Rupert and the patient's two sisters have recently discussed the possibility of stopping her fluids and nutrition since she has shown no improvement in nearly six years. Dr. Rupert concluded: "Family has accurate reason to believe that Judy would not want to prolong artificial feeding in her current condition based on their knowledge of her life goals."

The patient is single. Her mother is deceased; her father is still alive but uninvolved in her care. She has three siblings: a sister, Jerri, who has been her legal guardian since soon after the accident; a sister, Janet, who is also still involved, and who discusses management issues with Jerri; a brother who has not been involved in her care.

DISCUSSION

A feeding tube is medical treatment while voluntary eating by mouth is not. A feeding tube is sometimes used short term (e.g., in the post-op patient who is unable to swallow) and may be used long term (e.g., in a patient who wishes to survive but is permanently unable to swallow). A feeding tube is often used as a temporary measure (e.g., when a patient is unconscious from illness or injury) while other treatments or the passage of time clarifies the patient's prognosis. If the patient's condition does not improve to a level the patient thinks is acceptable, it is then ethically and legally permissible to accept the proven lack of benefit and to discontinue the artificially administered fluids and nutrition, with the expectation that the patient will die from the underlying problem, which will lead to dehydration. On the other hand, if it is believed that a patient would choose to be maintained via feeding tube in a permanent unresponsive state, it is ethically obligatory to honor that wish.

This patient has a devastating neurologic impairment from direct brain trauma and hypoxic brain injury. In either event, her six-year trial of therapy has far exceeded the accepted professional standard used to call her condition "persistent" (one month for **hypoxia**, twelve months for trauma). Her legal guardian and involved family co-**surrogate** are convinced that she would not want to be maintained in this state with this degree of certainty of nonrecoverability.

RECOMMENDATIONS

1. It is ethically permissible to discontinue artificially administered fluids and nutrition. The current literature suggests that this is best accomplished by abrupt cessation of all calories and fluids except for frequently moistening the patient's mouth. This avoids the potential wasting and/or edema that can accompany caloric restriction with continued fluid administration.

2. Before this is done, it would be preferable to do the following: (a) If a neurology consultation has not been done in the past two years, document clearly her diagnosis and prognosis. (b) All family members should be aware of the plans and should agree, even if reluctantly, to not contest the decision of her legal guardian. (c) Her caregivers should likewise be aware of the decision, the reasoning, and the plan. If any are uncomfortable participating in this **palliative care** plan, they should be excused from responsibility for her care.

FOLLOW-UP

A neurology consultant reaffirmed a diagnosis of **persistent vegetative state** with virtually no chance of improvement. Dr. Rupert met again with the family, and all agreed that they should request discontinuation of PEG feedings to honor their understanding of Judy's wishes. He met with the nurses caring for Judy and with the nursing home administrator. Her feedings were stopped and she died peacefully in nine days.

COMMENT

Discontinuation of chronic artificially administered fluids and nutrition is a huge decision. Such major decisions should not be made quickly or lightly, but after much deliberation and consultation with all the stake-holders — family, primary physician, nurses, consultants, administrators, and occasionally attorneys. If there is disagreement about the patient's previously stated wishes, the decision should generally be postponed until all the issues can be more fully explored. But in the end, the decision to continue or discontinue artificially administered fluids and nutrition is comparable to a similar decision for any other treatment modality.

Case 6.06

QUESTION

Is it ethically permissible to withdraw fluids and nutrition from this elderly man at his family's request while he is still improving from postoperative complications?

STORY

Ralph is an eighty-five-year-old retired carpenter who was fully active prior to this admission, caring for his home and for his wife who has **dementia**. Narrowing of the aortic valve of his heart, discovered on routine exam several months ago, recently began to cause him significant shortness of breath. He was admitted five weeks ago for surgical replacement of the valve, and he and his family were told before surgery that his surgical risk was "high." The surgery went well, but his post-op course has been complicated by prolonged **intubation**, pneumonia, wound bleeding, reintubation, and electrolyte imbalance. Decisions have been made and orders written for no resuscitation, no intubation, no dialysis, and no **total parenteral nutrition**. Despite his multiple complications, he has made slow, steady improvement. As recently as a few days ago he said, "I am going to a retreat [convalescent home] before I go home."

Two days ago he became unresponsive from poor kidney function leading to imbalance of his salts and fluids. This has been treated and his lab values are better. He is now awake but confused. He is currently receiving supplemental oxygen and nasogastric (NG) feedings because of persistent swallowing difficulties and inadequate oral intake. His care team view this as just one more complication that has been addressed and may be reversed. But today his family brought in his **advance directive** and asked that all life-prolonging treatment be stopped.

His standard durable power of attorney for health care, signed nine years ago, names his only daughter as his **agent** and one of his two sons as alternate. He chose the option for least treatment, which includes a request for no feeding tube. On the accompanying worksheet he said he valued "living an active and mentally alert life." In addition, he wrote, "anything less than a 75 percent chance of full recovery at my age (seventy-six) would not be acceptable," and "the older I get, the less I would want treatment."

I met with his daughter and one son. They describe their father as a very proud man who not only would not want to be confined in a nursing home or wheelchair, but also would be ashamed and embarrassed to be seen in such a condition. They are convinced that he agreed to risky surgery so that he could continue to care for his wife. When they told him several days ago that they would care for her, he said "good-bye" to each of them. They also say they have been talking with his physicians in the intensive care unit for two weeks about **limitation of treatment**, but have been encouraged to continue toward a goal of survival "for a few more days" on two occasions. They had been cautiously hopeful for some dramatic recovery, but his recent conversations with them and this last complication have convinced them that he does not want to continue even fluids and nutrition.

DISCUSSION

When a patient is no longer able to participate in decisions, we try to make a **substituted judgment**, that is, to do what the patient would want, based on the patient's written or spoken instructions or on an understanding of his or her values.

In this case, we have just learned that the patient has left clear written instructions and has named two family members to speak for him. After discussing the issues with his surgeon, they are convinced he has less than a 75 percent chance of achieving his goal of returning to independent function and of fulfilling his desire to care for his disabled wife. In addition, they are uncomfortable continuing full treatment because he indicated ten years ago that as he got older he wanted even less treatment. The only ethically justifiable reasons to continue treatment aimed at survival would be (a) if his stated goal is achievable or (b) if he had verbally indicated a change in his goals or values.

RECOMMENDATIONS

1. If his professional caregivers agree that Ralph has less than a 75 percent chance of achieving a full recovery, it is ethically permissible to follow his family's request to remove his feeding tube and give him comfort care.
2. If it is uncertain whether this 75 percent chance of recovery is feasible, it might be worthwhile to obtain a second opinion, perhaps from a rehabilitation medicine specialist, or to wait another day or two to see if the patient is able to discuss these issues.

FOLLOW-UP

After agreement among his family and professional caregivers, Ralph's NG feedings were stopped, he was given small amounts of morphine for comfort, and he died in five days.

COMMENT

Withdrawal of artificially administered fluids and nutrition from a patient who clearly has a dismal prognosis and is not improving is sometimes difficult. Doing so when the prognosis is still uncertain is even more difficult. But doing so in a case like this where the patient is showing signs of slow improvement is very unsettling for health-care professionals. Their response is often, "Give us a few more days to see if we can correct x" (or y or z, or x, y, and z). Families often remain optimistic through such trials but may become weary or may lose trust when the hoped-for improvement does not materialize.

When a family suddenly changes goals from survival to comfort care, professionals may be concerned about family fatigue and burnout, ulterior motives, etc. But the existence of written instructions from the patient, or a thorough discussion of the motivation and timing, may help to resolve such discomfort.

Case 6.07

QUESTION

Is it ethically permissible to honor this man's request to eat in light of his great risk for aspiration?

STORY

Greg, age forty-five, was diagnosed seven years ago with **Huntington's disease**. He has had the anticipated slow deterioration with abnormal muscular movements and some cognitive slowing, but prior to this hospitalization he was living at home, with major personal and medical care provided by his brother. He was admitted to the intensive care unit (ICU) three months ago with a life-threatening neck infection. At that time his family chose survival as a goal based on his functional capacity and bright outlook before his infection.

He has survived life-saving emergency surgery, several subsequent operations, an initial episode of cardiac arrest, prolonged ICU care on a **ventilator**, and multiple additional complications. He has responded to intensive therapy, has now stabilized, and is awaiting a bed in a nursing home near his brother's home. He has been fed primarily by a gastric tube, and now is able to tolerate a few ice chips to keep his mouth moist. He has had two swallowing studies, the most recent just two days ago after a trial of swallowing exercises. The speech-language therapist who performed this study notes that he has severe coughing with thin or thick liquids, and she believes he is at great risk of **aspiration**. For at least a month he has been asking for water, food, and beer. Yesterday he asked if he was allowed to refuse treatment and die. A psychiatry consultation has been requested; he is already on two antidepressants.

The patient is lying in bed, watching TV. He talks and smiles easily, and he exhibits erratic muscular movements typical of this disease. He clearly states his wish to eat and drink. He realizes he has a fatal disease that will likely take his life in the next few years, and he realizes he is at risk of aspiration and earlier death if he eats. He says he is discouraged, primarily about not being able to eat, but he denies depression and does not want to die. When I brought up depression, he mentioned that another brother (also with Huntington's disease) died by suicide about a year ago. He says, "He was different than me. He was depressed."

DISCUSSION

An adequately informed patient with **decision-making capacity** has the right to accept or decline any therapy, even potentially life-extending therapy. The patient is also free to accept or decline restrictions on activities of daily living, such as eating, even if this presents significant risk of morbidity or earlier mortality.

Depression with suicidal ideation often compromises a person's decision-making capacity. Life-endangering choices made by a suicidal patient require greater scrutiny than those made by a nondepressed patient. Sometimes the severity of the depression in a patient with a decent prognosis makes it ethically justifiable to override the patient's autonomous choice that presents a major risk. However, in patients who are terminally ill, a desire to participate in risky behavior does not necessarily mean they are suicidal. It may merely mean they have weighed the benefits and risks and have chosen, against medical advice (**AMA**), a course that puts them at some risk but gives them more benefit.

This patient appears to have made a rational choice for eating and drinking.

RECOMMENDATIONS

1. Unless it becomes clear that this man has a depression that can be improved with treatment, it is ethically permissible to allow him to accept the risk of eating and drinking, with due precautions.
2. It would also be appropriate to discuss **limitation of treatment** with this patient, for example, his wishes about deep suctioning, **intubation**, resuscitation, transfer to the ICU.

FOLLOW-UP

The psychiatry consultant found the patient to not be suicidal and agreed that he had the capacity to decide if he wanted to eat in spite of the risks. His care team met with him and his brother to explain the risks of eating, danger of needing reintubation and return to the ICU, etc. He appeared to understand, asked again to be allowed to eat, and said that if he did aspirate, he wanted full treatment including return to the ICU if needed.

When I returned to see him several days later, he was eating with delight, though choking frequently. When I asked if there was anything I could do for him, he said, "Six-pack!"

He was discharged to a nursing home about two weeks later, and three months later was reported to be eating with only modest difficulty.

COMMENT

In confronting significant irreversible disability from progressive disease, for example, advanced **dementia** or Huntington's disease, patients and clinicians are often faced with a trade-off between the pleasure of eating and the risk of aspiration. Not everyone agrees on how this trade-off should be handled. Some value the extension of life as paramount and would thus disallow eating to maximize the length of life. Others place a high value on the pleasure of eating and would be willing to risk potential shortening of life. This trade-off is not unlike that faced by some patients with advanced malignancy who could opt for another round of chemotherapy that has the potential to extend life for a few weeks or forgo it to have a better quality of life for a shorter time. Judgment about these trade-offs is value-laden and quite personal. I do not believe that any ethical principles, either secular or religious, mandate a particular choice.

The professionals caring for this man had invested their time and talents, along with tremendous resources, into pulling Greg back from the brink of death. They saw his request to eat as foolish since he had a major risk for recurrent aspiration and possible death. Their values, understandably, placed survival ahead of eating. The patient's values were different. In light of his good result, it is easy to retrospectively support the patient's choice. However, if he had suffered a major setback soon after beginning to eat, it would have been easy for the professionals to say, "I told you so."

Case 6.08

QUESTION

Is it ethically permissible to discharge this demented patient back to a nursing home with less than adequate nutrition? May we write a do-not-resuscitate order?

STORY

Hester is an eighty-two-year-old frail woman with mild Alzheimer's disease who was admitted to the hospital from her nursing home two months ago with fever and jaundice caused by a gallstone. She subsequently had her gallbladder removed with multiple postoperative complications that have been treated aggressively with several repeat surgeries, **ventilator** support, antibiotics, etc. She has improved but she is still being fed through a nasogastric (NG) tube because of inadequate oral intake. The NG tube is difficult to insert because her upper gastrointestinal anatomy is distorted due to a large hiatal hernia. Earlier her hands had to be restrained because she pulled at the NG tube. She now leaves it alone, though she constantly complains about it. She is nearly ready for discharge, but the nursing home from which she came is unable to care for her with the NG tube. Her care team is asking if it would be permissible to remove the NG tube so that she could return to the nursing home where she is known, since it is quite possible she will eat better in familiar surroundings. While this might compromise her nutritional status, they believe it might not be inconsistent with her very frail condition on admission. An alternative would be surgical placement of a permanent gastric tube (rather than a **PEG tube,** due to her anatomy).

Transfer records from the nursing home report that she was ambulatory and independent in all activities of daily living prior to this illness. I called the nursing home and learned that Hester never ate breakfast, ate one decent meal per day (sometimes two), and ate snacks in the night. Her weight had been steady (120-123 pounds) for the six months prior to this illness.

There is a durable power of attorney for health care form in the chart signed eleven years ago naming a nephew in Florida as her **agent.** In it she authorizes him to make decisions to withhold life-prolonging treatments only if there is "no reasonable hope of recovering the ability to think." This phrase is clearly defined as (1) "brain dead" or (2) "a hopeless and costly vegetative state." A nursing home form dated two years ago and signed by the patient requests resuscitation and transfer to the hospital for treatment of acute problems.

The patient is pleasant and interactive, but her answers are not always cogent. She says she was a corporate executive before she retired several years ago. She says she was active in athletics.

DISCUSSION

When previously competent patients lose the ability to make treatment decisions, we try to make a **substituted judgment**, that is, the decision they would make if they were able. The basis for this may be patients' written instructions about (a) what they would want or (b) whom they trust to make decisions for them (their agent) because of the agent's knowledge of their wishes or values. If patients have left no written **advance directive**, we try to reconstruct their wishes from those who know them best. Only when none of these is possible do we drop to the lower **best interests** standard where we choose what we believe most people in that situation would choose.

This patient has named an agent and has also left very clear instructions about what she wants done. For her current condition, she has clearly indicated in the past that she wants full treatment if needed. The "if needed" is a clinical decision.

RECOMMENDATIONS

1. **Limitation of treatment** orders (e.g., **do-not-resuscitate order**, do-not-intubate order, do-not-transfer order) should not be written for this patient, since they would be inconsistent with her previously stated wishes, unless her professional caregivers have reason to believe that a specific intervention would clearly not work.
2. All reasonable clinical measures should be taken to ensure adequate nutrition and hydration. It would be ethically permissible to do a trial removal of her NG tube to see if that (perhaps in conjunction with her return to the nursing home) would stimulate her to eat and drink. However, if objective measures demonstrate inadequate intake, whatever means are needed (long-term NG, surgical gastric tube) to give her adequate intake are ethically obligatory.

FOLLOW-UP

The patient's nephew, hospital physician, nursing home physician, nurse, social worker, and ethicist agreed in a conference call to complete a several-day trial without the tube in place, to see if she would eat. If her intake was inadequate, a surgical gastric tube would be inserted.

Her intake was deemed inadequate and she had surgery to place the gastric tube. She was then transferred back to the nursing home. She gradually increased her oral feedings and the gastric tube was no longer used, though left in place. Two months later she was discharged to the home of a close friend.

COMMENT

The hospital doctors and nurses were caring for a stranger, someone they didn't know, and they saw a frail woman with a diagnosis of **dementia**. They did not initially appreciate the quite acceptable quality of life she had experienced prior to admission. They had worked hard to pull her through a surgical crisis, but when she didn't bounce back as well as a younger person, they were ready to say, "We tried, but it looks like her chronic condition is too advanced." When those who knew her — her family and nursing-home caregivers — filled out the picture, they had a better appreciation of her situation and values and were then ready to pursue the goal of survival more vigorously.

Case 6.09

QUESTION

Is it ethically permissible to allow this elderly, disabled woman to refuse to eat or drink?

STORY

Nina is eighty-nine years old and is refusing to eat. She is a retired telephone operator who had a severely disabling stroke five years ago, leaving her unable to do anything for herself. Her husband, Willard, four years younger than she, chose to care for her at home rather than placing her in a nursing home. For the past five years he has pureed her food, crushed her pills, cared for her urinary catheter, cleaned up after her bowel incontinence, and used a mechanical lifting device to get her out of bed into a wheelchair once or twice each day so she could sit on their enclosed porch when it was sunny or watch her favorite TV quiz shows in the living room. He has had hired help for two hours most days, but for the other twenty-two hours a day he has provided her care, even sleeping on a couch in the dining room, which has been converted into her care room. She initially spoke a bit, but she has had multiple smaller strokes that have further impaired her motor abilities, now leaving her able only to stare and occasionally smile.

Six weeks ago Willard developed jaundice and was admitted to the hospital. Their three children, two from out of state, have taken turns trying to provide their mother with the same level of care while he was hospitalized. Unfortunately, he was found to have cancer of the pancreas that had spread throughout his liver. He died two days ago, and after Nina was informed, she stopped eating, clenching her teeth together and tightening her lips when she was encouraged to eat or drink.

Nina has been deeply religious, adhering to the Methodist tradition all her life. She was severely depressed during her menopause, but she told her family later that she decided against suicide because it was sinful. She completed a living will several years before her stroke and told Willard and her children that she never wanted to be on life support, or have a feeding tube, or be cared for in a nursing home.

Now, the day of their father's funeral, Nina's three children have been asked by her physician if he should insert a feeding tube. The children asked for an ethics consultation.

DISCUSSION

Most people consider feeding tubes to be medical treatment, and thus optional in some circumstances, to be used or not used depending on the patient's expressed wishes and values. A patient with **decision-making capacity** may refuse any treatment, even treatment that might postpone death. Decision-making capacity may sometimes be affected by medical, psychological, or social circumstances.

In this case, Nina has made previous statements indicating her understanding that a feeding tube is treatment, and she has expressed a personal aversion to having one. She is now in a situation where she could physically continue to eat if she desired, but because of her refusal to eat, a feeding tube is being considered. She has a strong religious belief that suicide is sinful, but it is not clear if she would consider refusal to eat in her current situation equal to suicide. Though she is terminally ill, and dying slowly of progressive neurological disease, she is not imminently dying and could conceivably live for several more months with adequate nutrition and hydration. Her acute grief is likely determinative in her decision to not eat.

RECOMMENDATIONS

1. It is ethically permissible to honor this patient's refusal of food and fluids.
2. However, she should be repeatedly encouraged to take fluids and nutrition. In addition, plans for ongoing care should be quickly made and presented to her in as positive a light as possible.

FOLLOW-UP

The patient continued to resist efforts to get her to eat or drink. She died five days after her husband died.

COMMENT

It is interesting to compare this case to Case 8.08, an eighty-five-year-old man who wanted to either actively take his life or refuse life-saving treatment soon after his wife died. In that case, treatment over his objection was felt to be justified. The difference between that and the current case is one of prognosis. With treatment he could likely survive for a prolonged period in a decent state of health. In the current case, the patient would continue to be severely disabled and would likely succumb to her progressive disease in a relatively short time.

Case 6.10

QUESTION

Is it obligatory to honor this dying patient's request for expensive total parenteral nutrition that may only marginally postpone his inevitable death?

STORY

Gene, age forty-two, is a disabled interior designer in the final stage of AIDS, which he contracted several years ago. His long-standing homosexual partner died of AIDS about two years ago.

Early in the course of his disease, Gene took medication, was reasonably healthy, continued to work part time, and cared for his partner until his death. In spite of continued medication, his disease has progressed. He now weighs only eighty-two pounds, less than half his healthy weight. He has had intermittent respiratory infections, but his primary problem currently is a gastrointestinal infection caused by the protozoan cryptosporidium, which gives him horrendous diarrhea and makes it impossible for him to take in more than a few swallows each day. He was readmitted to the hospital three days ago with dehydration, which has been corrected with intravenous fluids. A feeding tube would be of no benefit because pouring fluids and nutrition into his gastrointestinal tract would merely worsen his diarrhea. After some discussion with his long-standing physician, Dr. Sculley, Gene has requested **total parenteral nutrition** (TPN). He has asked that his parents and siblings not be notified of his critical condition. He has been estranged from them since they learned of his HIV diagnosis, confirming his gay lifestyle, which they had suspected.

Dr. Sculley has many patients with HIV, and he talks openly with them about their disease, treatment options, and likely outcomes. Gene recognizes that he is dying, and several months ago he requested "no resuscitation, no intubation, or ICU care." This seemed consistent with an acceptance that death was approaching, and his physician has clearly documented these requests. But paradoxically, Gene is now requesting TPN, which offers him very little potential for benefit.

DISCUSSION

An adequately informed patient with **decision-making capacity** is free to accept or decline any treatment recommended by his physician, even if his choice may shorten his life. This does not necessarily mean, however, that a physician is obligated to provide a requested treatment that will not work (i.e., is futile) or is outside the standard of care. When a patient makes such a request, it is important to try to find out the reason for the request and the patient's expectation.

In this case, TPN would likely have little benefit for this patient, though it would not be accurate to say that the treatment would be futile. It is not clear why the patient wants the treatment or what he expects it to do.

RECOMMENDATION

It is not obligatory to provide the requested TPN, but before declining, the physician should try to determine the patient's reason for this request, which seems at odds with his other decisions.

FOLLOW-UP

Dr. Sculley asked Gene why he wanted the TPN since he seemed otherwise resigned to his death and did not want other aggressive measures. He said he is practically penniless and does not want his family to have to pay his funeral expenses. He had qualified to receive government disability checks a few months ago, and if he could survive until he received one more check, he would have enough money saved to cover his cremation. He thought the TPN might make this possible. His physician began the TPN. He returned the next day and told Gene that he had found some AIDS funds that could be used for the last installment. (I suspect it may well have come from his own pocket.) Gene smiled and asked that the TPN be stopped. He died five days later.

COMMENT

This case illustrates that we must sometimes look beyond physiology in order to "do what is right." It also demonstrates why it is so important to find out why a patient makes a decision that seems to be outside expected boundaries.

Case 6.11

QUESTION

Is it ethically permissible to restrain and force-feed this patient with a serious eating disorder?

STORY

Louisa is a thirty-one-year-old schoolteacher with an eating disorder (anorexia/bulimia) of six years characterized by binge eating, induced vomiting (two to three times a week), laxative abuse, and vigorous exercise. She is five feet nine inches tall and currently weighs ninety-eight pounds. She has been increasingly fatigued and "unable to eat" and vomiting involuntarily for several weeks. She acknowledges that she has an eating disorder, but believes it would be good if she could lose another ten pounds. She has been seeing a new therapist for about two months, and was admitted for intravenous (IV) therapy four days ago when a medical evaluation showed a low potassium level in her blood, putting her at slight risk of a life-threatening cardiac **arrhythmia**. This electrolyte problem has now been corrected, but she is refusing to eat in spite of stating that she wants to get better. Her care team is asking about the permissibility of force-feeding her.

She has a history of over twenty years of substance abuse (many kinds) but states that she quit this pattern six months ago and has subsequently been in several rehabilitation programs. She also has a long history of depression, worse since her sister (and "best friend") died of suicide two years ago after a long struggle with mental illness (bipolar disorder). In addition, she reports recent bursts of energy, irritability, and insomnia. She made one suicide attempt (cut wrists) several years ago and now refers to it as a stupid and impulsive act. She currently denies a suicidal wish.

Louisa was raised in a family with four siblings and an abusive father. She is married and has a seven-year-old son. She reports that her husband has recently become more supportive of her.

The patient is alert and conversant. She states that she wants to eat and wants to get better, but she also wants to get out of the hospital now. When asked if tube feedings had been considered by the doctors or by her, she reported that she signed out of the last hospital when she was threatened with a tube. She says she does not want one because she is fearful that her repeated self-induced vomiting may have injured her throat, which might be further damaged by a tube. She says she has never seen a nasogastric tube, and would be willing to look at one and consider its use if it was felt to be the only way to correct her nutritional problems.

Anorexia/bulimia is a complex condition with physical and behavioral components, both of which require interventions. In addition, the malnutrition itself may adversely affect neurologic function and **decision-making capacity**. It is a chronic condition with a small but not insignificant mortality rate (5 percent of hospitalized patients), most often from severe electrolyte imbalance, or suicide. Criteria for hospitalization or nutritional support include failure to respond to outpatient treatment, life-threatening complications, and serious psychiatric comorbidity. The prognosis for recovery or survival is less good for individuals with severe psychiatric disturbance and for those whose onset occurs after adolescence.

DISCUSSION

Overriding a competent patient's refusal of a treatment felt to be in the patient's **best interests** is called "paternalism." Although fairly common in the past, such behavior is currently felt to be almost always inappropriate and unethical.

Paternalism may be justified in some unusual situations, however. While ethicists differ on the exact criteria for "justified paternalism," generally (a) there must be some defect in reasoning, either incompetence or irrationality; (b) there must be grave consequences (death or disability) of nonintervention; (c) the consequences of nonintervention must be greater than the consequences of intervention (loss of freedom, etc.); and (d) one must be willing to apply the chosen criteria universally.

In this case, (a) the patient appears to be competent, but she may be making an irrational choice (i.e., inconsistent with her stated goals of survival and recovery), and (b) it is not clear that forgoing tube feedings at this time will result in imminent grave consequences. In addition, (c) the consequences of intervention (loss of freedom, restraints, etc.) are probably of greater weight than the consequences of nonintervention (delaying her recovery). And finally, (d) I would be unwilling to recommend force-feeding for all anorexic patients at this stage of their disease.

RECOMMENDATIONS

1. Force-feeding this patient is not ethically permissible at this time. If she becomes a serious threat to herself and is felt to be a candidate for involuntary hospitalization, it could be reconsidered at that time.
2. She may be willing to receive information about, and even consider using, tube feedings at a later date if it is felt to be the only way to preserve her health or life.

FOLLOW-UP

Force-feeding by tube was not used during this hospitalization. Longer-term follow-up is not available.

COMMENT

Management of anorexia/bulimia can be very frustrating, especially to professionals less experienced in the treatment of this disorder. It is difficult to accept as unethical the provision of needed nutritional supplementation to a patient who refuses it, especially when this could be done with a fairly simple feeding tube. It is thus tempting to try to impose such therapy on patients with anorexia over their objection when they begin to show physical signs of danger. And indeed, this may be ethically justified if a patient is in danger of death or permanent disability.

But force-feeding is a stopgap measure that probably does little or nothing to correct the chronic disease. In addition, forcing this therapy on an unwilling patient is a serious ethical breach of professional obligation that may undermine the therapeutic patient-professional relationship. Thus it should be reserved for life-threatening situations.

*   *   *

Other Cases Involving Artificially Administered Fluids and Nutrition

Cases 7.01, 7.06, 7.08, 8.04, 8.07, 10.09, 12.04

References on Artificially Administered Fluids and Nutrition

Casarett, D., J. Kapo, and A. Caplan. "Appropriate Use of Artificial Nutrition and Hydration — Fundamental Principles and Recommendations." *New England Journal of Medicine* 353, no. 24 (December 15, 2005): 2607-12.

John Paul II. *On Life-Sustaining Treatments and the Vegetative State: Scientific Advances and Ethical Dilemmas.* Vatican City, 2004.

Lynn, J. *By No Extraordinary Means: The Choice to Forgo Life-Sustaining Food and Water.* Bloomington: Indiana University Press, 1986.

Orr, R. D., and G. Meilaender. "Ethics and Life's Ending: An Exchange." *First Things* 145 (August/September 2004): 31-35.

Sacred Congregation for the Doctrine of the Faith. *Declaration of Euthanasia.* Vatican City, 1980.

CHAPTER 7

Ethical Issues in Brain Failure

Families and professionals may struggle with treatment decisions when the heart or lungs fail, or when the kidneys or liver fails. They often want to know our best guess of whether that organ will recover function, or what can be done to substitute machines for permanently failed function. But when the brain fails, this often trumps consideration of all other organ systems. Many tough treatment decisions (and thus many ethics consultations) revolve around the issue of brain function, including how it functioned in the past, how it functions now, and how we think it might function in the future.

From a functional standpoint, it is important to recall that sentient functions (thinking, remembering, experiencing one's environment, etc.) take place in the "upper brain," the cerebral cortex. Physiologic functions that do not involve sentience (control of cardiovascular and respiratory functions, sleep/arousal, etc.) take place in the "lower brain," also called the brain stem.

Since most patients and families place such a high priority on brain function, in cases of serious dysfunction it is important to determine whether the brain can recover. Thus, whether the brain failure is reversible or irreversible is critically important.

Reversible Forms of Brain Failure

Coma is a state of total lack of upper brain function that may get better. The person looks asleep and is unconscious, unresponsive to stimulation, and also unaware. Coma may continue for a short or long (or very long) time. People in a coma usually have intact lower brain function so they breathe on their own, can maintain their blood pressure, etc.

Delirium is a state of partial impairment of upper brain function that is expected to get better. It may be caused by trauma, drugs, infection, or metabolic problem (imbalance of salt, water, sugar; temporary lack of oxygen), and is usually expected to improve when that problem is corrected. It is manifested by confusion, disorientation, and agitation. Delirium caused by trauma has a much more unpredictable course of improvement. **Encephalopathy** is another term often used to denote upper brain dysfunction that may or may not be reversible. The term may be preceded by a descriptor such as "hepatic" (caused by liver dysfunction) or "hypoxic" (caused by lack of oxygen).

The *vegetative state* is a condition of being awake but unaware (more below). It is almost always permanent but can improve in rare instances, so we must not totally discount that possibility.

Irreversible Forms of Brain Failure

Dementia is a generic term for permanent loss of some functions of the upper brain. It is most commonly caused by Alzheimer's disease but may also result from one or multiple strokes, traumatic brain injury, brain damage from lack of oxygen (e.g., recovery from near drowning, resuscitation). It may happen all at once (trauma, lack of oxygen), or it may develop gradually (Alzheimer's).

The vegetative state is almost always permanent, and is often called the **persistent vegetative state**, or even the permanent vegetative state (both are abbreviated PVS). The primary question is always, "how certain are we of its permanence?" In the PVS, the patient may look awake (eyes open) but is not aware of his or her surroundings. Some call it "eyes-open coma." The person usually breathes spontaneously without assistance, but is unable to do anything volitional and is incontinent of bowel and bladder.

The *locked-in syndrome* is a unique type of permanent brain dysfunction wherein the neural pathway that connects the upper brain and the lower brain does not work, usually because of a stroke. The thinking part of the brain is undamaged but disconnected. Thus the person is totally aware but totally paralyzed except for the ability to move his or her eyes upward (due to the location in the brain of the motor portion of this function). Communication by eye blinks is possible but difficult, especially so because the patient has lost all facial muscle tone, so the face is absolutely expressionless.[1]

The ultimate form of permanent brain failure is *death by neurologic criteria,* often called *brain death.* In this condition the entire brain, both the upper brain where we think and the lower brain that controls autonomic functions, shows total loss of function. When this condition is reached, total physiologic support can prevent further deterioration of the individual; the heart beats, the kidneys can make urine, the gastrointestinal tract can digest food, etc. Society has decided that this is equivalent to death so that organs can be retrieved for transplantation. The main ethics issue in brain death is what to do when the family or a **surrogate** fails to accept that this body is dead (it is, after all, warm, has good color, makes urine, has a blood pressure and pulse; it just looks comatose and is on **ventilator** support) and objects to the removal of organ support (not "life support" since the patient is dead).

Ethical Issues

In caring for patients with brain failure of any of the above types, or in doing ethics consultations, several important features recur.

Surrogacy

The patient cannot participate in treatment decisions. So, who is the appropriate proxy for a particular patient (see Case 7.08)? Is it someone who has been designated by the patient (an **agent** named in a durable power of attorney for health care)? Is it the next of kin? Does the state where the

---

1. A fascinating but sad and scary article appeared in the *Los Angeles Times Sunday Magazine* several years ago written by Julia Tavalaro, who had been locked in for twenty-eight years. But for the first many years, everyone thought she was in a PVS, and she was not treated nicely by some of the nursing home staff. When a therapist recognized her awareness, they developed a means of communication, and she subsequently published poetry and prose. She recounts her story in *Look Up for Yes* (New York: Penguin Books, 1997). Other moving accounts written by persons who are locked in are *The Diving Bell and the Butterfly,* by Jean-Dominique Bauby (New York: Vintage Books, 1997), and *How Will They Know When I Am Dead?* by Robert C. Horn III (Delray Beach, Fla.: GR Press/St. Lucie Press, 1997).

question arises have a surrogate law so that there is an automatic hierarchy, or is there no law so that we go by medical tradition?

Decision-Making Standards

How does the proxy make decisions? Do we have written instructions from the patient? Do those who know the patient best know what he or she has said, or do they know the patient's values (see Case 7.03)? How accurate are such **substituted judgments**? Do they really reflect the wishes of the patient? Does the proxy have a conflict of interest (see Case 7.09)? Is the demented person the same individual who wrote the **advance directive** several years earlier while healthy, or should we consider her or him to be a different person with potentially different values? If we don't have any idea about the patient's wishes or values, what is in the patient's **best interests**?

Prognosis

What is the likelihood that this brain dysfunction will improve? If it might, how fast and how much? How sure are we (see Case 7.11)?

Quality of Life

What is the likely maximal level of function? Will that be acceptable to the patient (see Case 7.02)? If we don't know the patient's values, would most people find this level of function to be acceptable?

Limitation of Treatment

If it is clear that the patient will never improve, or if we understand that he or she would find the likely level of maximal improvement to be unacceptable, which treatments must we continue and which ones are optional? If the patient is unable to take in sufficient fluids and nutrition to stay alive, must we use artificially administered fluids and nutrition, or is this optional (see Case 6.09)?

Place of Treatment

Does the patient require the services of an institution, or is the family able to care for the patient at home? Can the community supply services to make home care possible (see Case 7.04)? Will home care exhaust the family physically, emotionally, financially?

Research

Can we ethically do research on someone with no cognition or cognition that is impaired? Can we do research if it might help the patient? What about basic science research that might improve scientific understanding of the condition but will not help the patient? Who can give consent for research?

Let's look more closely at some of the more common causes of brain failure.

Cerebrovascular Accidents (CVAs, "Strokes")

One of the most common causes of brain failure is a stroke. A stroke is a sudden loss of partial brain function due to disruption of the circulation to a part of the brain; either a blood clot obstructs an artery or a blood vessel breaks, causing a hemorrhage. The symptoms come on over a period of minutes or hours. The only treatments that are effective in reversing the course of a stroke from a blood clot are "clot busters" given in the first three hours after the onset of symptoms. These, of course, cannot be given to patients with a hemorrhagic stroke (because clotting stops the bleeding that caused this type of stroke), but only to those with a stroke caused by a blood clot inside the artery. Sometimes the prognosis for a hemorrhagic stroke can be improved by surgically draining the area of hemorrhage.

The form and severity of brain dysfunction from a stroke depend on the location and size of the vascular accident. If recovery is going to occur, this usually begins in the first several days after the stroke but may not be complete for many weeks. Recovery or retraining is aided by physical, occupational, and speech therapy.

Strokes often lead to ethics consultations because of the difficulty of prognosis, uncertainty about the patient's wishes or values, and questions about therapy. The most common question, in my experience, is about the use or nonuse of a feeding tube, but may also involve questions about **cardiopulmonary resuscitation** (CPR) and use of a ventilator, dialysis, antibiotics, or other treatments (see Case 7.03). When such questions arise, it is sometimes helpful to focus not on the treatment modality but on goals: Which goals are possible (a medical decision)? Which goals would the patient want to aim for (proxy decision)?

Dementia

Another common form of brain dysfunction or failure occurs because of dementia. Of the many causes of dementia, Alzheimer's disease is the most common. It is a slow loss of cerebral function of unknown cause. It usually begins with forgetfulness and progresses to wandering, loss of social skills and motor function including incontinence, inability to feed oneself, inability to speak, inability to recognize others, and inability to swallow. The end stage can be a state of unawareness very close to the PVS. The course of Alzheimer's dementia is several years, typically eight to eleven. Loss of bowel and bladder continence is the most common reason for admission to a nursing home. The most common cause of death is infection, usually pulmonary or urinary.

Ethics consultations are often requested for patients with dementia, usually because the patient is somewhere along the slide toward unawareness and suddenly has an acute problem, most commonly an infection or a hip fracture. Questions arise about how aggressive to be in treatment: intensive care unit (ICU), ventilator, dialysis, CPR (see Case 7.02)? Sometimes the patient is still strong but unsteady or unreliable, and questions arise about the use of physical or chemical restraints; the latter term is used for sedatives given to restrict a patient's movement (see Case 7.01). At other times it is because the patient with Alzheimer's is nearing the end stage, and questions are raised about use of a feeding tube or about allowing the patient to continue to eat when he or she has a high risk of **aspiration** (see Case 6.02).

The Persistent Vegetative State (PVS)

Next to death by neurologic criteria (brain death), the most severe form of brain failure is the persistent vegetative state, in which upper brain activity (cerebral, or cortical, function) ceases totally but the brain stem continues to function. The patient is generally able to breathe and exhibits sleep-wake cycles. He or she will appear to be in a coma for a few hours and then the eyes will open for a time, but the eyes do not fix on anything or follow movement.

The persistent vegetative state may result from congenital malformations (e.g., **anencephaly**, holoprosencephaly);[2] from a degenerative process in a formerly normal brain (e.g., Alzheimer's dementia); from traumatic brain injury; or from nontraumatic brain injury (e.g., lack of oxygen during a cardiac arrest or a near-drowning episode). It is important to keep the cause of the PVS in mind because of its bearing on prognosis. The most important distinction here is that it takes much longer to have a clear idea of the permanence of the vegetative state following traumatic brain injury (many months) than it does for nontraumatic brain injury (days or weeks). In other words, there is a greater possibility of late improvement after a traumatic brain injury than there is after hypoxic brain injury sustained during a cardiac arrest.

The PVS was first described in 1972. The definitive description is a two-part Multi-Society Task Force report on the PVS published in 1994.[3] "Vegetative state"[4] is a descriptive diagnosis that merely says the patient has brain stem function but no cerebral function at the moment. The phrase "persistent vegetative state" means the patient has been in that condition for a period of time, so it is talking about past and present. This term was coined for the vegetative state that has persisted for at least thirty days. The idea was that if it persists long enough, we can assume it is permanent. Thus some say that PVS means *permanent vegetative state,* referring to past, present, and future; i.e., it is not only descriptive but also predictive. Everyone recognizes that these time limits are arbitrary, and that the potential for some improvement varies with the cause of the dysfunction and with the age of the patient (infants and children have more po-

---

2. Holoprosencephaly is the name given to a spectrum of developmental anomalies of the brain and face that result in moderate to severe mental retardation.

3. Multi-Society Task Force on the Persistent Vegetative State, "Medical Aspects of the Persistent Vegetative State: First of Two Parts," *New England Journal of Medicine* 330 (1994): 1499-1508, and "Medical Aspects of the Persistent Vegetative State: Second of Two Parts," *New England Journal of Medicine* 330 (1994): 1572-79.

4. Some people strongly object to the word "vegetative," believing it is equivalent to calling a person a vegetable. The derivation of the word is from Aristotle, who described three forms of life: rational — capacity for choice of one's principles; animal — capacity for representation and action; and vegetative — capacity for nutrition and reproduction.

tential for late improvement than adults). As a result, some **neurologists** prefer to require ninety days for nontraumatic causes and twelve months for traumatic causes before considering the condition to be permanent.

Understanding these distinctions is important because the acronym PVS is sometimes used incorrectly. Not infrequently I get a consultation request from a young physician in the ICU who says, "This patient had a cardiac arrest three days ago and is now in a PVS." This is incorrect. The patient may be vegetative but cannot by definition be in a persistent (or permanent) vegetative state. The BIG question in this and many cases is, "How sure are we that the patient will never regain cognition?" In truth, the thirty-day time limit set by the formal definition is completely arbitrary, as would be extended time limits of three, six, or twelve months. The authors of the Multi-Society Task Force report reviewed the literature thoroughly and concluded that very rarely patients in a clearly and carefully diagnosed PVS may have some delayed improvement, though usually the improvement is minimal (resulting in a **minimally conscious state** [MCS]). A rehabilitation specialist from England has published two studies suggesting it may not be as rare as we all think.[5] This would suggest that decisions to limit therapy in PVS patients may be a self-fulfilling prophecy. However, we do know that the vast majority of patients in the PVS — in fact, almost all of them — can remain that way for many years if they continue to receive good nursing care, fluids, and nutrition. The longest recorded survival was over thirty years.

It is not uncommon for a patient to be in a coma after some severe brain insult, then after a few days or weeks to open his or her eyes. The clinicians may be distressed to see that the patient has no apparent awareness — and is vegetative, their worst fear. On the other hand, family members see the eyes open and are greatly encouraged that the patient is getting better. The clinicians want to consider limiting treatment and the family wants to get more aggressive with rehabilitation therapy (see Case 7.07).

Ethics consultations for patients in the PVS usually involve these questions: Early on, how certain are we of the diagnosis (have we waited long enough?), or, later on, which treatments are obligatory and which are optional?

---

5. K. Andrews, "Recovery of Patients after Four Months or More in a Persistent Vegetative State," *British Medical Journal* 306 (1993): 1597-1600; K. Andrews, L. Murphy, R. Munday, and C. Littlewood, "Misdiagnosis of the Vegetative State: Retrospective Study in a Rehabilitation Unit," *British Medical Journal* 313 (1996): 13-16.

The Minimally Conscious State (MCS)

The MCS is a condition of neurologic function just a little above the PVS. The patient in an MCS has some cognition, that is, some awareness of environment. Some patients merely respond to painful (or pleasurable) stimuli, so we know they are sensate. Others are able to indicate yes or no or say a few words. There is no clear demarcation between MCS patients and patients with more function who are merely said to be neurologically impaired. The MCS is usually the end result of some type of brain injury, either trauma or metabolic. The patient often starts in a coma and gradually emerges into the MCS by showing withdrawal from physical stimulation, or possibly showing awareness when spoken to. Occasionally a patient moves from coma to PVS and then on to MCS; that is, the vegetative state may have been persistent, but clearly was not permanent.

When it is clear that the patient is in an MCS rather than a PVS, the questions may take on a different flavor. In the PVS the patient is not aware, so delaying definitive decisions about treatment will not cause the patient any suffering. The result may be difficult for families, and may involve great cost. These burdens may be considerable, but they do not directly affect patient suffering (see Case 7.08). But in the MCS, the patient has some awareness, so he or she may suffer from continued treatment or, on the other hand, may experience pleasure from continued life.

One of the basic questions that often arises in doing ethics consultations on patients in a PVS or MCS involves the concept of personhood. These patients are clearly still alive (as opposed to those who meet the neurologic criteria for death). Some would say, however, that they have lost their personhood and so are as good as dead, or even worse than dead because of the ongoing potential for suffering for them (MCS) or their family (PVS). Some philosophers have suggested changing the definition of death (again) to accept the idea of "neocortical death" (as opposed to whole brain death); that is, if the upper brain has permanently lost function, the person should be considered dead. This would include individuals in a PVS, neonates with anencephaly, and elderly folks with end-stage dementia. This utilitarian argument has some appeal since it could result in more organs for transplantation and major financial savings from not providing ongoing support. However, it is unseemly to call someone "dead" who is breathing spontaneously.

Life is biological. Personhood is psychological, social, and spiritual.

The philosophical debate will likely continue, but in the meantime clinicians, ethics consultants, clergy, and family consider these individuals to be alive — though severely impaired, perhaps to the extent that there is no moral obligation to prevent their deaths if we have a clear understanding of their values.

Let's now look at some ethical dilemmas encountered in patients with brain failure.

Case 7.01

QUESTION

Is it ethically permissible to restrain this patient with dementia to keep his nasogastric drainage tube in place over his objection?

STORY

Tom is an eighty-eight-year-old retired farmer who has had mild-moderate **dementia** for some time. His wife died many years ago and he had been living with his daughter, Maureen, until he fell and broke his left hip six weeks ago. He underwent surgical repair in spite of multiple medical problems (including oxygen-dependent chronic lung disease, **anticoagulation** for cardiac **arrhythmia, congestive heart failure**). The admission note says he did not have decisional capacity, and consent for surgery was obtained from his daughter. He had a somewhat rocky postoperative course, including an ileus (lack of motility of his intestines causing painful abdominal distension from gas) treated with decompression tubes through his nose and through his rectum. He slowly improved.

While awaiting a nursing home bed for long-term care, he fell and broke his other hip, which was repaired ten days ago. He has now developed **sepsis** and another bout of ileus. He refused a nasogastric (NG) drainage tube, though he gave consent for a rectal decompression tube two days ago. At a management conference with family that day, his poor overall prognosis was discussed, but Maureen was certain that he wants to live if possible, based on an earlier conversation in which he told her he wanted full treatment. After the conference she was apparently able to convince him to consent to the NG tube. However, since then he has repeatedly said he wants it out, has pulled it out, and has said he didn't care if he died as a result. His nursing caregivers are increasingly uncomfortable about restraining him in order to leave his NG tube in place over his protests and have requested an ethics consultation.

The patient appears alert, is tugging at his restraints, and is asking for a drink of water. He is unable to engage in meaningful conversation about his condition, his wishes (other than that he clearly wants the tube out), or his future. His chart indicates that he is **full code status**. There is no **advance directive** in the chart.

Dr. MacIntosh believes the patient can recover from his current ileus, though his long-term prognosis is not good because of his many medical problems. In addition, she feels his cognitive state between crises is good and he appears to enjoy life at that time. She shares the nurses' concerns about the restraints, and her goal is to remove the NG tube as quickly as possible, hopefully in two or three days.

DISCUSSION

Involuntary treatment over the objection of a patient is rarely justified. It may be justified, using **surrogate** consent, in situations where the person appears to have some deficit of understanding or deciding, serious harm is likely without the intervention, and the probable benefit from intervention outweighs the harm of nonintervention.

In this case, the patient has been diagnosed with dementia and was judged to not have the capacity to consent at the time of admission. His ileus is unlikely to be corrected without the NG tube, leading to a worsening of his condition, significant discomfort, and possible death. There is a good chance of reversal of the ileus with use of the tube, though his longer-term prognosis remains poor.

It would not be ethically justified to use burdensome treatment over this patient's objection if it had very little chance of improving his situation. However, since the tube appears to be resolving the acute situation, and since the patient is reported to have stated a goal of survival in the recent past, it is ethically justified to leave the tube in place over his objection (and in spite of his current statement that he doesn't care if he dies) if there is no other way to adequately treat his condition.

RECOMMENDATIONS

1. It is ethically justified to temporarily restrain this patient in order to accomplish his recently stated goal of survival. Supplemental measures should be sought to minimize his discomfort and distress.
2. Effort should be made to remove the NG tube and the restraints as soon as is clinically prudent.
3. If his condition should deteriorate such that survival is unlikely, it would then be ethically problematic to continue the unwanted treatment.

FOLLOW-UP

After the consultation, Tom's nurses were less uncomfortable with keeping him in restraints to allow the NG tube to continue draining his upper gastrointestinal tract, even though he continued to ask that it be removed. His bowels began to function on the following day. Two days after the consultation, the tube was removed and he was allowed to drink and subsequently to eat. One week later he was transferred to a nursing home for continued convalescence.

COMMENT

It may seem intuitive that health-care professionals should treat a patient with effective treatment in order to save the patient's life, even when he or she objects. This seems especially appropriate when the patient is cognitively compromised. And thirty years ago it would have been done without a second thought. However, the evolution of thought over the past generation has changed the knee-jerk response.

Physicians in the past were overly paternalistic, doing what they thought best for the patient, even over the patient's objection. This has been modified in recent years by the prominence given to patient autonomy. In some respects this shift in locus of decision making from physician to patient is ethically appropriate and makes perfectly good sense. However, in other situations the (new) knee-jerk response of not treating anyone over his or her objection seems strange. The request for ethics consultation from Tom's nurses reflects this shift. They really wanted to treat him but were uncomfortable forcing treatment on an unwilling patient. Thus, ethical reflection and analysis were very appropriate.

Case 7.02 ————————————————————————————————————

QUESTION

Is it ethically permissible to not use lifesaving surgery for this man with dementia?

STORY

Will is a seventy-six-year-old man with Alzheimer's disease and hypertension who developed rapidly progressive paralysis of his right side after shoveling light snow three days ago. An early head **CT scan** showed a large (one and one-half inch) **intracranial hemorrhage** in the left side of his brain with extension into the ventricle (fluid-filled cavity in the center of the brain). He initially remained awake, though confused and combative, but has now been sleeping for more than thirty hours after his last dose of mild sedation. Although his repeat CT scan yesterday showed no change in the size of the hemorrhage, Dr. Moses, his **neurologist**, believes this somnolence may indicate increased **intracranial pressure**. Will was unable to participate in a test of his swallowing capacity yesterday and is receiving intravenous (IV) fluids. **Limitation of treatment** orders were signed the day after admission for no resuscitation, no **intubation**, and no surgical drainage procedures. His family requested ethics consultation because they wanted to talk about options for his current and future management. They are particularly concerned about their decision against a surgical drainage procedure.

I met with his wife, Ida, and their only son. They have supplied a living will signed by the patient years ago, and a durable power of attorney for health care document signed fourteen months ago in which he named his wife as his **agent** and checked the option on the standard form requesting no life-prolonging treatment, including feeding tube, if he is unable to think and act for himself.

The patient had been a marine as a young man and enjoyed his career as a financial planner. He sold his business ten years ago and has enjoyed his retirement (woodworking, tennis, daily Mass). He was diagnosed with **dementia** two years ago but experienced early symptoms for about four years prior to that. He has continued to deny having any problems, but he has slowly become more easily confused, agitated, and insecure, though he continued to accompany family on outings. His self-care has deteriorated from his earlier fastidious self. He and his family are devout Roman Catholics.

His father died at age sixty-eight, several days after a stroke. When his father-in-law, in his late nineties, suffered deterioration last year, he encouraged his wife to agree to "no heroics," preferring that he be allowed to die with dignity and without machines.

DISCUSSION

When treatment decisions must be made for a person who is no longer able to participate, we attempt to make a **substituted judgment**, that is, the decision the patient would make if able, based on a written **advance directive**, previously spoken wishes, or values expressed through previous treatment decisions for self or others.

In this case the patient was already on a slowly deteriorating pathway of dementia. He has left written instructions indicating he would not want aggressive measures if it is unlikely he will be able to recover sufficiently to think and act for himself. Though prognosis is always somewhat uncertain just a few days after a stroke, the fact that he has continued to deteriorate rather than to improve suggests to his physicians and his family that he meets those criteria. His caring family members are in agreement that they want to honor him by honoring his wishes.

RECOMMENDATIONS

1. If it seems quite unlikely to his physicians that this patient would be able to recover sufficiently to think and act for himself even if maximal therapy were used, it is ethically permissible to shift treatment goals to comfort care and not perform intracranial drainage or other procedures designed to postpone his death.
2. If he fails a swallow test or is unable to complete the test, it would also be ethically permissible to discontinue IV fluids, to offer fluids or nutrition by mouth, and to give good mouth care.
3. If he has no significant improvement in the next twenty-four to forty-eight hours, it might be appropriate to have a **palliative care** consultation to assist the family with posthospital plans.

FOLLOW-UP

The patient's wife and son were in agreement, earnestly seeking to "do the right thing" on the basis of their understanding of the patient's wishes and the tenets of their Catholic faith. I prayed with them for wisdom and peace.

The patient remained unresponsive for the next two days and did not appear uncomfortable. Comfort measures were chosen over lifesaving interventions. A palliative care consultation was obtained. The family kept a bedside vigil. Will died quietly four days after the consultation.

Several weeks later his wife expressed gratitude for both the consultation and my willingness to pray with them.

COMMENT

It might have been possible to save Will's life. If measurement of his intracranial pressure had confirmed the suspicion that it was elevated, decompressive surgery could have been done to reduce the pressure. His family based their decision to not intervene on two things: (1) the site and size of the hemorrhage made it quite clear that he would be left with significant residual dysfunction; and (2) his progressive dementia had already decreased his activity and enjoyment of life and had caused him significant distress; this was likely to worsen before he moved on to the "contented demented" picture of late Alzheimer's disease. Had either not been the case, I suspect Will's family would have opted for life preservation.

I often seek God's guidance in situations that are not clear. When talking with families in distress, I am often tempted to ask to pray with them, but in a secular setting this must be done cautiously by nonclergy. I almost always inquire from family members about the patient's faith tradition and practices, and sometimes about their own. When it seems appropriate, as in this case, I am comfortable asking if they would like me to pray with them.

Case 7.03

QUESTION

Is it ethically permissible to honor the family's request to withdraw support from this patient who suffered a recent stroke when her surgeon recommends continuing treatment?

STORY

Eleanor is a sixty-three-year-old woman who collapsed while teaching pre-schoolers in Sunday school three days ago and has been found to have a large left **intracerebral hemorrhage** with extension both into the subarachnoid space (fluid-filled space between the brain and the skull) and the ventricle in the center of her brain. She had emergent surgical evacuation of the blood clot, and her level of recovery is minimal, as expected, but she is still slowly improving. She is on minimal **ventilator** assistance to help her breathe, and she is making some purposeful movement. In spite of this, she is felt to have a very poor prognosis. Dr. Plumbly believes her best possible outcome would be survival with right-sided paralysis and difficulty with both speech and comprehension. On examination, she is **intubated**, having what appears to be seizure activity, and she withdraws from any physical contact.

The patient has no written **advance directive**. After a family conference yesterday (husband, two daughters, sister), a **do-not-resuscitate order** was written. On the basis of her previously expressed wishes, her family also requests withdrawal of her current support, a request her surgeon feels is premature. He would prefer to **wean** her from the ventilator, and he would be less uncomfortable accepting a decision to not reuse it if she should deteriorate again. He is somewhat concerned that the family may be making this choice because the patient has no health insurance.

The patient has been disabled for ten or twelve years from arthritis, and for the past few years has been able to walk only short distances with a cane, using a wheelchair most of the time. She has been in a lot of pain, including significant headaches, but she has avoided physicians for twenty years. Her family reports that she has said for twenty years that she did not want aggressive treatment, and she specifically did not want to be on life support, even short term. They believe the basis for this request is (a) a strong religious (Pentecostal) belief that God is in charge and will decide whether she lives or dies, and (b) a significant aversion to being touched by anyone. She has been cared for at home by her husband, but insists on maintaining as much independence as possible because she does not want to be a burden. Some in the family believe she would have refused the surgery that has already been done, and all agree she would not want her current level of support nor to be dependent on others even if her stroke had a less pessimistic prognosis. They also believe she would find rehabilitation therapy to be intolerable because of the necessity for physical touch.

There is one other daughter who is flying in from out of state. Family members present have had little contact with her, but believe she might opt for continued treatment.

DISCUSSION

When a patient is seriously ill, it is important to discuss goals of therapy and the appropriateness of each modality with the patient or a **surrogate**. While most often the agreed-upon goal is survival and recovery, some patients choose to limit therapy to avoid certain modalities or certain outcomes. While family or professional caregivers may not always agree with the patient's values, goals, or specific requests, it is important to recognize that the patient's choices should most often be honored. In the absence of a written advance directive, the patient's choices can usually be learned by talking with family or those who know the patient best.

When a patient so chooses, it is ethically permissible to change goals from survival to comfort care. When that decision is made, each treatment modality should be reviewed to see if its goal is comfort or survival. There is no ethical, legal, or professional difference between withholding and withdrawing a treatment, although it is often psychologically easier to withhold than it is to withdraw.

While financial considerations cannot be totally ignored, they should rarely be determinative in choosing treatment goals.

In this case, the patient has been handicapped for many years by pain and immobility, and she now has a poor prognosis for survival and a very poor prognosis for recovery from a major stroke. She has clearly stated that she would not want the current level of treatment and that she would find survival in a more dependent condition to be intolerable.

RECOMMENDATIONS

1. If her family are in agreement that she would want to change treatment goals to comfort care, it is ethically permissible to do so. This is true even if she is still improving and might survive, but with more disability. It would be more problematic if she had a reasonable chance of returning to her baseline condition, but that does not appear to be the case here.
2. It would be wise to await the arrival of her other daughter to see if true consensus exists or she has a different perspective.

3. If a decision is made to withdraw support with the expectation that the patient will die, she should be given adequate sedation and/or analgesia to ensure her comfort.

FOLLOW-UP

Her level of support was continued after the consultation. The other daughter, Rachel, arrived from out of state that evening. She said she did not adhere to the family's Pentecostal faith, that she had been virtually estranged from them for three years after she chose to live with a man over their objection. At the same time, paradoxically, she said she was the only one who truly knew her mother's values and wishes, and she was sure she would want to live regardless of her prognosis. She was very agitated, weeping, pacing, cursing. She kept asking, "Why in God's name did this have to happen to her?"

I acknowledged her frequent reference to God and asked if she would like me to pray with her. She jumped at the opportunity and clung tightly to my hand as I sought God's wisdom, guidance, and peace. After the brief prayer, a "peace that passes all understanding" came over her.

The following morning the entire family, including Rachel, met with the neurosurgeon. After a review of her condition, all were in agreement to withdraw support, even though the surgeon recommended continuing for a few more days. She was disconnected from the ventilator.

A short time later the family's pastor arrived, and held hands and prayed with all members of the family — all members except Rachel. She had climbed over the bedrails, and was hugging her mother and whispering in her ear. Eleanor died surrounded by this display of love.

COMMENT

It is not uncommon for "the family outlier from out of state" to arrive in the midst of crisis and offer an opinion at variance with the opinions of those who appear closer to the situation. It is possible to speculate about this: different life path leading to different values; guilt about noninvolvement; financial issues; estrangement; etc. It is important to discuss the different perspective, to try to learn if there is a legitimate cause for the different opinion. Most often, however, the hidden agenda remains hidden.

In this case the division seemed to involve some different faith-based values, perhaps including some guilt on Rachel's part about choices she had made. I was frankly a bit surprised by her eagerness to seek God's guidance, but then not so surprised when her antipathy and emotion changed suddenly after the brief encounter with God.

Case 7.04

QUESTION

Is it ethically permissible to allow this man to go home when he appears to be unaware of his poststroke disabilities?

STORY

Ernest ("Ernie") is a seventy-four-year-old man who was admitted three weeks ago with confusion and was found to have had a left temporal lobe **ischemic** stroke (i.e., from a blood clot obstructing an artery rather than from a hemorrhage) that has left him with difficulty speaking and a denial of illness typical of a stroke in this particular part of the brain. He has been **anticoagulated** during this admission. He is now medically stable and does all his self-care. Neuropsychological testing last week found significant language deficit plus diminished comprehension and awareness of his illness. Using sluggish speech, he maintains that he feels well, that there is nothing wrong with him, and that he is able to and wants to go home. In hospital, he has frequently refused medications and blood testing, making his anticoagulation control difficult. His professional caregivers are concerned that his deficits make it unsafe for him to live alone and care for himself, and have recommended that he go to a nursing home to allow greater supervision of his medical needs.

He has a past history of diabetes, coronary artery disease, prostate enlargement, and irregular heart rhythm. Dr. Burns, his primary physician for many years, reports that Ernie has previously always been conscientious about his medication and that his social situation is unique. He has lived at the same motel for nine years, supporting himself with a pension and part-time work doing dishes at a nearby restaurant. He has quite a network of social support — friends at the motel and restaurant have looked after him, have visited him in hospital, and are said to be willing to give even more supervision if he returns to the motel. His only relative is an elderly sister who also wants him to return to the motel. She is willing to assume responsibility for his financial affairs, but she is unwilling to petition for guardianship because she had a bad experience doing the same for another brother in the past.

Dr. Burns feels it would be unsafe for him to return "home" because of his significant change in attitude, specifically his lack of cooperation in the hospital with medication and lab tests. His concern is not so much about the patient's personal physical safety (falling, wandering, etc.), but more about his irregular taking of medication for multiple medical problems. The process for public guardianship has been initiated with the recognition that a long waiting list exists even if the court decides to appoint a guardian. However, he was evaluated yesterday by the psychiatric consultant for the Office of Public Guardian, who feels he does not qualify for guardianship because he has manageable risk and adequate social support.

DISCUSSION

A patient who retains **decision-making capacity** may accept or decline all treatment recommendations, that is, the patient is allowed to judge regarding risk and benefit. When a patient lacks such capacity, another must act as a **surrogate,** and should choose what he or she believes the patient would want (a **substituted judgment,** using the patient's values to balance risks and benefits) or, when that is not possible, make a decision that appears to be in the patient's **best interests,** which generally means using the values of most people who might be in this situation. When a patient is compromised neurologically or psychologically, it is often difficult to determine whether the patient has decision-making capacity. This determination is a clinical judgment without an objective gold standard.

If we were sure this patient had the capacity to make decisions, we would allow him to accept the increased risk of going home as long as he understood the potential consequences of failure to take his medication. If we were sure he lacked this capacity, we would probably go to court to impose a protective living situation over his objection. However, his decision-making capacity is borderline and is compromised by his denial of illness and change in attitude toward health care. Thus we should try to use what we understand to be his values in making a decision about letting him go home versus going to court to impose restricted living on him.

RECOMMENDATIONS

1. Further attempts should be made to see if individuals from his network of friends at the motel or restaurant are willing to supervise his medications and ensure his follow-up with Dr. Burns. If this can be arranged, it would be ethically permissible to discharge him with the understanding that failure of these arrangements, or failure of the patient to cooperate with the arrangements, might necessitate a petition for guardianship. If this plan is followed, a separate benefit/risk judgment should probably be made about the anticoagulation.
2. If the above suggested supervisory arrangements cannot be made with some confidence, then a decision must be reached by those who know him best (Dr. Burns, his friends at the motel and restaurant, his sister) about whether his values have been such that he would be willing to accept increased risk of medical complications in order to be able to return home.

FOLLOW-UP

The patient continued to refuse nursing home placement. About two weeks after the ethics consultation, he was discharged back to the motel on his preadmission medications, but without anticoagulation. His healthcare professionals recognized that not being anticoagulated placed him at somewhat increased risk of having a recurrent stroke, but protected him from potentially life-threatening complications from anticoagulation without adequate monitoring. This arrangement worked well for a few weeks, then began to deteriorate.

Three months later he was readmitted with a slow lower gastrointestinal hemorrhage and anemia. He was transfused and the bleeding stopped, and he felt well. Another ethics consultation was requested about the permissibility of restraining him because he wanted to leave the hospital **AMA** (against medical advice); he became violent with hospital staff on two occasions. A psychiatric consultation this time found that he clearly lacked decision-making capacity and that it was unsafe for him to live on his own at the motel. The patient was held in the hospital against his will, sometimes requiring the use of restraints and security personnel.

I wrote the following second report.

DISCUSSION

Restraining or treating patients over their objection is ethically troublesome and should not be done without adequate moral justification, for example, (a) if their choices are irrational (not compatible with their chosen goals) or (b) if they lack decision-making capacity and their choices are likely to harm them seriously. A determination of the presence or absence of decision-making capacity is a clinical judgment, and it includes the requirement that patients understand their own condition. In the past it was not uncommon to assert that patients had this capacity if they agreed with the doctor but lacked it if they disagreed; this paternalistic assessment is not an adequate measure of decision-making capacity.

It is paradoxical to accept as valid the consent of this patient without capacity before doing invasive procedures (endoscopy, transfusion) that entail known risk, but to decline to accept his refusal of continued hospitalization when discharge carries an unknown risk. Because his stroke includes a "denial of illness" deficit, by definition he is incapable of full decision making. In spite of this he had been functioning for several weeks in a supportive environment. Thus, his lack of capacity may not alone be adequate justification for restricting his freedom. Perhaps he perceives the hospital environment as threatening, exacerbating his agitation and rendering him less functional.

RECOMMENDATIONS

1. It is ethically justifiable to temporarily restrict this patient's freedom to protect him while trying to optimize his level of function. To protect his self-determination, every effort should be made to restore him to his baseline function and situation. It may not be possible to predict his ability to live again in his prior situation without a short-term trial.
2. If it becomes clear that he will not be able to safely function in that environment, or if it is tried and does not work, it would be ethically permissible to arrange assisted living or nursing home placement, even over his objection.
3. Since the outcome is so uncertain, it is appropriate to pursue guardianship while efforts at restoration are under way. His guardian could then participate in discussions about whether a trial of semi-independent living is worthwhile.

FOLLOW-UP

After spending five weeks in the hospital, Ernie's condition improved; he had no further bleeding and became more cooperative. No private or public guardian could be found (he qualified for the latter, but none was available due to short staffing). He was released back to the motel with Visiting Nurse Association supervision.

At the motel he gradually refused to allow the visiting nurses to assess or visit him. Ten months later he became mildly ill at home, refused readmission, suddenly deteriorated, and died.

COMMENT

Most health-care professionals like to see situations wrapped up in nice, neat little packages. But life is not always neat. Less than ideal alternatives sometimes need to be accepted or even sought.

Ernie had been living in a unique community for many years before his stroke. While some might assess this as less than ideal, it worked well for him and, in fact, evoked an altruistic concern in his neighbors, who might well have ignored his plight. The challenge arose when he needed more help. His unique community rose to the occasion, though providing far from what his health-care professionals thought was optimal.

Case 7.05

QUESTION

Please help with management plans for this patient who is refusing recommended workup, therapy, and nursing home placement.

STORY

Margine is a seventy-three-year-old woman with a history of breast cancer, which was known to have spread to her bones and thus be incurable when she received treatment five years ago. This resulted in a fracture of her left hip last year requiring short-term nursing home placement. She has been living at home. She began intermittent vomiting a few weeks ago, and an outpatient upper gastrointestinal series showed gastritis and a mass outside the stomach suspicious for malignancy. She refused **CT scanning** at that time, saying she was "too sick."

She was admitted to the hospital seven days ago with dehydration, and she requested a **do-not-resuscitate order** on admission. She has accepted intravenous fluids but has intermittently refused both further testing and medications. Her caregivers feel that she needs more treatment and that she clearly needs nursing home care. They predict she will have recurrent and worsening stomach symptoms. She twice refused to talk with the psychiatry consultant yesterday.

She is divorced, and has no children and no guardian. Her primary physician, oncologist, and social worker report that she has a long history of intermittent confusion, paranoia, and erratic and irrational behavior, including refusal of help from visiting nurses, failure to show up for scheduled physician appointments and lab tests, etc.

I spoke with the patient. She says she wants treatment and is willing to accept whatever is needed except nursing home care ("they nearly killed me last time"), and says she will be going home when she is strong enough. She says she will have help from visiting nurses as well as friends and neighbors, though she was unwilling to give names and seemed paranoid when asked.

DISCUSSION

Patients with **decision-making capacity** have the right to make their own treatment decisions, even decisions that will compromise their health or lead to avoidable death, as long as they understand the consequences and alternatives. This "rule" becomes problematic, however, if patients are inconsistent in their decisions or are making irrational decisions. An "irrational decision" is one that is not consistent with their own values (e.g., "I want to live, but I don't want you to amputate my septic gangrenous leg"). In such cases, it is occasionally ethically justifiable to override decisions with life-threatening consequences.

In this case the patient is frequently inconsistent in her decisions (refusal of labs, later consent) and occasionally irrational (says she wants to survive but refuses testing or treatment that would enhance that goal). Overriding a patient's right to refuse treatment is a serious ethical breach and should be considered only if the patient's decision would lead to imminent death or disability and there is no alternative acceptable to the patient.

RECOMMENDATIONS

1. It is ethically permissible to continue to try to persuade this patient that she needs more treatment and nursing home care. It might be helpful to have her meet with three or four professional caregivers (including someone from the Visiting Nurse Association) and those she expects to provide home care, to present a united front to her of the need for nursing home care. Care must be exercised that persuasion doesn't become coercive.

2. If there is even a small possibility of successful management at home, it would be ethically permissible to discharge her home with as many services in place as possible to allow her to prove herself. If it should not work, this would force the issue of a long-term-care placement.

3. If neither of these situations comes to pass, and she remains in the hospital, it may be necessary to seek a court-appointed guardian with authority to impose involuntary nursing home admission.

FOLLOW-UP

She was discharged home three days later with her ex-husband agreeing to help her. She had to be readmitted two days later with diarrhea. When this was under control, she agreed (very reluctantly) to temporary nursing home placement.

Case 7.06

QUESTION

Please assist with making plans and setting goals for this patient in a vegetative state.

STORY

Habib is a forty-eight-year-old, previously healthy Saudi man who suffered a cardiac arrest at home seven weeks ago. His teenage daughter began **cardiopulmonary resuscitation**, and paramedics continued; rhythm and perfusion were eventually restored in the emergency department. He may have had a seizure during or just after the resuscitation. He was admitted to the intensive care unit (ICU), and it soon became clear that he had suffered severe brain injury from lack of oxygen. Repeated neurology evaluation has determined that he is now in a **persistent vegetative state.** He has had a **tracheostomy** done and a permanent feeding tube surgically placed.

The patient has been dependent on a **ventilator** for most of the seven weeks, failing several attempts at **weaning,** but three days ago his oxygen saturation was maintained without ventilator support. Plans are under way to move him out of the ICU in a few days. He has repeatedly demonstrated metabolic instability (abnormal cardiac rhythms, fevers) felt to be precipitated by brain dysfunction rather than by intrinsic heart disease or infection. Both the need for ventilator support and this instability suggest to the **neurologist** that his brain damage is widespread, including his brain stem as well as his cerebral cortex. Ethics consultation was requested to assist with plans for management of anticipated complications. The patient and his family are Muslim.

The patient left no written **advance directive.** His wife has been his proxy and has applied for guardianship (the court hearing is in one month). She told the ICU staff early in his admission that he would not want to be maintained in this condition if there was no prospect of improvement. However, she has been continually optimistic in spite of hearing his very poor prognosis, and she has become increasingly antagonistic with the ICU staff. She has resisted any discussion of **limitation of treatment,** and she believes he is able to respond to her via eye blinks. She requested a second opinion from an outside neurologist. This neurologist agreed with the ICU team that the patient is nonresponsive to voice or noxious stimulation; demonstrates brain stem function only, without any cortical function; and has a prognosis for meaningful recovery that is nearly zero.

I met with the patient's wife and sister (who has traveled from Saudi Arabia to be here with her brother and sister-in-law), along with the ICU physician, nurse, and social worker. The patient's wife and sister are insistent that full treatment continue. They prefer that he remain in the ICU, are resigned to the need to move him out to the ward, but want him returned to the ICU if he has complications after he is on the ward. His wife says it is "too soon" and she is not ready to "give up." When reminded of her earlier statement about his wishes, she says he would not want to "give up" this soon. She clearly said she didn't believe the dismal prognosis she has heard from everyone here. She has spoken by phone with a specialist in

Europe who told her that Habib's prognosis was in doubt until a minimum of six months had passed. She is convinced that more should be done for him, and she says she will never consent to nursing home care for him.

DISCUSSION

When a patient is no longer able to participate in treatment decisions, we turn to a proxy for help, usually a relative who knows the values and wishes of the patient. The proxy is expected to provide **substituted judgment**, that is, to authorize treatments the patient would request if the patient were able. Such substituted judgment should be based on a written advance directive, the patient's previously stated wishes, or an understanding of his or her values.

With a very high degree of certainty, this patient's physicians expect him to remain in a persistent vegetative state. His caring wife has been advocating for his care and says she believes he would agree that it is too soon to "give up." She has received a different prognosis from a physician who has not seen the patient; this physician may be basing his conclusion on traumatic head injury data rather than data from patients who have suffered brain injury from lack of oxygen. Though many Muslims have a strong belief in the sanctity of human life, and follow a mandate to preserve life whenever possible, this religious belief does not seem to play a large part in the current difference of opinion.

RECOMMENDATIONS

1. It is ethically permissible to continue full treatment on the basis of the patient's wife's statement that this is what she believes he would choose at this point.
2. She should be periodically updated on his condition and prognosis. When she comes to the point of believing he would want to change treatment goals, this should be done.
3. It would be permissible to write limitation of treatment orders over her objection only if continued treatment is clearly physiologically futile (i.e., it just plain will not work), or if he shows signs of awareness in the future and continued treatment would cause him unrelievable suffering.

FOLLOW-UP

For the next three months the patient moved in and out of the ICU several times (**sepsis**, pulmonary emboli, heart failure). He died from recurrent sepsis on full support, about four months after the initial event.

COMMENT

Families are at a terrible disadvantage when two professionals give different prognoses for their loved one. Almost invariably, they are willing to accept the better prognosis over the more dismal prediction. And if the primary caregivers are the ones giving the poor prognosis, the family may worry that these caregivers are not doing everything possible or are more concerned with allocation of expensive resources than with their loved one's care.

Sometimes the reason professionals arrive at different prognoses is a matter of personal clinical experience (or inexperience), or where they trained, or what journals they read. Sometimes, especially when prognosticating is done at a distance, it is because they have been given inaccurate information.

Regardless of the source, since prognosticating is an inexact science, we will always have to deal with differences of predicting. And the assessment accepted by the patient or **surrogate** should lead to a decision based on those values. Only when a requested treatment is clearly futile is it ethically permissible for professionals to decline to provide it.

In an era when the cost of health care is so high, and professionals are urged to preserve health-care dollars, it is easy to look back at this case and say that the hundreds of thousands of dollars spent on Habib's care for the final three months of his life were "wasted." But an assessment of such matters depends on whether one is taking a clinical ethics perspective (as here) or a health policy perspective. Quite different indeed.

Case 7.07

QUESTION

Should this man in a vegetative state continue to receive vigorous treatment or should his treatment be limited to honor his previously expressed wishes?

STORY

Dr. Granger is a fifty-seven-year-old professor of anatomy at a medical school who six weeks ago collapsed on the street with a heart attack. He received **cardiopulmonary resuscitation** from a bystander; paramedics transported him to the emergency department; and his heart was successfully resuscitated. He required **ventilator** assistance for two weeks but was successfully **weaned**. However, he has not awakened, and it is now clear that he has suffered severe brain injury from lack of oxygen. He has had aggressive treatment of several medical problems, and currently is stable.

He has been unresponsive since his cardiac arrest. His neurological status has changed over time; he was initially comatose but now he opens his eyes and has sleep-wake cycles. The neurology consultant has recently concluded that he is in a **persistent vegetative state** (PVS) with virtually no chance of significant improvement.

The patient's only previous significant encounter with ill health was about three years ago when he fell down stairs, breaking his leg and his cervical spine. He chose not to stabilize the neck fracture with a halo cast in spite of some disagreement among his physicians about management. He felt the risk of destabilization was small, and he would leave the outcome to God. Thus he chose not to be burdened with the cast.

His wife, Cathleen, a retired nurse, describes him as a very patient, unselfish servant. He is a deeply religious Christian and believes strongly in the sovereignty of God in regard to illness outcomes. He has no written **advance directive** and has not talked about his treatment wishes if critically ill, but he has said on several occasions that he does not want to be a burden to his family. Their six children are supportive and are looking to their mother to act as **surrogate** for their father.

Cathleen is quite realistic about his current condition but continues to be hopeful because she sees signs that she thinks represent gradual improvement such as opening of his eyes, longer periods of wakefulness, apparent fixing of his eyes on the TV screen, etc. She thinks that if the patient were able to participate in decisions about his care now, he would press on with therapy as long as there was any chance of further improvement. She feels that he would not want to "exist without living" if his current condition proved to be his maximal level of recovery.

DISCUSSION

When persons are no longer capable of participating in treatment decisions and have left no written instructions, we make decisions using **substituted judgment**, trying to reconstruct their thoughts and wishes based on our best understanding of their wishes and values.

When the degree of certainty is high that patients will not improve to a condition they would find acceptable, it is ethically and legally permissible to limit treatment, either by withholding or by withdrawing modalities that are merely postponing an otherwise inevitable death.

In this case, in spite of a clearly bleak prognosis from the **neurologist**, the patient's wife is not yet convinced of the irreversibility of his condition. She believes the patient would choose to continue treatment until there is a higher degree of certainty that he will not improve, though she is even more certain that he would choose to limit or even withdraw treatment if this should become clear.

RECOMMENDATIONS

1. It is ideal in situations like this to follow the patient's wishes regarding treatment. With no advance directive or prior statement from the patient, his wife is in the best position to help us determine what those wishes would be.
2. Once there is consensus about the irreversibility of his condition, it would be ethically permissible to consider **limitation of treatment** such as withholding of interventions for new medical crises or withdrawing organ support (including artificially administered nutrition and hydration) while continuing good nursing care.

FOLLOW-UP

The patient stabilized and was transferred to a long-term care facility. He had no awareness and was thus unable to participate in a rehabilitation program. About six months after his cardiac arrest, his wife accepted the irreversibility of his condition. She was unwilling to consent to withdrawal of his artificial feedings but requested instead that he not be treated with antibiotics when he next developed a pulmonary infection. This happened about two months later, and after several days of good **palliative care**, he died.

COMMENT

Prognostic data may be convincing to health-care professionals. It is sometimes less than persuasive to those who love the patient and cling to optimism. Such optimism may be fueled by misinterpretation of physical signs, as in this case. When the doctors saw the patient open his eyes without any awareness, this convinced them that he was in a PVS. However, his wife saw this as a sign of improvement, and she was thus unwilling to consent to limitation of treatment, even though she knew this is what he would want if the doctors' dismal prognosis was in fact true.

Case 7.08

QUESTION

Is it ethically permissible to discontinue the feeding tube in this young man who has been in a persistent vegetative state for five years?

STORY

Irving was a young engineer when he sustained multiple injuries, including a severe head injury, in a motorcycle accident five years ago. After several weeks of intensive care, his other injuries had healed but he was declared to be in a **persistent vegetative state** (PVS) by his **neurologist**. Rather than place him in a nursing home, his loving family took him home, still hopeful that he might show even some minimal awareness.

They have now cared for him for nearly five years, and he has not required any hospital readmissions. He is fed via **PEG tube**, kept meticulously clean, turned frequently to prevent skin breakdown, and his urinary catheter is changed regularly. Care is provided by both parents, two siblings, and several volunteers from their Jewish community.

Different members of the family have come to the conclusion at various times that his condition is permanent. Prompted by public discussion of legal proceedings about a woman in a PVS, there has been family conversation for several months about stopping his feedings but considerable reluctance to take this huge step. I was asked by his sister to meet with the four family members in their home.

Everyone in the family understands that Irving's condition is permanent, that the improvement they had hoped and prayed for is not going to happen. All agree that he would not want to be maintained in this condition — he had been an active sportsman, concerned about his physical prowess and appearance. They have talked with their rabbi and have been told there is no Jewish prohibition to stopping tube feedings in a case like this. His mother worries "what the neighbors will think happened" since he has been "healthy" for the five years since his accident. She is not certain she can tell them the family stopped feeding him.

DISCUSSION

Artificial administration of fluids and nutrition by feeding tube is recognized to be medical treatment, morally different from feeding by mouth. Feeding tubes are often used after accident or injury, with the anticipation that the patient will recover or improve. If it becomes clear that the patient will not improve to a level of function he or she would find satisfactory, continued administration of fluids and nutrition is considered optional, comparable to other treatment modalities that may be given on a trial basis.

Whether to continue artificially administered fluids and nutrition for a person who is permanently unaware is a very personal choice. This choice should be made by those who know the patient best, based on the personal and religious values of the patient. If a decision is made to discontinue tube feedings, it remains morally imperative to continue to give good mouth care and even to offer fluids to see if the patient is able to swallow reflexively.

In this patient, all who know him firmly believe he would choose to stop tube feedings. There is some reluctance to do so based on social concerns. Continuation of tube feedings in this patient would not cause him any additional harm since he is unaware of his surroundings.

RECOMMENDATIONS

1. It would be ethically and legally permissible to discontinue artificially administered fluids and nutrition in this patient on the basis of the understanding that he would not want to receive such treatment.
2. If this is done, he should continue to receive frequent mouth care, and should be offered small amounts of fluid to see if he is able to take it in.

3. For the sake of family unity, it would likewise be ethically permissible to continue the tube feedings until there is full agreement on removal and on how to inform the neighbors.

FOLLOW-UP

Tube feedings were continued for another six months. Slowly Irving's mother came to agree with the rest of the family that feedings must be stopped to honor his values and their understanding of his wishes. This was done, and he received hospice care for eleven days before he died. The family was open and frank with the neighbors, who were supportive of their decision.

COMMENT

Discontinuation of artificially administered fluids and nutrition continues to be a contentious issue for some people, because of their understanding of moral requirements within their faith tradition. This move should never be made lightly or hurriedly, and usually should be preceded by spiritual counsel from knowledgeable clergy.

Case 7.09

QUESTION

Should the tube feedings be stopped in this man who is "locked in" after a recent stroke at the insistence of his wife (who is also his designated agent)?

STORY

Jeffrey is a fifty-one-year-old business executive. Three days ago he had a sudden devastating stroke that has left him "locked in," that is, he is awake and aware, breathing on his own, but totally paralyzed except for the ability to raise his eyes. He is clinically stable, is being fed by a nasogastric (NG) tube, and is receiving antibiotics for a small pneumonia that resulted from **aspiration** of stomach contents at the time of the stroke.

Cathy, his forty-two-year-old second wife, has been insisting for two days that the antibiotic and NG tube be discontinued and that he be allowed to die. She bases her request on an **advance directive** (a copy of which is on his chart) signed by Jeffrey several years ago that names her as his **agent**, and requests that he not receive treatment if he is unable to make his own treatment decisions and is unlikely to recover the ability to think and act for himself.

Cathy does not work and has been a housewife since they married fifteen years ago. She spends many hours a day on the Internet and has recently met a man with whom she has been corresponding for several weeks. She told the hospital social worker that she and Jeffrey have had an open marriage and that she had just introduced her new friend to Jeffrey when he had his stroke.

I met with the patient, his wife, his brother, and his nurse. Cathy immediately tried to dominate the meeting, getting right down in Jeffrey's face, telling him that we were there to discuss his feeding tube and that she would get a lawyer to support his written wishes if the hospital staff was unwilling to stop his feedings. I asked her to remain quiet while I spoke with Jeffrey. His facial muscles were flaccid resulting in a total lack of expression. We were able to establish a code for yes and no responses via his eye movements. He understood his condition and that it was almost certainly permanent. He further understood that efforts could be made through rehabilitation services to enhance his communication and improve his quality of life, and that he could likely be sustained for a very long time in this condition. He demonstrated some ambivalence about the feeding tube, and seemed to want more time to think about his goals and wishes. His brother appeared to be intimidated by Cathy.

DISCUSSION

When a patient sustains a major permanent change in physical ability but retains **decision-making capacity**, it is not uncommon for the patient to find the new quality of life unacceptable and to thus decline life-extending treatment. Before acceding to this understandable decision, it is imperative that the patient be given reliable specific information and time to think about the future. The patient should be fully informed about the potential for rehabilitation, and ideally should be encouraged to meet others who have a similar condition and are satisfied with continued existence with the disability.

A patient's written advance directive is an important vehicle to communicate one's wishes about treatment, but unless it specifies otherwise, it does not take effect until the patient is unable to participate in decisions.

When a patient with decision-making capacity appears to be pressured by others toward a specific decision, this pressure should be countered with a thorough explanation to the patient (and to the one applying the pressure) about patient autonomy.

In this case, the patient has suffered one of the most devastating types of permanent neurological disabilities possible. It is understandable for him to find the quality of his new life to be intolerable. Unfortunately, there are very few survivors in this condition to meet with him. This places an added burden on his professional caregivers to portray to him the best possible outcome from continued treatment.

RECOMMENDATIONS

1. It should be repeatedly reinforced with the patient that the ultimate decision about continued treatment is his, but if he declines treatment, this request will not be honored until staff and family have spent adequate time and effort showing him his potential.
2. Full rehabilitation consultation should be carried out as soon as possible, including psychological and social support services.
3. Counseling should be offered to the patient and his wife about their relationship and interactions.
4. Someone else (his brother?) should be encouraged to be involved in his ongoing care, with the hope that he can be a patient advocate.

FOLLOW-UP

Two days after the consultation, I returned to have a conversation with Jeffrey alone. He expressed a wish to continue to receive treatment and to go to rehab. I called Cathy to inform her, and she was furious that I was interfering with her responsibility as his wife. She insisted that I was "off the case" since my services were no longer desired.

Jeffrey was transferred to the rehabilitation hospital about one week after the ethics consultation, and discharged home five weeks later. His obituary appeared in the newspaper three weeks after discharge.

COMMENT

This consultation presented the very difficult challenges of a devastating medical condition and a dominating spouse who may well have had another agenda. It is not known if Jeffrey succumbed to a new complication of his condition, reached a valid decision to stop his tube feedings, or was badgered into that decision by Cathy.

Case 7.10

QUESTION

Is it permissible to continue treatments insisted upon by some family members for this woman who is "locked in" when it is reported by other family that the patient had previously declined?

STORY

Jesse is a fifty-four-year-old woman with a history of hypertension and diabetes. She had her first of several strokes about five years ago, has been totally disabled for three or four years, and has been quadriplegic and essentially "locked in" for some time. Ten days ago she was transported to the hospital with respiratory depression and a change in her sputum color to green (suggestive of a new pneumonia). She was **intubated** in the emergency department for respiratory failure. She is being treated for a pneumonia caused by a type of bacteria that is resistant to most antibiotics, and she is slowly improving. On admission, it was felt the respiratory depression was potentially reversible, and full therapy was instituted with the goal of returning her to her baseline status. However, two days ago the pulmonary consultant said he felt the patient would probably require long-term ventilatory support. Her daughter, Belinda, is her primary caregiver, and she has now requested continuation of full therapy and is reported by staff in the intensive care unit (ICU) to have "unrealistic expectations." The patient is currently being evaluated regarding the feasibility of home mechanical ventilation.

Jesse has received twenty-four-hour care at home by Belinda, one of eight children. Her other children occasionally help, but Belinda prefers to provide full care herself because she doesn't think others are as careful or as competent as she in giving the needed care. Jesse is fed via gastric tube, and she communicates by eye movements. She has had frequent admissions for pulmonary and urinary infections. During an admission about three months ago, Jesse and Belinda talked with the hospice admission coordinator while considering a change in treatment goals.

Her primary physician, Dr. Edelstein, reports that Belinda has expressed varied desires about level of treatment, and those have been based on "the patient's **best interests**" (including her quality of life, degree of pain, etc.) rather than on a **substituted judgment**. There is on the chart a durable power of attorney form naming Belinda as her **agent** for financial affairs, but it does not include health-care decisions.

Her children describe the patient as having been an energetic and happy woman who had been a good single mother before her illness and disability. They believe her quality of life as a disabled person has been satisfactory to her. However, several of her children report that she has stated in the past that she did not want to be kept alive on "life support."

On examination, the patient responds to verbal stimulation and moves her eyes on command. She is currently on a **ventilator**, intravenous antibiotics, tube feedings, insulin, and other chronic medications.

DISCUSSION

When a decision must be made about the use or nonuse of burdensome technology to postpone death, that decision should be made jointly by the patient (or **surrogate**) and medical professionals. The ranking for preferred patient/surrogate input is: (1) the patient with **decision-making capacity**, (2) the family of a patient without decision-making capacity based on the patient's previously written or spoken wishes (substituted judgment), and (3) the family of a patient without such capacity based on the patient's presumed best interests. Professional input should include both the current care team and the primary professional caregiver if they are not the same individual.

In this patient, a previous consideration of hospice care would suggest that the patient might in some circumstances prefer comfort care without aggressive interventions to postpone death. The choice for aggressive treatment at the time of this admission is understandable and justified because of the presumed reversibility of the situation. Now that her condition has been assessed as likely irreversible, however, the goals and options need to be rediscussed.

RECOMMENDATIONS

1. If home mechanical ventilation is feasible, an effort should be made to restore the patient's decision-making capacity by eliminating sedation, optimizing her metabolic condition, etc. If she can communicate via eye blinks that she understands her condition and her options, her choice for or against home ventilation should be honored. If home ventilation is not feasible, there is less pressure to have this conversation with the patient.
2. A family conference should be arranged to include the patient, as many family members as possible, representatives of her current care team, and her primary physician. At the conference, they should be informed about the available options and made aware of the possibility of recommendation 1, and everyone's views of the patient's values and best interests could be sought and subsequently implemented if recommendation 1 is not feasible. An ethics consultant could also be present at, or even facilitate, this conference.
3. Belinda should be offered as much help as is available through agencies and resources.

FOLLOW-UP

Four days later the patient coughed and dislodged the **endotracheal tube**. She appeared comfortable and was clinically stable, so the tube was not immediately replaced. The following day a management conference was held with the family, the ICU team, and the home mechanical ventilation admission coordinator. After considerable discussion, the following was agreed upon as a continued management plan: (a) continued aggressive nutritional support and treatment of infection in an effort to return to her baseline condition; (b) rediscussion with the patient about "life support" to learn her wishes now that she has experienced short-term intubation and ventilation; and (c) if the patient reaffirms her previous statement against "life support," (a) will be continued but a **do-not-resuscitate order** and a do-not-intubate order will be written.

One week later the patient had returned to her baseline condition and was discharged home.

COMMENT

This is another example of the limits of prognostic ability. While the pulmonary specialist felt that **weaning** from the ventilator was not likely, her daughter remained optimistic. The professional caregivers were concerned that Belinda's optimism was "unrealistic" and might lead to a type of care that the patient had previously said she would not want. In such situations, it is best to move slowly in order to avoid premature, irreversible decisions. Legitimate questions remain about deciding how slowly to move, how long to wait, when optimism is truly unrealistic, etc.

Case 7.11

QUESTION

Please advise about further management options when the family of a patient who is brain dead is unwilling to accept the diagnosis.

STORY

Aasmaa is a thirty-nine-year-old East Indian woman who was well until about one week ago when she developed swelling of her ankles and fatigue. Four days ago she began to vomit, became lethargic, and had a series of seizures although she has no prior seizure history. She was transported to the emergency department and was found to be pregnant (unknown to her family), but the fetus was dead and the patient was in full-blown eclampsia.[6] She suffered a cardiac arrest in the emergency department, was resuscitated, and had a normal head **CT scan**. She was admitted to the intensive care unit (ICU) and almost immediately spontaneously delivered a stillborn infant of about thirty weeks' **gestation**. Later that day she had further neurological deterioration, probably from **herniation of the brain stem**.

Her clinical exam the following day was consistent with death by neurologic criteria, and this was confirmed by a cerebral blood flow study (it

6. Eclampsia is an uncommon life-threatening complication of pregnancy manifested by hypertension, seizures, and coma.

showed no flow in the arteries to her brain) and an **electroencephalogram** (EEG) (it was flat, indicating no electrical activity in the brain). The family was notified at 4:15 P.M. that she was dead, but they requested a repeat EEG the next day. Repeat EEG and repeat clinical exam the following day were unchanged. The family has refused to allow disconnection of organ support believing that she will miraculously recover.

The patient's husband is a professor of biology and they have a six-year-old daughter. The patient's sister, an obstetrician from New Jersey, has flown in to assist and states that she has seen patients recover from eclamptic coma after several weeks. The patient's brother also resists withdrawal of support because his wife and child survived near-death situations of an unknown type several years ago and are now healthy. The patient and her family are Hindu.

DISCUSSION

The clinical criteria for death by neurologic criteria are clear, and there is both professional and legislative agreement on their use. Once death has been declared with the highest possible degree of certainty, professionals caring for the patient have no further clinical obligation to that person except respectful treatment of the dead body. Occasionally the family of a patient who meets these criteria resists withdrawal of organ support, especially when the illness or injury leading to death has been unexpected or when cultural or religious beliefs do not recognize death until the heart stops. In such situations we generally allow a brief period of family accommodation while further discussion and explanation encourage them to accept the tragic facts.

All U.S. states define "brain death" using the wording of the Uniform Determination of Death Act.[7] New Jersey and New York are the only states that have an exception clause that disallows the declaration of death by neurologic criteria if a family objects on the basis of cultural or religious belief.

While statutory law in this state is clear on this issue, there is case law precedent that requires judicial review before withdrawal of organ support

---

7. "An individual who has sustained either (1) irreversible cessation of circulatory and respiratory functions, or (2) irreversible cessation of all functions of the entire brain, including the brain stem, is dead. A determination of death must be made in accordance with accepted medical standards."

from a neurologically dead patient over the objection of a family. This hospital has a new policy that allows physicians to withdraw organ support from a person who has been declared dead by neurologic criteria over the objection of family. It is recognized that this is at variance with state case law, but the policy has not been subjected to review by the courts.

In this case the clinical situation is clear. It is not yet clear if family resistance is solely due to their experience with critical illness or whether there are religious or cultural aspects as well. In addition, since her sister is a physician from New Jersey, she may have the perception that brain death is a flexible concept because of that state's statutory definition.

RECOMMENDATIONS

1. The professionals involved in the care of this patient should be consistent in their approach to the family and in the words they use. The patient is "dead" (not "brain dead"); she is on "organ support" (not "life support"); the plan is to disconnect the organ support very soon.
2. The family should be offered further education on death by neurologic criteria as well as compassionate support from social workers and chaplains. In addition, an effort should be made to clarify the reason for their resistance.
3. If they are not persuaded in the next twenty-four hours, perhaps a conference should be held tomorrow to include the family, the ICU attending physician, the neurology consultant, the obstetrics consultant, and the ethics consultant. If the family's resistance continues, the medical team's options are to (a) seek a court order to withdraw support, or (b) withdraw support based on clinical facts and hospital policy. Advice should be sought from hospital legal counsel about the preferred course of action.

FOLLOW-UP

The patient's sister responded that the family does not have religiously or culturally based reasons to resist a diagnosis of death by neurologic criteria. The day after the consultation, the patient's sister spoke on the phone with a **neurologist** who, she said, concurred with the family that it is premature to withdraw support. The ICU physician requested a formal consultation from that neurologist, and it was scheduled for the next day. However, hemodynamic deterioration (severe blood pressure fluctuations) began before this could be accomplished. The patient's family at that point began to recognize the finality of her condition, and her sister agreed to the withdrawal of support. However, the day that agreement was reached was not a good day for the patient to "die" for religious (Hindu) reasons. Support was continued for another twelve hours, but she had no blood pressure in spite of maximal doses of three drugs to sustain it. Her heart stopped while she was on full support.

COMMENT

It is not unusual for family members to doubt the diagnosis of death when they see their loved one in the ICU, breathing (because the **ventilator** is breathing for him or her), warm, having good color, making urine, with a blood pressure and pulse. It takes considerable education, along with compassionate support, to help families in such situations to realize the finality of death; thus the common practice of allowing families a "reasonable time of accommodation." Discussion continues over what is reasonable in such situations.

While it might seem more compassionate to continue support in such a patient, this exacts a tremendous cost in human and clinical resources, as well as a psychological toll for professional caregivers who realize they are working intensely to maintain physiologic homeostasis (stability of many variables, including blood pressure, pulse, blood levels of several chemicals) in a situation where there is absolute certainty of no improvement because the patient's total brain is dead. Thus the common hospital policy of mandating an end point based on physiologic **futility**.

In these situations, it is important to be (or to become) aware of cultural or religious beliefs or practices that might modify one's approach and/or require additional counsel, and to recognize the potential for different perspectives based on various state laws.

*   *   *

Other Cases Involving "Brain Failure"

Cases 3.02, 4.03, 5.02, 5.09, 6.01, 6.02, 6.03, 6.04, 6.05, 6.08, 6.09, 8.05, 9.11, 10.04, 10.05, 10.06, 10.09, 10.11, 10.12, 11.01, 11.05, 11.09, 13.03, 13.04, 14.01, 14.02, 14.09

References on "Brain Failure"

Bauby, J. *The Diving Bell and the Butterfly.* New York: Vintage Books, 1997.

Bernat, J. *Ethical Issues in Neurology.* 2nd ed. Boston: Butterworth-Heinemann, 2001.

Glannon, W. *Bioethics and the Brain.* Oxford: Oxford University Press, 2006.

Jennett, B. *The Vegetative State: Medical Facts, Ethical and Legal Dilemmas.* Cambridge: Cambridge University Press, 2002.

Mitchell, C. B., R. D. Orr, and S. A. Salladay, eds. *Aging, Death, and the Quest for Immortality.* Grand Rapids: Eerdmans, 2004.

Purtilo, Ruth B., and Henk A. M. J. ten Have. *Ethical Foundations of Palliative Care for Alzheimer Disease.* Baltimore: Johns Hopkins University Press, 2004.

CHAPTER 8

Ethical Issues in Mind Failure

Currently in medicine, we distinguish between problems of the brain (cared for by specialists in neurology) and problems of the mind (cared for by specialists in psychiatry). Traditionally we have thought of the former as "organic," that is, caused by some physical disorder of the brain, and the latter as "functional," that is, caused by some nonphysical malady. However, it is difficult to draw a clear line between what I have called "brain failure" in the preceding chapter and what I refer to here as "mind failure." Both include disorders or disability in thinking.

As science advances, we are learning that many psychiatric disorders do in fact have a biologic basis, whether genetic, chemical, or something else (e.g., some depressions, schizophrenia). In the future I expect that these two chapters will have to be combined, or disorders of brain function will have to be classified on some other basis.

Some of the issues involved in caring for patients with psychiatric illness are very similar to those encountered in patients with **delirium** or **dementia**, as outlined in the introduction to the preceding chapter. Other issues are unique to this part of medical and nursing care. The most common psychiatric diagnoses that raise ethical issues are psychosis, depression, and substance abuse.

A very common question in caring for psychiatric patients deals with their capacity to make decisions (see Case 8.01), especially decisions about treatment for their condition. Thus questions of competence and capacity are prominent, and are not always easily answered. While psychiatric illnesses probably have more clearly defined diagnostic criteria than most other conditions, many of the criteria are subject to individual or variable interpretation. On occasion it may not be completely clear to everyone involved if the patient meets the criteria for a specific diagnosis or not. But it is perhaps even more important for us to realize that the presence of a particular psychiatric diagnosis, for example, schizophrenia or depression, does not automatically mean that the patient lacks the capacity to make treatment decisions. And as we have already discussed, the criteria for decisional capacity are deceptively vague in some instances.

One of the issues encountered frequently in patients with mental illness is involuntary hospitalization (see Case 8.03). Until the middle of the twentieth century it was not very difficult for a physician or family member to admit someone to a mental hospital over his or her objection if that person was acting in a bizarre manner. This was most often for the patient's own good, but was sometimes abused by individuals who merely wanted to remove the patient from a social setting or restrict his or her ability to act.

In the 1960s and thereafter, rules and laws were changed to protect the autonomy of persons with mental illness. In most jurisdictions it is now possible to hospitalize a person involuntarily only if he or she is a danger to self or others — for protection. This may be done for only a short time, typically for three days, based only on the signature of a physician. If the person is felt to be a continuing danger, it can be extended only by a judge after a court hearing. The measures used during the initial period of involuntary hospitalization may involve isolation, restraints, or other measures that understandably increase fear and resistance in the patient who does not fully comprehend the situation.

Involuntary treatment of the psychiatric condition (distinct from involuntary hospitalization) is another matter entirely. Treatment is directed at the mental illness itself, and is not so much a matter of protection but of therapy. Such involuntary therapy most often cannot proceed without a court order. And again, such measures may include injections, electroconvulsive treatments, or other measures deemed very threatening by the patient. As a result of this enlightened approach to the care of patients with mental illness, many people who clearly have conditions that could be improved with treatment resist or refuse treatment and continue to live in a state considered by most to be a condition of impairment (see Case 5.06).

One of the recurring issues in caring for patients with mental illness is suicide. It is very common for individuals with severe depression or with psychosis to try to take their own lives. For decades, one of the major functions of psychiatry was to prevent suicide by assessing patients for suicidal risk and protecting them from themselves when this seemed like a real possibility. Such prediction of human behavior can be very difficult, and it often is in the forefront of questions about involuntary hospitalization or treatment.

In addition, in recent years philosophers, psychiatrists, and other physicians have discussed the concept of "rational suicide." Are there situations where voluntarily taking one's own life is the rational thing to do? Perhaps with painful terminal illness, or with depression that is resistant to all forms of therapy? In some settings psychiatrists are now being asked, not whether a person's suicidal thinking is dangerous, but whether that thinking "makes sense." This is more evidence of the dominance afforded to patient autonomy in modern culture. This also generates more difficult assessments for many people of faith, particularly those who always consider suicide to be immoral. This dilemma will be addressed in Cases 8.04, 8.05, and 8.12.

It is sad, but true, that a psychiatric diagnosis often carries with it a sense of stigma. A diagnosis of schizophrenia makes a person "abnormal" in a sense that a diagnosis of diabetes does not. Even though we continue to learn more about the biochemical causes or mediation of mental illness, laypersons and many medical professionals continue to attribute such illness to a character flaw and failure to improve to a lack of the will. Some of this stigmatization begins because such individuals have to be treated differently when they react differently to interpersonal encounters. But there is often a snowball effect of unusual behavior, diagnosis of "abnormal," recommendation for treatment, patient resistance, involuntary treatment, increased unusual behavior, etc. This potential makes these patients particularly vulnerable and increases the professional and societal responsibility for their care. It also increases the potential for ethical dilemmas.

The treatment of patients who are chemically dependent or addicted, whether to drugs or alcohol, raises these and other issues, especially because of the frequently added dimensions of the patient's lack of truthfulness and the intervention of law enforcement. In caring for and addressing ethical issues in these patients, it is critical to make some distinctions. Chemical dependence means that without the chemical, the patient will predictably have withdrawal symptoms that are physiologically mediated. Addiction, on the other hand, is the compulsive psychological and physiological dependence on a substance that extends to the individual's lying or breaking of laws to obtain the substance. Pseudoaddiction may occur if a patient is given a medication with the potential for dependence, feels he or she is not receiving enough to control the symptoms adequately, and uses the techniques of the addict to obtain more.

Let's now look at some cases where psychiatric illness led to ethical dilemmas and ethics consultations.

Case 8.01

QUESTION

Is it ethically permissible to proceed with scheduled surgery on this woman who has lost the capacity to give consent?

STORY

Katie, age thirty-six, was at thirty-seven weeks' **gestation** in her first pregnancy when the baby unexpectedly died in utero. Labor was induced twelve days ago. Delivery was difficult and she sustained a large laceration extending from her vagina into her rectum. This was repaired immediately after delivery. Three or four days postpartum the repair broke down causing fecal soiling and incontinence. She was caring for this problem at home and was being seen daily by her physician for wound care. Secondary repair was scheduled for tomorrow, probably under spinal anesthesia.

Two days ago Katie exhibited signs of recurrent psychosis leading to voluntary admission to a locked psychiatry ward. She has a history of bipolar episodes,[1] which required two hospitalizations in the past six years. Her current diagnosis is mixed manic state. She is confused and disoriented, and her psychiatric caregivers believe she does not have the capacity to give valid consent for surgery at this time. She is on medication and is somewhat more relaxed according to her social worker and her husband. It is anticipated that she will need from ten to fourteen days of inpatient psychiatric care. She is now unable to care for her perineal wound and she cannot be discharged until it is repaired or she has regained the psychomotor ability to care for it at home.

The timing of secondary repair of her perineal wound is elective. The tissue is now ready, and repair could be done at any time. It could even be postponed for an extended period, which would likely result in wound clo-

---

1. Bipolar disorder, formerly called manic-depressive illness, is a cyclic mood disorder manifested by periods of overactivity (mania) or depression, with or without psychotic features, usually with periods of normal activity and mood between episodes.

sure with rectal incontinence; the muscle repair to restore continence could be done at a later date. Though this would likely give an acceptable surgical result, comparable to repair now, it would entail ongoing fecal incontinence that might in turn require an extended hospital stay.

Dr. Putnam, her obstetrician-gynecologist, reports that he had a presurgery consent discussion with Katie and her husband, in the presence of his office nurse, three days before her psychotic break. At that time both she and her husband gave consent and were eager to proceed with the scheduled repair. The patient was not asked to sign a consent form at that time, and there was no discussion about what type of anesthesia would be used. Her inpatient psychiatric social worker reports that during her psychiatric admission process the patient told her about the scheduled surgery, even recalling the day it was to be done.

Dr. Putnam believes it would be in her **best interests** to proceed with surgery now rather than waiting for repair at a later date.

DISCUSSION

Valid surgical consent is a process of communication between patients and their physicians. For consent to be ethically valid, patients must have the capacity to give consent, they must be given adequate information, and they must be free of coercion. A signed informed consent form merely documents that the process has been accomplished.

In this case, a valid consent discussion has taken place. Subsequent to that, one element of the ethical requirements has disappeared in that the patient no longer has the capacity to repeat the discussion or sign the consent document. With the availability of several witnesses to the adequacy of that consent discussion, the absence of a patient signature does not invalidate the discussion.

RECOMMENDATIONS

1. It is ethically permissible to proceed with surgery as planned unless the patient's psychiatric caregivers believe this would be detrimental to her current condition or recovery.
2. The physician and the nurse who were present during the consent discussion should document in her chart the content of the discussion and the patient's response.
3. It would be ethically permissible for her husband to sign the consent

form as her proxy. Prior to doing this, he should talk with the anesthesiologist and give consent for whatever type of anesthesia he believes his wife would choose.

4. Any questions about the legality of this documentation should be addressed to Hospital Risk Management.

FOLLOW-UP

The physician and nurse documented the earlier consent discussion. Katie's husband was allowed to sign the surgical consent. Surgery was done with a good result.

COMMENT

Prior to the 1970s, patients with mental illness were often deprived of basic human rights, like the right to consent, and were often treated over their objection. The rise in prominence given to patient autonomy at about that time led to tighter rules and laws that have made it much more difficult to treat mentally incapacitated patients who decline treatment unless they can be clearly shown to be a danger to themselves or others. In most cases this shift from paternalism to autonomy has proven beneficial to patients. However, in some instances it has led to patients with florid psychosis, occasionally causing them great torment, to be legally free from unwanted interference.

Had Katie not had the consent discussion before her psychotic break, it would not have been legally or ethically possible to operate until either (a) she was able to give consent or (b) it was ordered by a court after full review, even though that delay would have entailed weeks or months of mess and inconvenience. This consultation revolved around the difference between valid consent (an ethical determination) and informed consent (a legal doctrine that is not complete until documented).

Case 8.02

QUESTION

Is it ethically permissible to accept a family's request for limitation of treatment for this man with chronic schizophrenia because they perceive his quality of life to be poor?

STORY

Reggie is a sixty-two-year-old man who was admitted to the medical intensive care unit (ICU) yesterday with altered mental status and dehydration. On admission, his mother and brother requested no aggressive treatment or diagnostic interventions because of his long-standing poor quality of life. A **do-not-resuscitate order** and an order prohibiting **intubation** were written, but upon reflection, his physician is uncertain if this is appropriate. The patient's electrolyte and fluid abnormalities are being corrected, but his mental status has not returned to baseline, and it is not clear if this will be possible. He has been found to be jaundiced and to have an enlarged liver and lymph nodes as well as a lesion on a chest X-ray that is suspicious for malignancy.

Reggie has been disabled from schizophrenia for many years. Members of his family report that he is delusional and actively hallucinates much of the time, but he generally cares for himself and calls them when he has needs. His ex-wife receives his disability checks, buys groceries, and looks out for him. His mother and his brother live nearby and are also involved in his life.

On exam, he is sleepy but arousable. He is oriented to person and place, but not to time. It is not possible to have a meaningful conversation with him about his treatment wishes.

DISCUSSION

Making a **limitation of treatment** decision based on poor quality of life is a very personal and subjective assessment. It is very difficult for a **surrogate** to declare a patient's baseline quality of life to be so poor that life-prolonging therapy should not be used. There are, however, some clinical situations where almost everyone would agree that future quality of life is so poor that limitation of treatment is appropriate. This requires a high degree of clinical certainty.

In this case, the patient was recently quite functional and had a quality of life that appears to have been satisfactory to him without evidence of suffering. While it may be tempting to believe that a psychotic patient has a poor quality of life, there is no way for a surrogate to know what the patient perceives. In addition, his current illness has been inadequately evaluated, so an accurate prognosis cannot be known.

RECOMMENDATIONS

1. It is not ethically appropriate to accept this patient's family's request for limitation of treatment on the basis of their assessment of his poor baseline quality of life. These orders should be rescinded until his prognosis is clarified.
2. If it is determined that he has a poor prognosis for recovery or even survival, it would be ideal to try to restore his **decision-making capacity** in order to involve him in treatment decisions. If this is not possible, there should be a conference with as many family members as possible to make a **best interests** decision for him. Limitation of treatment may be appropriate based on poor prognosis when it is not appropriate based on poor quality of life.

FOLLOW-UP

After several diagnostic tests were performed, it was determined that Reggie had cancer in his lungs, which had spread to many areas of his body and was incurable. It was determined that the cancer cell type was not likely to respond to chemotherapy or radiation. On the basis of this prognostic information, there was consensus that a goal of comfort care would be in his best interests. He was discharged to a nursing home for hospice care.

COMMENT

It is often tempting for family members and even for professional caregivers to judge that a patient's quality of life is unacceptably low. This may be based on the patient's mental capacity (or incapacity), physical disabilities, advanced age, or a combination of these. However, quality of life is very subjective. Two individuals with seemingly equivalent problems may judge their lives quite differently — one accepting and coping, the other miserable and complaining — so it is difficult to have any objective accuracy in such assessments. In addition, numerous research studies have confirmed that patients consistently rate their quality of life better than do either family members or professionals. For both of these reasons, decision-makers are cautioned to not be too quick to adversely judge a patient's quality of life, and to generally take a positive view unless there is reasonable evidence from the patient for the opposite.

This patient's family had expended an amazing amount of time, effort, and resources to look after him. Most chronically psychotic patients are not so fortunate. The family may (or may not) have been understandably weary of this duty. Their initial response of "keep him comfortable but no heroics" turned out after further investigation to be an appropriate decision, but their stated reason did not give adequate ethical justification.

Case 8.03

QUESTION

How should we treat someone who has proven that she is untreatable? Is it ever permissible to say that a patient in this circumstance is terminally ill and further treatment is futile?

STORY

Tammy, age twenty-three, has a history since childhood of behavioral and mental health problems, most notably frequent self-harm (trauma, bites, deep cuts), threats of suicide, and violence toward others when restrained (hitting, biting), all complicated by substance abuse. Her current diagnosis is borderline personality disorder,[2] but she also has some features of bipolar disorder and antisocial personality disorder.[3]

She has had countless involuntary (and some voluntary) hospitalizations; in the past several years her annual days of hospitalization have ranged from 94 to 280.

Tammy is described by her mental health caregivers as engaging, entertaining, and giving much of the time (she has trust funds, but limited access), but she is not reliable and frequently dishonest. She seems to suffer from internal stormy impulses, sometimes driven by voices. It is not clear to what extent her actions are volitional. Because of the intensity of her vi-

---

2. Borderline personality disorder is a condition in which the person's attitudes toward and relationships with others undergo dramatic and often rapid changes, ranging from dramatic dependency to violent attacks. Persons with this diagnosis often lead lives of tumult and chaos.

3. Persons with this disorder (sometimes called "sociopaths") are unable to sympathize with others and have no respect for laws, rules, or the rights of others.

olence, she often needs physical restraints, and indeed, she sometimes requests to be restrained. However, her usual pattern is to become docile soon after admission. She usually demonstrates postviolence remorse.

She has had two children, one as a teenager and one three years ago. She realized she would be unable to parent, so she placed them up for adoption. Interestingly, she had no episodes of self-harm while pregnant.

Tammy has been under the care of county mental health services for several years. Several living situations have been tried — group homes, prolonged hospitalization, supervised community living. Several approaches have been tried to deal with her violence — active intervention, downplay, encouraging voluntary admission, etc. She seems to understand the rules and does all she can to thwart them. Her caregivers have concluded that they are unable to cure or control her, so they seek a reliable systems-response aimed at protecting others from her violence and protecting her from self-destruction.

DISCUSSION

It may be helpful to compare physical and mental illness vis-à-vis prognosis and obligation to treat. A few physical illnesses are curable (e.g., infections), many are controllable (e.g., diabetes). Some are relentless but can be slowed (e.g., some malignancies). In a number of conditions treatment is unable to alter the course of the disease, but we may be able to provide symptom control or assistance with quality of life (e.g., **amyotrophic lateral sclerosis**, **dementia**, some malignancies). Most disease processes have fairly predictable courses, though many have the potential for unpredictable crises (e.g., coronary artery disease). In some of these, treatment may forestall the inevitable crises.

Management of some incurable physical conditions can be very frustrating as long as the goal is cure or control. Management of these conditions can be rewarding if the focus is shifted to palliation, comfort measures, and enhancing quality of life. Treatment of many physical conditions can become exasperating if the patient is unwilling or unable to follow recommendations for treatment known to be effective (e.g., the noncompliant patient with diabetes or alcoholism).

In all these situations, however, our professional obligation is to continue to provide treatment that has a reasonable chance of working. For the noncompliant patient, that includes treating episodic crises, even though we know they could have been avoided. It is ethically permissible to refuse to provide "futile" treatment. However, that word has generated much discussion. It applies only to a treatment that clearly will not work — physiologic **futility**. The word "futility" should not be used to refer to treatments that are "not worth it" (high patient burden or cost with small chance of efficacy). In attempting to quantify futility, Lawrence Schneiderman includes treatments that "have not worked in the last 100 patients."

But even more important than quantification is an understanding that it is impossible to declare a treatment to be "futile" unless a clear goal has been identified. For example, if a permanently unconscious patient develops renal failure, some would say dialysis is futile. It may be "inappropriate," it may be a poor use of resources, and it may be futile in terms of recovery of cognition; but it is not futile in terms of postponing death.

In this patient, a multitude of treatment options has been tried that might reasonably be hoped to control her behavior, all without apparent success. However, the measures used have prevented her from taking her life or seriously harming others. Thus currently employed measures may seem "futile" vis-à-vis cure or control, but they cannot be deemed futile if the goal is postponing what seems like her inevitable self-destruction.

RECOMMENDATIONS

1. It would be appropriate to search for other treatment options that have not yet been tried for this patient. (The mental health team was reluctant to consider my suggestion of demon possession and had no resources for exorcism.)
2. It would not be ethically permissible to consider continued treatment of this patient to be "futile."

FOLLOW-UP

The patient's situation remains essentially unchanged several years after the consultation.

COMMENT

Continued treatment of a patient can be very frustrating for health-care professionals when they see no sign of improvement. It is then tempting to call the treatment futile — it just isn't working. However, it is necessary to consider the goal of treatment when making such an assessment.

A diagnosis of demon possession has little credibility in the medical profession. I have no personal or professional experience with this phenomenon and have no qualifications to diagnose or discuss it, but if any patient fits my layman's picture of demon possession, this would likely be the one.

Case 8.04

QUESTION

Is it permissible to allow this woman to take her life by not eating and drinking when she is not terminally ill and claims not to be depressed?

STORY

Mrs. Costello, a woman in her late seventies, lives with her husband in the independent living section of a facility that also has nursing home beds for its residents. She has repeatedly told Dr. Franklin, her long-standing primary physician, that she wants no life-extending therapies. She is mobile, alert, and in good health except for two problems. Macular degeneration in both eyes, present for several years, has progressed to blindness. Though her husband leads her to meals and activities, she says her life is miserable because of the blindness ("I hate my life," she says). She also has coronary artery disease. Two years ago she initially refused recommended therapy, but later consented to a therapeutic intervention to relieve the frequently recurring severe pain. She subsequently regretted that decision, wishing she had not had treatment so that she might die. Yesterday she had a recurrence of chest pain and, though it resolved quickly and spontaneously, she adamantly said, "That's it. I am ready to die. I will stop eating and drinking as soon as I can be moved to a nursing home bed" (so her husband doesn't have to provide care during her dying process). Her husband generally defers to her and supports her choice on this. She has steadfastly refused psychiatric evaluation for depression in the past or an offer of antidepressants. Dr. Franklin is convinced she is not depressed and is comfortable with her choice, but he and the nursing home are asking for assistance in responding to this request.

DISCUSSION

After prolonged debate, there is a strong professional and judicial consensus that artificially administered fluids and nutrition (AAF&N) are treatments, and thus optional. There is a growing consensus, though not unanimity, that there is no obligation to provide AAF&N when a person is unable to ingest adequate amounts and is terminally ill or severely cognitively impaired (advanced **dementia; persistent vegetative state**). These are not suicides.

It is also accepted by many that a person who is terminally ill and close to death may voluntarily stop eating and drinking when he or she believes the burdens of continued life exceed the benefits. Some consider this to be "rational suicide." In these situations, there is a professional obligation to offer fluids and nutrition and to provide good mouth hygiene, but there is no obligation to forcefully administer fluids and nutrition if the patient is unable or unwilling to swallow.

A person who is not terminally ill who takes his or her life by voluntary dehydration is clearly committing suicide. Some believe all suicide is irrational (based primarily on professional grounds) or immoral (based primarily on religious grounds). Many would accept "rational suicide" by someone who is terminally ill, imminently dying, with unrelievable symptoms, but would consider all other suicides irrational. A few would argue that sometimes suicide by a non–terminally ill person may be "rational" if the person deems the quality of his or her life unsatisfactory. By this they usually mean it is understandable or acceptable rather than implying a moral judgment.

Adequately informed patients with **decision-making capacity** are free to accept or decline any offered treatment, so persons trying to end their life by dehydration would generally be free to decline feeding tubes and intravenous fluids. A good case can be made for involuntarily feeding patients with a treatable depression, but many find it difficult to justify force-feeding those who are not clearly depressed but have decided their quality of life is below their acceptable threshold.

A (California) legal precedent on this question was set in the case of Elizabeth Bouvia, a young woman with severe cerebral palsy and painful arthritis who requested admission to a hospital "to commit suicide" by dehydration. She was instead admitted to a psychiatric ward and was force-fed. A lower court refused to support her request (1983), but the California Court of Appeals found in her favor (1986). When her pain was adequately

239

treated and she was befriended, she chose to eat and remains alive twenty years later.

Providing medical or nursing oversight during this process would not be assisting with a suicide. Assisting with a suicide, not legally permitted in this state, involves providing the means for the hastened death (e.g., a lethal prescription). Though oversight is not strictly illegal, many professionals have moral scruples about providing this because of the unsettled discussion about "rational suicide." If they so choose, they may decline involvement on the basis of professional autonomy regarding matters of conscience.

In this case, the patient has made an assessment that her life is not worth living as a blind person. Though she may claim to be making a rational choice, that choice is sufficiently outside the societal norm (i.e., most blind persons do not take their own lives) to raise serious questions. In addition, though she may not appear to her caregivers to be clinically depressed, her statement of loathing her life likewise raises questions.

RECOMMENDATIONS

1. It is not ethically impermissible[4] to accede to this patient's request for medical and nursing oversight while she takes her life by voluntary dehydration if: (a) she has been adequately assessed and treated for depression or another condition that might be affecting her decision (e.g., something causing other treatable symptoms) and (b) all feasible efforts to enhance her quality of life have been exhausted, including aids for the blind.

2. If any of her professional or personal caregivers are morally uncomfortable with providing care for her during her suicide, they should be excused, and her care should be transferred to others who are willing to provide the requested care.

3. The facility could also decline to provide oversight on either moral, policy, or regulatory grounds (the latter because she may not qualify as a patient who needs what is called a "skilled bed").[5]

4. I purposely chose the wording "not ethically impermissible" rather than "ethically permissible" to indicate that professional standards may support this, but I personally find this action ethically troubling.

5. Beds in nursing homes are usually categorized by funding agencies so that some are for patients who need chronic care that can be provided by professionals with a lower level of training, and others are for "skilled" patients who need short- or long-term care that can only be provided by registered nurses.

FOLLOW-UP

Dr. Franklin met several days later with the patient, her husband, and the facility administrator. The administrator told Mrs. Costello that her suicide by voluntary dehydration might cause trouble for the facility and for Dr. Franklin. After further discussion, she said she didn't want to cause trouble for anyone, so she would not follow her plan. Dr. Franklin will use our recommendations to insist on psychiatric evaluation or assessment by the State Association for the Blind before he honors a future request from her.

COMMENT

Most, but not all, people of faith in the three monotheistic faith traditions consider the intentional taking of one's life to be an immoral affront to the sanctity of human life. Our secular society has for a very long time accepted that suicide is an irrational act that should be prevented when possible. The concept of "rational suicide" has been raised intermittently for centuries, at least since the time of Seneca, a first-century Roman stoic philosopher. The advent of technological innovations that can forestall death has raised questions about the patient's right to stop treatment.[6] This in turn, along with the dramatic rise in personal autonomy, has brought front and center the rediscussion of rational suicide, and indeed the morality and legality of assisting a person in carrying out this lethal act.

In this case, the utilitarian concern raised by the nursing home administrator caused the patient to change her mind. This line of reasoning is clearly not the moral high ground, and it is not clear whether the result suggests some ambivalence on her part or whether she was such a thoughtful soul that she was unwilling to cause difficulty for others. Often patients determined to take their own life will be thoughtful of others, but their commitment to the goal of death is more often paramount.

---

6. This right to refuse treatment (or the right to be left alone) is often misrepresented as a "right to die." This is incorrect. There is no right to die. If there were, then there would be a concomitant duty to help a person to die if he or she wanted to exercise that "right" but was unable to do so unaided.

Case 8.05

QUESTION

Does this patient with early dementia have a "right to commit suicide"?

STORY

George is a sixty-five-year-old man who worked as an engineer for many years, resigning last year when he realized he was beginning to lose his memory. He reports that he decided as a young adult he would end his life if he ever faced the prospect of deterioration to the point of needing to be "warehoused." He would, however, accept treatment for a life-threatening disease (cancer) or be willing to live at home with a disability (stroke). He came to his decision after watching his grandfather die in his nineties after many years of **dementia**, after watching his father die in his eighties after a few years of dementia (including two years in a nursing home), and especially after watching his mother die with **amyotrophic lateral sclerosis** while begging her family to end her life. Though George recognizes that his symptoms are mild, he is concerned that his dementia may progress rapidly, and he doesn't want to wait until he gets beyond the point of being able to take his own life. He greatly fears loss of the ability to communicate and also does not want to be a burden on his family.

He reports that his decision is supported by his second wife of fifteen years, and by his two daughters, who are to arrive today from out of state. He had a son who died of suicide several years ago.

Two days ago George and his wife visited his primary physician to ask if he would come to their home to pronounce him dead and sign a death certificate saying it was a natural death. He indicated that he already had in hand the pills he needed to take his life. His physician declined, and when he understood the imminence of the plan, he reported George to a local mental health agency, because of his obligation to protect a patient from self-harm. They persuaded George to accept voluntary psychiatric admission. He has now been evaluated by the inpatient psychiatric team, which finds him to be articulate, intelligent, logical, and unwavering in his decision. He smiles freely, does not have a depressed affect, but has some signs and symptoms that may be somatic manifestations of depression (insomnia, weight loss, lack of energy). He exhibits mild memory loss, but for both recent and remote events, not only for recent events as might be expected with dementia. The differential diagnosis is early dementia versus depression.[7] Further testing would include neuropsychiatric testing, brain imaging by **MRI**, and a trial of an antidepressant, but the patient declines these.

DISCUSSION

Though our society does not recognize a "right to suicide," a spectrum of beliefs exists about ending one's life. A few suicide advocates argue for an inviolable right to end one's life based on a belief in radical autonomy. Most who support a right to suicide recognize a societal need to protect individuals from self-destruction before they have adequate treatment for a reversible condition such as depression, but would defend the depressed patient's right to suicide if treatment proved to be not satisfactory to the patient. The majority in our society concur that most (some would say all) suicides are "irrational" and should be prevented if possible, even if this requires involuntary treatment. Many, however, argue in support of "rational suicide," defined as the logical choice of people who want to avoid intolerable physical suffering (pain, shortness of breath) for themselves or suffering of others (also called "surcease suicide"). Such "intolerable suffering" is by definition subjective; some would include intolerable psychic or existential suffering.

It is notoriously difficult to prevent "rational suicide" in functional patients who are privately committed to this goal but are able to convince those around them that they are not at risk for taking their own life.

The patient in this case is asking to be left alone to pursue his plans for what he considers a rational suicide. However, his rationality must be questioned because: (a) he acknowledges that depression may look like dementia but denies this could be so in his case, and (b) he admits that if he does have dementia, it is in an early phase, but he will not accept a four-to-eight-week trial of antidepressant therapy.

7. Differential diagnosis is the process that a physician goes through, thinking of all the possible conditions that might account for the patient's signs and symptoms. In this case the physician thinks the way the patient appears may be because he is in the early phase of dementia, or he might instead be suffering from depression. This is an important differential because the latter is treatable in most cases, but dementia cannot be reversed.

RECOMMENDATIONS

1. This patient should be encouraged to consider further evaluation or a trial of an antidepressant. It might be possible to enlist his family to assist with this persuasion. If he continues to refuse, it would be ethically troublesome to release him if his caregivers continue to believe he is at risk for suicide.

2. It would likewise be ethically troublesome to force unwanted treatment on this patient, so if he cannot be persuaded to accept the recommendation, he may require prolonged involuntary admission unless he is able to convince his caregivers that he is no longer a suicide risk.

FOLLOW-UP

George's daughters arrived and were supportive of his position. They were also convinced that he had dementia. Though they did not want to overlook any correctable cause of pseudodementia (other conditions that may look like dementia, e.g., depression), they wanted him to go home and have whatever workup or therapy he needed as an outpatient. He said he might postpone his plan for some time since he understood that he was in the early phase of dementia, and he consented to a six-week trial of antidepressant. He was discharged with follow-up plans in both the psychiatry clinic and the memory disorder clinic. His daughters were to stay with him for four weeks and provide other oversight when they had to leave. About two weeks later it was reported that the patient died out of state.

COMMENT

In retrospect, it seems likely that this patient was committed to his own death, and that he said what was expected of him in order to be released from hospital oversight. It is difficult, if not impossible, to detect or predict this, especially if the patient has family or friends who are willing to collude with him.

Case 8.06

QUESTION

Is it ethically permissible to honor the request of this depressed patient's surrogate to discontinue life support when she has a survivable condition?

STORY

Bonnie is a forty-eight-year-old woman with a long history of psychiatric disability (depression, borderline personality, suicide attempts) and medical problems (diabetes, hypertension, migraine headaches). Last evening she sent a "good-bye" e-mail to a friend. He called 911 and the paramedics found the patient minimally responsive with several empty pill bottles that had contained antidepressants and tranquilizers. She was transported to the emergency department, where she was **intubated**, and then transferred to the medical intensive care unit. After she was treated for a critical cardiac rhythm disturbance, her condition stabilized. It is anticipated she will make a full recovery.

She lives in her own apartment and is reported to have intentionally distanced herself from her family. She completed an **advance directive** three years ago in which she named a friend, Jennifer, as her **agent**, selecting from a list of several options the following instruction: "If I suffer a condition from which there is no reasonable prospect of regaining my ability to think and act for myself, I want only care directed at my comfort and dignity, and authorize my agent to decline all treatment (including artificial nutrition and hydration) the primary purpose of which is to prolong my life."

The patient's agent has requested that her **ventilator** support be stopped and that she be allowed to die, believing this is what the patient would choose. When it was pointed out to the agent that the condition described in the document did not currently exist (i.e., no reasonable prospect of regaining the ability to think and act for herself), she became angry, feeling certain the patient had not properly understood the document and that she would expect not to be treated with "life support" in her current state.

DISCUSSION

Patients, especially those with chronic disability, often write an advance directive either stating what treatments they would or would not want should they become unable to participate in treatment decisions, or naming an agent to speak on their behalf, or both. An agent is morally and legally bound to try to follow the patient's wishes as he or she understands them.

A suicide attempt, whether deemed irrational (most) or rational (occasionally), is almost always viewed as a situation where the patient's prior written or verbal requests for **limitation of treatment** may be overridden. This is virtually always true if the condition is survivable, but may be modulated if the person's condition is thought to be nonsurvivable.

In this case, the patient has a valid advance directive in which she has named an agent and given instructions. However, the conditions offered in the document do not pertain; that is, there is an excellent prospect that she will return to her baseline condition. In addition, her suicidal action negates her prior request for limitation of treatment.

RECOMMENDATIONS

1. It is not ethically permissible to accede to this agent's request to withdraw life support from this patient for the two reasons outlined above.
2. If the patient should suffer an unanticipated complication that makes her prognosis for survival very dismal, this request should be rediscussed.

FOLLOW-UP

Though in restraints, the patient somehow managed to remove her **endotracheal tube**, and she breathed adequately without mechanical assistance. She did not require reintubation, but she did need restraints for a short time. She was subsequently transferred to the psychiatry service on an involuntary basis for continued treatment.

COMMENT

A person takes on a very serious task when completing an advance directive, and that person's agent likewise has a very serious responsibility to see that the person's wishes are carried out. When the agent requests something different from what is written, the physician may have a difficult time deciding which is truly the patient's wish. In this case, even if the agent were able to convince the physician that she knew what the patient really meant, her request would be trumped by the precedent of temporarily setting aside the wishes of a suicidal patient when her condition is reversible.

Case 8.07

QUESTION

Is it ethically permissible to follow this patient's previous request for no artificial feeding when her current condition may be self-induced?

STORY

Darla, age thirty-two, has a history of diabetes, substance abuse, depression, and **Huntington's disease**. She was admitted seven days ago, unresponsive, with an extremely low blood sugar. She has been treated intensively but has not awakened. Neurology workup has been negative for a correctable cause, and the presumptive diagnosis is insulin-induced hypoglycemic **encephalopathy**, possibly self-induced.[8] She has spontaneous movements of all four extremities and her eyes are open but do not fix on any object, and her only response is to painful stimulation (e.g., pinching or pressure over a sensitive nerve). **Limitation of treatment** orders have been written (no resuscitation and no intubation). She is currently maintained on intravenous fluids and mild sedation. A neurology note written yesterday indicated a poor prognosis for significant improvement. Though some late improvement from such a **minimally conscious state** is not unknown, it occurs only very rarely.

She was diagnosed with Huntington's disease over ten years ago, but the manifestations of this devastating disease are so far quite subtle in her

---

8. Her severe brain dysfunction (encephalopathy) was brought on by low blood sugar (hypoglycemia) from an excess of administered insulin, and this may have been self-induced.

case. Her father is fifty-nine, has had this same diagnosis for many years, is in a nursing home out of state, and is reported to be unresponsive. The patient last visited him about four years ago and has been increasingly depressed about her future since that time.

She has had a long history of depressive episodes and substance abuse, with several hospitalizations, some for intentional suicidal overdoses of medications or drugs. She has also had several episodes of low blood sugar, but has responded quickly to treatment each time.

The patient has not completed a written **advance directive**. Her mother, stepfather, and primary physician all report that she has said on several occasions that she would not want to live on life support, would not want to be cared for in a nursing home, and would not want a feeding tube.

DISCUSSION

When a patient is no longer able to participate in treatment decisions, we generally use **substituted judgment** to learn the patient's wishes and values: we try to do what the patient would choose if he or she were able. This may be accomplished by reading the patient's written statement or talking to those who know the patient best. Artificially administered fluids and nutrition are considered medical treatment, and as such are optional; whether to use them or not is based on an understanding of the patient's wishes.

Almost always we honor the previously expressed wishes of a patient who has lost the capacity to participate in treatment decisions. One of the few circumstances where overriding such expressed wishes is felt to be justified is if the patient has attempted suicide and has a reasonable chance of recovering to a condition of reasonable quality of life with continued treatment.

In this case, the patient has a history of repeated suicide attempts, and in fact, her current situation may have resulted from such an act. However, standard treatment has failed to return her to a quality of life she (or most people) would find acceptable. The expectation that this might be achieved with continued support is very small and diminishing with time.

RECOMMENDATION

It is ethically permissible to honor this patient's previously expressed wish to not be maintained with artificially administered fluids and nutrition if there is a reasonable degree of certainty that she is unlikely to recover significant cognitive function.

FOLLOW-UP

Over the next several days, further testing and consultation were undertaken to gain as high a degree of certainty as possible about her prognosis. There were further conversations with extended family, including her brother, a Baptist minister, who came from out of state. When it was concluded that there was no further treatment that might return her cognition, there was consensus among her professional caregivers and her family to withdraw her feeding tube. This was done, she continued to receive good nursing care including mouth care, and she died in eight days.

COMMENT

The analysis and these recommendations here are different from those made in Case 8.06. Even though this patient's current problem was likely the result of a suicide attempt, discontinuation of treatment was deemed justifiable because her best possible outcome was so bleak. This would not have been the case if her prognosis had been better. If she had a reasonable chance of regaining some degree of cognition, even if she might require nursing home care (which she had said she would find intolerable), it would have been ethically obligatory to continue treatment.

Not everyone would agree with the consensus reached in this case that it was acceptable to discontinue this patient's feeding tube. A minority of people of faith, and even a few health-care professionals, do not consider artificially administered fluids and nutrition to be treatment and thus they consider continuation to be morally obligatory. See chapter 6 for further discussion of this important dilemma.

Case 8.08

QUESTION

Is it ethically permissible to continue to restrain this grieving man in order to treat him over his objection?

STORY

Gaston is eighty-five years old and is in the coronary care unit, in restraints, being treated with intravenous medication while shouting, "Just leave me alone and let me die!" He had been in good health until about a year ago when he found a lump in his neck. This was biopsied and found to be a low-grade malignancy of the lymph nodes that had a good chance of being cured with several months of chemotherapy. He began the recommended therapy but stopped about halfway through when his wife was found to have an incurable cancer of her rectum. He had been providing hospice care for his wife at home for the past several months.

Eight days ago he was admitted to the hospital because of dehydration from vomiting and diarrhea. Four days ago, while he was in the hospital, his wife died. His gastrointestinal symptoms cleared, but he was scheduled to go to a convalescent home yesterday for several days of therapy to improve his strength and mobility before he returned home. As his physician was writing the transfer orders yesterday morning, the patient told him that he had tried to strangle himself the night before using the tie to his bathrobe, but he had been unable to pull it tight enough. His nursing home transfer was canceled, and instead a psychiatrist talked with him. The patient agreed to transfer to the hospital psychiatry ward.

Less than twenty-four hours after transfer he developed a life-threatening abnormality of his heart rhythm, and he was transferred to the coronary care unit over his objection. His condition is now stabilized, but he is still objecting loudly.

I spoke with the patient, who said he would still take his life if he were able (by shooting himself, by jumping out the window), and that he saw no reason why the doctors were treating him for a heart condition when he didn't want treatment in the first place, and he was dying of cancer in the second place. He said he had nothing to live for now that his wife was dead. They had married late in life, had emigrated from France, and had no friends or family. He said neither he nor his wife followed any faith tradition, and he had no moral scruples against taking his life.

The consultant spoke with the patient's cardiologist and learned that his rhythm disturbance was under control and that he would merely have to take oral medication to prevent its recurrence. He spoke with the oncologist who had treated the patient's cancer a year ago and learned that the patient was probably already cured, but this could be nearly ensured by his receiving the remainder of his chemotherapy.

DISCUSSION

Some would consider suicide by a person who is terminally ill, suffering, and imminently dying to be rational, but almost everyone considers suicide by a person in the early phase of a life-threatening illness to be irrational. Likewise, only the rare professional would decline to prevent suicide in a person who is recently bereaved.

In this case, the patient's understanding of his condition vis-à-vis his malignancy is incorrect. In addition, his wife (and only friend, according to him) has just died, so he is grief stricken.

RECOMMENDATIONS

1. It is ethically permissible to temporarily protect this man over his objections, even if this requires involuntary readmission to the psychiatry service.
2. His oncologist should talk to him again to clarify his condition and prognosis.

FOLLOW-UP

I told the patient I was going to tell his doctors that it was permissible to treat him over his objections. He reacted with anger. It was further explained to him that (a) his prognosis was much better than he thought, and (b) grief was difficult. Though most people come to a place of recognizing that life will never be the same, they are able to accept that continuation of an adjusted life is acceptable. After he was helped with the initial stages of his grief, and after he had a clearer understanding of his future, if he continued to feel he did not want treatment for his heart condition, he could then choose to discontinue the heart medication.

The patient was transferred to the psychiatry service, received counseling and medication, and three weeks later, about to be discharged, he thanked the physicians and nurses for sticking with him and helping him through his crisis.

COMMENT

Some physicians or ethicists might be uncomfortable promising this patient some degree of control in the not-too-distant future. Certainly we are obligated to protect patients from impulsive decisions that may be detrimental, but once their condition is stabilized, our responsibility diminishes. We may disagree if patients choose to stop a medication (or decline surgery, or whatever might be recommended for their well-being), but there are limits to our ability and authority to exert control over their lives.

Some interesting similarities and differences exist between this case and Case 6.09. Both patients were acutely grieving and were making choices that would end their lives soon. This man has a reasonable prognosis, whereas the woman in 6.09 would continue to have a severely compromised function with a great likelihood of more strokes. It is these differences that led to different recommendations.

Case 8.09

QUESTION

Is it ethically permissible to accept this depressed patient's refusal of evaluation of a suspected malignancy?

STORY

Edith is a seventy-eight-year-old woman who has been chronically depressed for eleven or twelve years, since the death of her husband. She has attempted suicide twice and has had two psychiatric admissions. She has been under the psychiatric care of Dr. Watson for about eighteen months. Because she had exhibited recalcitrant symptoms of depression and increased preoccupation with suicide, Dr. Watson persuaded her to be admitted three weeks ago for electroconvulsive therapy (ECT). She is felt to retain **decision-making capacity** and has consented to ECT three times per week; her affect may have improved somewhat, but she remains suicidal.

During her admission exam she was found to have a large, hard, irregular mass in her right breast that is fixed to the chest wall and has overlying skin redness and swelling. She says it has been present for many years and "is not cancer." Surgery consultation agrees that this is almost certainly malignant, but the patient has refused any further evaluation. Her care team has requested ethics consultation, asking if her refusal should be honored in light of the severity of her depression.

The patient lives independently in an assisted living situation. She has two sons and a sister, but she has been estranged from them for several years.

The patient is alert and conversant. She tried to dismiss discussion of the breast lump, but readily lets me examine her breast. The mass is as described above. When I asked her why she didn't want it evaluated, she said first, "It's not cancer," and after my assertion that it certainly looked like cancer, she said, "Good. Then it will kill me." I said it might very well be slow-growing and would probably not take her life in the near future, but we could have a better idea with a mammogram and biopsy. When I then asked if she would like this information, she consented to both mammogram and biopsy.

DISCUSSION

Patients who retain decision-making capacity are generally free to decline medical interventions, even those that might preserve life. Debate is ongoing over whether suicidal depression precludes this right of self-determination. Clearly there is a societal mandate to protect a depressed person from self-injury and suicide. However, it is less clear whether a depressed person should be allowed to decline treatment necessary to prevent imminent death (e.g., **ventilator** support for respiratory failure) or for possible remote death from disease (e.g., evaluation and treatment of suspected malignancy). The obligation to intervene over a patient's objection decreases as the imminence of harm decreases.

This patient is being protected from suicide while being treated for depression. She does not have an imminently life-threatening medical condition that requires urgent treatment. She probably has a malignancy that may threaten her life in many months or years. Though early diagnosis and treatment of breast cancer may improve the prognosis, her breast mass does not appear to be early since it is already fixed to the chest wall. Therefore, there would appear to be little or no medical advantage to seeking judicial imposition of unwanted investigation and treatment at this time. She has tentatively consented to appropriate workup of this problem.

RECOMMENDATIONS

1. If the patient's tentative consent persists and her caregivers continue to believe she is capable of giving valid consent, it would be ethically permissible to proceed with workup and treatment.

2. Since her breast lump presents no imminent hazard to her life, it would be ethically troublesome to impose unwanted investigation or treatment if she should revoke her tentative consent. In that event, she should periodically be encouraged to reconsider her refusal of medical recommendations as her depression improves. Even if her depression does not improve, if attempts at persuasion by professionals or family are not successful, it would regrettably be most appropriate to honor her refusal and offer her good symptomatic treatment.

FOLLOW-UP

Mammogram and biopsy were done while the patient was in hospital for the ECT. These tests confirmed the diagnosis of advanced breast cancer that was not curable. She declined treatment but said she would reconsider this decision at a later date.

COMMENT

It is very frustrating when a health-care professional encounters a patient who is unwilling to pursue investigation or treatment that would seem to be in her **best interests**. It is doubly so if the patient is also depressed, especially if her refusal appears to be based on her assumption that nonintervention will lead to her death. The question whether it is ethically justified to intervene over her objection revolves primarily on the imminence of harm from nonintervention, and the likelihood of being able to treat the patient's depression and hopefully persuade her to accept recommended testing and treatment.

Case 8.10

QUESTION

Is it ethically permissible to continue to prescribe narcotics for this patient who admits to their misuse?

STORY

Jimmy is a thirty-four-year-old man who has been paraplegic (total paralysis of both legs, but with some residual sensation) for fifteen years since receiving a gunshot wound in his thoracic spine during gang warfare. He has had multiple infections (in his lungs, liver, skin) during this time, and specifically has been troubled by several large and deep decubitus ulcers[9] of his sacral area and on his left hip. These ulcers have caused him significant pain for which opiates[10] have been prescribed intermittently in the past. He has now been in hospital for the past six days to address the worsening ulcers and to improve his pain management. He has a history of "drug-seeking behavior," so his pain management has been under the exclusive care of the pain service for the past six months. It is reported that he told someone in the pain clinic a few weeks ago that he sometimes trades his prescription medication for street drugs.

The patient lives in his mother's home, along with a sister, a brother-in-law, and a baby. The inpatient ward team (nurses, aides) reports that the home is a "crack house" (source of information unknown), further motivating the pain service to switch him to nonopiate analgesics.

His current home-care nurse, however, tells me it is a nice house in a decent neighborhood, and that it is always neat and clean — except for the patient's room, which is always filthy. His mother has told the nurse that she would like to improve his hygiene, but he refuses to allow this and occasionally threatens to hit her. She says she loves him and no one else would be able to care for him as she does. She denies that he uses, or even has access to, illegal drugs.

I met with the patient. He was surly and uncooperative. When I raised the issue of drug diversion, he became angry, said it was a lie, and threatened to have his "home boys" kill me and whoever told me that. He said he had never used any illicit drugs except marijuana.

---

9. A decubitus ulcer is a pressure sore. These skin ulcerations are not infrequent in a patient who is immobilized, especially if he has diminished sensation, and especially if he is unwilling to follow a meticulous schedule of being turned to avoid prolonged pressure in the same location.

10. Opiates are a class of analgesics that have the potential for dependence or addiction, thus also the potential for abuse. Codeine and morphine are included in this class.

DISCUSSION

The ethical tension in this case involves the physicians' duty to relieve the patient's pain and their legal obligation to avoid being involved in illicit use of prescription drugs. Where their primary allegiance lies is dependent on the likelihood that the information about misuse of prescription drugs is true.

If the information cannot be traced, or if on review it appears to have been a flippant remark possibly made to impress the hearer, it would appear that the duty of pain relief overrides this tenuous suspicion. If, on the other hand, the remark was reliably heard and appeared to be true to the hearer, or if there is other evidence to raise the suspicion of diversion of prescription narcotics, then the physicians have an obligation to restrict their prescribing and pursue this suspicion.

RECOMMENDATIONS

1. The patient should not be discharged until this suspicion is investigated.
2. The veracity of the allegation needs to be further investigated by the patient's physicians or by someone skilled in substance abuse. If there appear to be grounds for the suspicion, substance abuse professionals and/or legal authorities should confront the patient.
3. Perhaps a management conference (to include his primary physician, home care nurse, pain management professionals, hearer of the comment in question, mother, and possibly other family members) would help to clarify the issues. An ethics consultant would be willing to participate in such a conference.

FOLLOW-UP

Investigation led his clinicians to suspect the patient was either misusing the prescription drug himself or, more likely, giving or selling it to someone else for recreational purposes. Under the direction of the pain service, his oral medication was switched to methadone, which has minimal abuse potential, and arrangements were made for home delivery of daily medication.

COMMENT

Some of the more challenging ethics consultations have involved providing prescription medication for patients with a history of substance abuse.

Physicians generally do want to provide what is best for their patients, but they also do not want to contribute to the clinical and societal problem of drug abuse.

Case 8.11

QUESTION

Are we obligated to continue to use aggressive treatment for this alcoholic patient with a poor prognosis who has been noncompliant with treatment?

STORY

Rudy is a fifty-two-year-old man with end-stage liver disease from alcohol abuse. He was recently in the hospital with liver failure and hepatic **encephalopathy**. He was discharged home two days ago, but was unable or unwilling to eat or take his medications (including lactulose, a laxative to keep his bowels clear to prevent recurrence of the liver failure). He became increasingly lethargic, and his visiting nurse sent him back to the emergency department yesterday. There his family was given the choice of re-admission for continued full treatment or return home with hospice care. They chose readmission for one more effort at restoration of function. He was admitted with **full code status**, and a nasogastric tube was inserted for administration of lactulose. The admission note indicated a plan to redis-cuss treatment goals with the patient if he became able to converse. Some of his professional caregivers are uncertain about appropriate goals or modalities in this patient with a poor prognosis who has bounced in and out of hospital. He is improved today.

The patient has no written **advance directive**. He has reportedly always requested full treatment in the past when the question has been raised, apparently basing this choice, at least to some extent, on a doctor in Texas telling him five years ago that he would be dead in six months, so he questions dire prognoses.

The patient lives at home and is cared for by his wife with considerable help from visiting nurses and his two siblings. They have three teenage children at home.

I met with the patient, his wife, his sister, and his brother. He is fairly alert (the best he has been in a week, according to his wife). He said, "I am not ready to give up yet." He is willing to accept a nasogastric tube if it is needed short term to try to improve his mental status, but he does not want to use this or any other tube or machine to keep him in a state of unawareness. Everyone agreed that the current goal of treatment is to restore his function sufficiently so that he can go home. If that is not working, all agreed, including the patient, to shift goals to comfort care. The patient is also willing to give his doctors some discretion to use or not use specific modalities based on their assessment of chances of achieving his goal.

DISCUSSION

Patients with **decision-making capacity** should participate as much as possible in the setting of treatment goals, and often in decisions about the use or nonuse of specific treatment modalities. When they are no longer able to participate, their written or previously spoken wishes should be honored. If their condition deteriorates so that their goals or wishes are not achievable, there is no moral obligation to continue those specific treatments.

RECOMMENDATIONS

1. This patient has stated a goal of survival as long as he is not suffering and is able to meaningfully interact with others. He is willing to shift goals from survival to comfort when it becomes clear that this goal is no longer possible.
2. Full treatment to optimize his mental function is appropriate. This includes trying to optimize posthospital care as well.
3. If the patient does not do his part to sustain that goal, that is not sufficient reason to ignore his stated goals; i.e., if he slips into a coma again from willful failure to take his medications, rescue attempts should still be used until they are clearly not working.
4. If or when it becomes clinically clear that it is no longer possible to return him to the level of function he seeks, **limitation of treatment** orders may be discussed with his family and written without his explicit consent.

FOLLOW-UP

He became much more alert over the next few days, able to walk alone and speak clearly. Plans were made for him to go home on lactulose, but he was already talking about trying to reduce the dose after he got home. He wanted to know if he could come back to the emergency department if he gets worse again. I strongly recommended against his changing the dose. He was discharged.

COMMENT

Patients who are addicted to alcohol not infrequently decline recommended treatment. This is troubling, especially if they say they want to live as long as possible. Health-care professionals must sometimes be reminded of their obligation to focus on trying to achieve the goal of patients (survival), even when patients' actions seem to go counter to that goal. The professional should also remind patients of this discrepancy and encourage them to do what appears to enhance their goal.

Case 8.12

QUESTION

What are the ethically permissible treatment options for this man who has consistently expressed a desire to "not be here," and has now made a serious attempt to end his life?

STORY

Jack is a seventy-eight-year-old retired pharmacist with multiple health problems, including painful arthritis, spinal stenosis, and atrial fibrillation; he also has a cardiac pacemaker in place. He has lived in a small house in the country for many decades. His wife died of cancer six months ago. According to his son, he has been threatening to commit suicide for many years because of chronic pain that has not been ameliorated by several medications.

Yesterday the patient acted on those threats. He first rubbed a refrigerator magnet over the area in his chest where his pacemaker sits in an attempt to cause it to malfunction. When this was unsuccessful, he ingested forty-five digoxin tablets (a medication to control his heart rate; it has a high toxic potential, manifested primarily by abnormal cardiac rhythms). He lost consciousness within ten minutes, woke up three to four hours later, and vomited several times. The first thing he said on waking was, "I took forty-five pills," pointing to the bottle beside him. The rest of the day he steadfastly refused to let his family (two sons, one daughter) make any intervention. They are all devoted to him and acceded to his request with great sadness, feeling he was making a sad, but rational, choice because of his chronic unrelieved pain and his loneliness after their mother's death.

This morning the patient felt miserable, and one of the children called his primary physician to report the overdose. The patient agreed to the physician's recommendation to be taken to the emergency department. His serum digoxin level was found to be markedly elevated into the severely toxic range (patient's level was 8.9 nanograms per milliliter; therapeutic level is 1.0–1.5; toxic level is greater than 2.0) and his electrocardiogram showed a markedly abnormal rhythm. He was immediately treated with a drug that binds the digoxin to render it inert until it can be cleared from his system. It is not yet clear if the patient has also suffered a myocardial infarction (heart attack) or whether his **arrhythmias** are all attributable to his digoxin toxicity.

The patient is garrulous and demanding, upset that his suicide attempt was not successful and angry that he is now being treated against his will. His children are torn. They would like him to live longer, but are so supportive of him and so understanding of his terminal frustration that they are inclined to accept his suicide as both rational and inevitable.

DISCUSSION

In contemporary Western society, patient autonomy has been accorded dominance over the other principles of medical ethics — patients have a right to make treatment decisions, and they can accept or refuse any recommended treatment. The dominance of this principle is always questioned and usually overridden when patients try to take their own lives. Some physicians and ethicists, however, are willing to support patient autonomy even in suicidal patients if they believe the patient's reasoning is "rational," that is, consistent with the patient's goals. Others always consider a suicide attempt to be an irrational choice.

This patient has consistently asserted for several years that the quality of his life resulting from multiple medical problems is not satisfactory. He managed to carry on as long as his wife was alive, but has struggled daily for the past six months to retain a sense of purpose and achieve pain control. His family has struggled even more, trying to be supportive of the father they adore, help him to achieve his goals, and maintain their own equilibrium. The threat of suicide has been looming over them all week, and yesterday's attempt has both exhausted them and left them feeling helpless and hopeless.

RECOMMENDATIONS

1. Since this patient's suicide attempt has induced a potentially reversible condition, it is not ethically permissible to accept his refusal of lifesaving treatment.
2. If his condition stabilizes, repeat efforts at pain control should be initiated. Perhaps consultation from Pain Service or Palliative Care would be of benefit.
3. After his pain is better controlled, it might be appropriate to offer grief counseling or to reevaluate him for a treatable depression.

FOLLOW-UP

After a few days in the hospital, the patient's toxic condition was under control and he was convinced by his children to accept the recommended short stay in a convalescent home. He was admitted to a local nursing home under the care of a **palliative care** specialist. He was initially uncooperative and unpleasant. He consented to further treatment of his pain, though he was angrily skeptical that it could be improved. However, within seventy-two hours of transfer, adjustment of his analgesic medication gave him the first extended period of comfort and natural sleep that he had experienced in several years. His disposition improved dramatically over the next two weeks, and he was discharged home in much better spirits.

COMMENT

Ending one's life may seem like "the only thing to do" when no relief from intolerable symptoms seems available. However, most people really do want to go on living. They choose death only when the prospect of living as they are, or as they anticipate being in the near future, is unacceptable.

Most people of faith reject the option of suicide and thus support and encourage efforts of the medical practitioners, counselors, and clergy to address the intolerable symptoms. See "Comment" on Case 8.05.

Case 8.13

QUESTION

Is it ethically permissible to limit treatment in the aftermath of a suicide attempt?

STORY

Tim is a sixty-four-year-old man with a long history of complex regional pain syndrome, a condition of chronic unrelenting pain that is often only minimally relieved with standard and extraordinary pain treatments. In addition, he has multiple medical problems related to toxic inhalation some years ago when he was working as a military medic, and severe debilitation (minimal sleep, poor mobility even in a wheelchair). He attempted suicide by shooting himself in the mouth. The end result, however, was a severely damaged jaw with relative sparing of his vital structures.

The patient completed an **advance directive** six years ago, including a "living will" with the standard wording,[11] and a treatment directive that named his wife as his health-care proxy.

At the time the consultation was requested the patient was sedated and his airway had been **intubated** for protection, so he was not able to participate in decision making. Subsequently, though, he awakened and repeatedly and consistently requested **extubation**. When the ethics consultant arrived in the intensive care unit, the patient had been extubated and was breathing without assistance.

The patient at that time was reporting significant pain, and a pain specialist had recommended a mixture of two potent analgesics that were new

---

11. "If I suffer a condition from which there is no reasonable prospect of regaining my ability to think and act for myself, I want only care directed to my comfort and dignity, and authorize my agent to decline all treatment (including artificial nutrition and hydration) the primary purpose of which is to prolong my life."

to the patient. Over the years he had developed a tolerance for opioid analgesics. At that point the patient was unable to take part in substantive conversation regarding goals of care.

The ethics consultant met with the patient's wife. She described years of chronic pain, met with minimal responsiveness from the medical system and implicit (and sometimes explicit) accusations of drug-seeking behavior. She describes him as sleeping only intermittently, "pacing" at all hours of the night in his scooter, unable to find a comfortable position, and generally not enjoying life at all (as he once did, to the fullest). She strongly requests only comfort measures be offered at this time.

DISCUSSION

There is a "presumption of rescue" in the immediate aftermath of a suicide attempt. Because our culture does not generally accept the notion of "rational suicide," such an attempt is de facto evidence that the patient lacks **decision-making capacity**, and any **substituted judgment** from family or friends might reflect the incapacitated patient's mind-set as well. The dominant ethical consideration thus becomes doing what is best for the patient, and full treatment is indicated.

Most commentators would agree that after the sequelae of the suicide attempt have been treated, the patient's decision-making capacity can be assessed and **limitation of treatment** at that point might be an option. It has been argued, though, that certain other considerations might permit limitation of treatment even in the immediate aftermath of such an attempt:

- characteristics of the underlying depression (i.e., intractable and long-standing, rather than transitory and potentially treatable)
- extrinsic factors influencing the probability of improvement (e.g., additional medical procedures necessary to remedy the effects of a traumatic suicide attempt)
- level of surrogate's certainty as to what the patient would have wanted (e.g., an advance directive composed well in advance of the attempt)
- amount of psychic pain involved in asking the patient to make the decision (e.g., realizing his attempt failed, accepting the increased health problems incurred by the attempt itself, etc.)[12]

12. R. C. Macauley, "The Role of Substituted Judgment in the Aftermath of a Suicide Attempt," *Journal of Clinical Ethics* 18, no. 2 (2007): 111-21.

This case is the exception to the rule, in that it meets all these criteria. The primary basis for moving toward an exclusively palliative course is not the suicide attempt but rather the long-standing and intractable pain the patient is experiencing. In that respect, a shift of goals toward palliation would have carried the same weight had it been made *before* the patient attempted to end his life.

The primary goal at this point should be the patient's comfort, which means aggressive symptom management and limitation of burdensome interventions (such as intubation or **cardiopulmonary resuscitation**, if they were to become necessary). In addition, patients with decision-making capacity can refuse any treatment, even one that is life-sustaining, and if they lack capacity their **surrogate(s)** can refuse it on their behalf. Since artificially administered nutrition and hydration is considered a medical treatment, the patient or his surrogate (if he lacks capacity) may refuse this as well.

RECOMMENDATIONS

1. It is ethically permissible to shift goals to comfort care, which would include orders specifying no cardiopulmonary resuscitation, electro-shock, intubation, dialysis, etc.
2. It is ethically permissible to withhold artificially administered nutrition and hydration, based on the refusal of the patient (or, if he lacks capacity, his surrogate).
3. The goal of care at this point is pain control. If this is not achievable with analgesics alone, the use of sedatives in the context of intractable suffering (i.e., "palliative sedation") may be necessary.

FOLLOW-UP

The patient died peacefully four days later, after having a restful, pain-free night from treatment with opioids and a sedative.

COMMENT

In this case, the patient's suicide attempt was a cry of desperation signaling that he was unable to cope with his chronic condition. His physicians and therapists had tried valiantly for a long time to relieve his symptoms, but had failed. Thus, limitation of treatment with the expectation that he would likely die could be justified in this case where it could not in most cases of attempted suicide, e.g., Cases 8.08 and 8.12, where other things can be done to address the patient's condition.

* * *

Other Cases Addressing Psychiatric Issues ("Mind Failure")

Cases 3.07, 3.08, 3.11, 4.02, 4.08, 4.09, 5.05, 5.08, 5.11, 5.12, 6.07, 6.11, 7.05, 14.01

References on "Mind Failure"

American Psychiatric Association Ethics Committee. *Opinions of the Ethics Committee on the Principles of Medical Ethics.* 7th ed. Washington, D.C.: American Psychiatric Publishing, 1995.

Bloch, S., P. Chodoff, and S. A. Green. *Psychiatric Ethics.* 3rd ed. Oxford: Oxford University Press, 1999.

Browning, D. S., T. Jobe, and I. S. Evison, eds. *Religious and Ethical Factors in Psychiatric Practice.* Chicago: Nelson-Hall, 1990.

Green, S., and S. Bloch. *An Anthology of Psychiatric Ethics.* Oxford: Oxford University Press, 2006.

PART III

CHAPTER 9

Ethical Issues Involving
Cultural and Religious Beliefs

As was mentioned in chapter 1, on ethical foundations, treatment conflicts often arise because of different perspectives, different experiences, different relationships, different emotions, or different loyalties. But the conflicts that seem to generate the most intense discussion are those based on different cultural or religious beliefs. In some situations the conflict arises because the patient's values lead him or her to refuse a treatment that has been recommended by the professionals. The paradigm here is the refusal by Jehovah's Witness patients of most blood products. In other situations the conflict arises because the patient's (or family's) values lead to a requested treatment that the professionals consider inappropriate. This includes families who are waiting for a miracle, those who say that "God will decide," and several other situations.

We sometimes use the term "culture" rather loosely. Let me propose for the sake of our discussion that culture is the complex range of beliefs, values, and attitudes shared and perpetuated by members of a social group. An individual's culture contains many components, including race, ethnicity, language (even dialect), geographic origin, history, art, literature, folklore, food, customs, and of course, religion.

Let me give a simple personal example of cultural differences. A friend of mine, native to New England, had been a missionary in South America for several years. After he returned on deputation, I was talking with him one-on-one. He stepped closer to me, and I stepped back a bit. This dance repeated about three times before he broke into a smile and explained that in South America personal space is smaller than in North America. If different perceptions of personal space can cause misunderstanding and perhaps mild discomfort, think of how misunderstandings about health and sickness, life and death, and life after death can contribute to conflicts in health care.

The cultural beliefs and values of non-Westerners may require using a different standard for **surrogates** from what is accepted in our Western culture (see Case 9.01), and may imply different rules about disclosure of information (see Case 9.03). Also, cultural differences may include beliefs that are unfamiliar and even uncomfortable to health-care professionals in North America (see Case 9.02). Sometimes it is possible to compromise in situations where cultural beliefs would require different management than the North American standard (see Case 11.07).

Religion is one of the major components of an individual's culture, and religious beliefs often lead a person to refuse or request specific treatments. Religious beliefs should sometimes trump personal preferences (autonomy-based) or shared ideals (community-based). This is because they are more than culturally determined; they are transcendent, that is, derived from divinity. Sometimes these derived beliefs are codified in the sacred writings or teachings of a faith tradition (see Case 9.11), and sometimes they are claimed as a personal revelation directly from Yahweh, God, Allah (see Case 9.07).

Admittedly, many evil beliefs and horrific actions have been attributed to religion — from the Inquisition, to slavery, to the Ku Klux Klan, to ethnic cleansing, and beyond. But these distortions of revealed wisdom do not invalidate all religious belief. An individual coming from an anthropocentric (person-centered as opposed to a theocentric) worldview could seriously question the validity of religious beliefs that lead individuals or groups to such horrible ends. But in the name of tolerance, these same individuals who view autonomy as the summum bonum should at least be willing to consider religious beliefs rather than dismissing them out of hand. While not determinative, religiously based claims should not be automatically dismissed as mystical, nonscientific, or irrelevant.

Let me propose that religiously based claims that, when compared to orthodox beliefs of the individual's faith tradition, appear to be idiosyncratic or unique to the claimer should be accorded the same weight as autonomy-based beliefs. As a second tier, if the claim comports with the beliefs of a sect or denomination but not necessarily with those of one of the major monotheistic religions (e.g., the Jehovah's Witness beliefs about avoiding blood products), it should be given more weight than an idiosyncratic or autonomy-based claim. And finally, if it is consistent with a doctrine of one of the major faith traditions, it may sometimes deserve trumping weight.

I recognize, and continue to struggle with, the differences between religiously based decisions adults make for themselves and those they make for their children. I do not have a quick or easy answer. But I do know that my religious beliefs are very important to me. And I would be loath to have a physician or an ethicist or a judge say, "Your beliefs do not count. You cannot care for your children as you see fit but must do it as we see fit." Yes, I have (reluctantly) followed the societal mandate and sought a court order to impose transfusion on an infant of Jehovah's Witness parents, but only after encouraging the attending physician to go the extra mile to try to preserve the family beliefs if there was any way possible, even if that entailed some risk to the child of a prolonged stay in the intensive care unit, or other nonlethal complications.

Cultural beliefs are important because they are part of an individual's shared heritage. Religious beliefs are important because they are (sometimes at least) transcendent. Let us look at some real-life clinical situations where differing cultural or religious belief led to ethics consultation.

Case 9.01

QUESTION

How aggressive should we be in further management of this Korean man with very poor prognosis? Who is his appropriate surrogate?

STORY

Mr. Kim, age sixty-four, and his second wife (of eight years) are Koreans visiting relatives in the United States. Six weeks ago they were involved in a single-car accident in which Mr. Kim was seriously injured but his wife was unhurt.

Mr. Kim was admitted alert and oriented with multiple injuries including a closed-head injury and a severe crush injury of the chest. The day after the accident his condition deteriorated and a head **CT scan** showed evidence of bleeding into the brain with increased pressure on one side. This pressure was reduced with surgical drainage, but after surgery he was in a coma, had loss of muscle tone on his right side, and required a **ventilator** to help him breathe.

In the intervening six weeks he has had multiple medical problems, including generalized infection, pneumonia, seizures, and cardiac **arrhythmia**. He has had a **tracheostomy** and placement of a permanent feeding tube. He has now been off the ventilator for two weeks and is receiving oxygen by mask, but he has persistent pneumonia with copious secretions, which has put him in the intensive care unit (ICU). He is on two antibiotics and has no fever at present. His neurological status has remained unchanged for the past few weeks with a stable Glasgow Coma Scale of 6.[1] He is somnolent and responds only to pain, but occasionally has spontaneous movement of his left side. Three weeks ago a specialist in rehabilitation medicine said he might be a candidate for intensive rehabilitation if his medical conditions stabilized. If this should happen, his long-term neurological outcome remains uncertain, but almost certainly involves significant disability. The ICU team recommends a **do-not-resuscitate order** (DNR order) be written, believing more aggressive treatment would be inappropriate if his condition should deteriorate further.

The social worker reports that the patient's wife is younger than he and is not close to his family. She is staying with friends and has filled out papers indicating intent to stay in the United States, making him eligible for Medicaid. Mr. Kim's only son from his first marriage visited from Korea for a few days, but has returned home.

When approached by the ICU team about further management options, Mrs. Kim was uncertain of goals and preferences and wanted to consult with others. The physicians and nurses requested an ethics consultation for guidance in decision making for this patient.

I spoke with the patient's wife using a local Korean physician as translator. She said the patient is a retired business executive and would not want to be a burden on his family or on society. She realizes that he is currently suffering. She was unable or unwilling to say what she thought he would choose in such a situation. Mrs. Kim says she has great respect for the doctors involved in the care of her husband and she trusts them to make the right decisions for her husband. When asked how she would feel if the doctors decided not to be aggressive in treatment of further complications, she did not directly answer. She wishes that she were not being asked to make such heavy decisions for him.

---

1. The Glasgow Coma Scale is a measure of brain function often used serially in head injury patients. The maximal score is 15, the minimum score is 3. A score of 6 indicates a severe brain injury, though it is not useful in predicting long-term outcome.

With Mrs. Kim's permission and in her presence, I spoke on the phone with Pastor Pang from the Korean church Mrs. Kim has been attending in the United States. He said that in Korean culture the eldest son is responsible for caring for parents and his decisions take precedence over those of the wife, especially a second wife. He said he had advised Mrs. Kim to request continued treatment, hoping for a miraculous recovery, since the patient is not a believer.

Mrs. Kim reported the following day that she had spoken by phone with her husband's son in Korea and he told her it was all right for her to make medical decisions with the advice of Pastor Pang. When she told him that the pastor was advising continued aggressive care, he encouraged her to follow that advice.

DISCUSSION

Decisions for a patient without **decision-making capacity** should be made by the **surrogate** after hearing adequate information about diagnosis, prognosis, and treatment options from the patient's care team and after counsel from supportive people in the surrogate's life. Surrogates must use their best judgment of what the patient would desire if able to communicate. If we have no indication of what the patient would want, as might be the case with a younger wife of only eight years, the decision should be made using the **best interests** standard — a standard that is much more difficult to determine.

By Korean cultural mores, Mr. Kim's son is responsible for his care, but he agrees to allow Mrs. Kim to make decisions. She prefers not having to make these decisions and is looking to a pastor for advice. He, in turn, is advising aggressive care, hoping to allow time for a physical miracle to occur, and allowing time for a spiritual discussion and decision.

RECOMMENDATIONS

1. Since (a) the patient is not imminently dying and might continue in his current condition for some time, since (b) he has a small chance of further neurological improvement, and since (c) his current suffering is not extreme, it is ethically permissible to follow the pastor's advice for the near future and aggressively treat treatable complications.
2. If, however, a new situation develops that the ward team believes is not remedial, there is no moral obligation to provide futile therapy, and

aggressive management of such a condition could ethically be withheld. For example, if two or more physicians believe the patient could not survive a cardiac arrest, it would be permissible to enter a DNR order after appropriate documentation of the reasoning behind it and after informing his wife.

3. I do not believe there to be an obligation to provide medically unreasonable care to a patient in order to allow time for a miracle. My understanding of God's miraculous interventions is that they are not dependent on our actions, but are truly supernatural.

FOLLOW-UP

The patient was given continued full treatment for another four weeks. He had no neurological improvement and developed an overwhelming infection. The ICU team recommended withdrawal of life-sustaining treatment at that time. Mrs. Kim and Pastor Pang consented, and the patient died.

COMMENT

In caring for patients from another culture, we must avoid automatically using our cultural standards in determining who has the appropriate authority to make decisions for an incapacitated patient. In some situations we may need to protect a patient whose known wishes or best interests are being overruled by the surrogate. But in situations with a poor prognosis and unknown patient wishes, it is appropriate to look to the culturally determined surrogate for guidance.

Prolonging treatment that seems inappropriate to professional caregivers may be permissible in some situations, for example, if conditions (a) through (c) mentioned above apply. Spiritual counsel from clergy of a similar faith background may (or may not) help sort out our obligation to patient or family. This is often more difficult if the patient and his family have differing beliefs.

Case 9.02

QUESTION

Is it permissible to honor a request from this dying Gypsy's husband that ignores the basic principles of surgery?

STORY

Maria is a thirty-one-year-old Gypsy woman from eastern Europe who came to the emergency room three weeks ago with abdominal pain. The cause was not immediately clear, and she was admitted for observation by Dr. Newman, the surgeon on call. He detected some distrust and suspicion from the patient's husband, several friends, and relatives who accompanied them, and from the man introduced as the tribal chieftain. After three days of nonspecific findings on physical and laboratory examination, Maria suddenly worsened, suggesting that she had some life-threatening abdominal condition. When Dr. Newman spoke with her husband and the tribal chieftain, they very reluctantly gave consent for exploratory surgery.

The surgery revealed that her appendix had been situated in an uncommon position, behind her colon, making the diagnosis of appendicitis difficult. The inflamed appendix had perforated and formed an abscess, and the abscess was now leaking, causing extensive peritonitis. Much of the inflamed and dead tissue was removed and a surgical drain was placed. When her husband and the chieftain were informed of her very serious condition, they became hostile and threatening.

Over the next two and one-half weeks, Maria experienced just about every conceivable complication: respiratory failure, **sepsis**, pneumonia, further abscesses requiring two more surgeries with placement of multiple drains, and abnormal bleeding. Then her kidneys began to fail. This morning, when told that everything possible was being done for her but that it looked as if she would probably die, the chieftain loudly insisted that her multiple surgical drains be removed. Dr. Newman requested an ethics consultation because honoring this request would eliminate the very slim chance that Maria might survive.

DISCUSSION

In North American society, when a patient is incapacitated, the physician seeks a **surrogate** decision-maker and turns to family, most commonly the spouse, for consent to treatment. In some societies the authority for such consent is deferred to or shared with others, for example, a tribal chieftain, as in this case. This unusual arrangement does not present a problem in this case because the husband is present and is not only willing but also anxious to follow the wishes of the chieftain. It is not clear, of course, that the patient would make this request if adequately informed about the likely outcome.

Again, the standard in our society is that the patient's autonomy (or the surrogate's **substituted judgment** for the patient's autonomy) generally trumps. But not always. If the request or refusal falls outside the appropriate standard of care, the physician may seek a second opinion and may even consider trying to impose treatment contrary to the request.

In this case the surgeon is pretty certain the patient will not survive regardless of what is done. He knows the family is hostile and threatening and would like to not inflame the situation any further. In addition, there is the issue of professional liability; if he removes the drains as requested, he might be blamed for contributing to the patient's death if he is sued for malpractice.

The ethics consultant met with Maria's husband and the tribal chieftain to make sure they understood her condition and the consequences of their request to remove the drains. He asked them why they wanted the drains removed. They stared incredulously, as if it should be obvious, and said, "If she dies with extra holes in her body, her spirit will escape and have no place to live. That is worse than death." Further discussion led to the compromise outlined in the recommendations below.

RECOMMENDATIONS

1. It is appropriate to leave the surgical drains in place.
2. Equipment to remove the drains and close the drain sites should be maintained at her bedside at all times, and house staff on duty should be informed of the urgency of recommendation 3.
3. If and when her heart stops, the drains should be removed and the drain sites closed within five minutes.

FOLLOW-UP

Maria's condition did not improve. A **do-not-resuscitate order** was placed on her chart. She lived for another forty-eight hours. When her heart stopped, an intern was summoned to pronounce her dead and to remove the drains and sew closed the several drain sites. This was accomplished in less than five minutes. Her husband and the chieftain were distressed at her death but seemed content with the process.

COMMENT

As in Case 9.01, it was appropriate to allow a nonrelative surrogate to play a role in this patient's decision. It was not problematic here, since her husband was willing to share this role.

Whenever a patient or surrogate refuses recommended treatment or requests treatment felt by the professional caregivers to be inappropriate, it is imperative to determine the reason for the refusal or request. The answer to this question may reveal some serious misunderstanding, or, as in this case, it may reveal differing cultural beliefs or values.

Case 9.03

QUESTION

Should we (may we) tell this Hispanic man his prognosis over the objection of his family?

STORY

Jesus is a fifty-four-year-old Hispanic man from Guatemala who was admitted one week ago for treatment of **congestive heart failure** and evaluation of thrombocytopenia.[2] He first became ill over two years ago, at which time he migrated to the United States to live with family and to receive medical treatment. He was found to have an underlying malignancy of his bone marrow (multiple myeloma), very poor heart muscle function, poor kidney function, and depression. He is alert and communicative, but he speaks only Spanish.

---

2. Thrombocytopenia means a low number of blood platelets, small components of blood that are an important part of the coagulation process. Thrombocytopenia generally results from poor bone marrow function, and it places the patient at risk for abnormal bleeding.

Dr. Ashwal, his medical resident, reports that his prognosis for survival is six months or less, but the patient is not aware he is dying because the family does not want him to be told. They say it would make him more depressed and he would not want to know. Dr. Ashwal believes that the patient has a right to know his diagnosis and prognosis and that he has an obligation to inform him.

DISCUSSION

The past thirty or forty years have witnessed a marked shift in Western medicine from the vast majority of physicians not telling patients when they were dying to the vast majority telling patients about their terminal diagnosis and prognosis. The consensus in our society today is that patients have a right to know such information. In addition, most physicians feel more comfortable with the informed patient who participates in his treatment decisions. However, the patient's right to know does not automatically translate into a duty to inform.

A very small minority of patients still prefer more paternalistic health care, may not want to know their diagnosis and prognosis, and may want their physician to make the treatment decisions without their input. Such patients tend to be older or from cultures that do not emphasize individual self-determination as American culture does. Thus patients also have a right to be uninformed.

It is possible that this family is right, that the patient does not want to be told of his prognosis. However, it is also possible that the family does not want the patient to know because they expect it would make their communication with him more difficult. The morally significant item is not what the family thinks the patient wants to know, but what he himself wants to know.

RECOMMENDATIONS

1. The ward team should communicate with the patient's primary physician to see if the patient has been informed about his diagnosis and prognosis and whether he has indicated that he does not want to know this information.
2. If the ward team thinks the patient may have incomplete information and does not learn that he has specifically requested to remain uninformed, (a) they should tell the family that they want to give the pa-

tient the opportunity to ask questions but they will not force unwanted information on him; and (b) they should approach the patient
(through a medically trained, nonfamily translator, but preferably
with family present) with open-ended questions such as: What is your
understanding of your illness? Do you have any questions about your
treatment? Would you like your family to continue to make treatment
decisions, or would you like to participate? Is there anything else you
would like to know from us?

3. If it is learned from the primary physician or from the patient that he
   does not want to be informed about his diagnosis or prognosis, the
   chart should be clearly marked with this information. While it is difficult to honor such a request in a large teaching hospital setting, it may
   be workable in this case because of language limitations.

FOLLOW-UP

The patient's primary physician reported that the patient had been under
the care of a Hispanic oncologist who had told him that he had an infection in his bone marrow that required periodic regular treatment with intravenous medication. He was not aware of his prognosis. Dr. Ashwal sat
down with the patient, with his family present, and through a hospital
translator told him about his current test results and status and asked him:
(a) "Has anyone told you what to expect from this disease?" His answer:
"No." (b) "Do you want to know what is likely to happen or would you
rather just wait and see what happens?" Answer: "I'd rather wait and see."
(c) "Do you want your family and doctors to continue to make treatment
decisions, or would you like to be consulted?" Answer: "You can talk with
them."

COMMENT

When faced with situations like this, we may be tempted to feel culturally
superior, believing we have advanced to a higher plane. However, the role
of family in protecting patients from bad things, including bad news, is an
important cultural value that we shouldn't ignore. It is probably true in
those situations, as it was in our own culture prior to the changes in the
1960s, that patients really do know or suspect their poor prognosis, but if
they do not expect to be informed, it is culturally arrogant for us to force
this information on them.

There may be an occasional situation where major decisions must be made with significant trade-offs of survival, disability, etc., in which we should strongly encourage patient participation. But if the patient indicates a desire for others to make such decisions, we should honor that choice.

Case 9.04

QUESTION

Should we go to court to prevent this Samoan man's family from taking him home against medical advice?

STORY

Tuiasosopo is a thirty-nine-year-old Samoan agricultural worker who was admitted seven weeks ago after two weeks of headache with intermittent nausea and vomiting, and blindness for the twenty-four hours prior to admission. He was found to have cryptococcal meningitis[3] and has been treated with two standard antibiotics for this uncommon infection (amphotericin given intravenously and flucytosine by mouth). Initially he improved gradually, witnessed in weekly testing of his spinal fluid and considerable improvement in his mental status. He was nearing the end of his six-week course of treatment when, one week ago, he suffered a stroke. This precipitated vomiting that precluded retention of his flucytosine for several days. The spinal fluid test has subsequently worsened, and his mental status is again severely depressed. It is suspected that his body may not be adequately fighting this infection because of underlying immunosuppression,[4] but no explanation for this has been found.

The patient has lived in this country for two years, is married, and has one child, a six-month-old son. He has been employed as a farm worker but has no health insurance. He has qualified for emergency Medicaid cov-

---

3. A life-threatening infection around the brain, in this case caused by an encapsulated yeast rather than by the more typical bacteria or virus.

4. A decrease in the body's ability to resist or fight infection; can be caused by many things including illness (e.g., diabetes), infection (e.g., AIDS), drugs (e.g., steroids).

erage for this hospitalization only. He has a large and supportive extended family. A brother (with whom the patient and wife live) is the family spokesperson.

The patient started asking to go home early in his course of therapy. He consented to stay because Medicaid declined to cover home intravenous therapy. He was receptive to conventional therapy but did refuse his fifth weekly spinal tap. When told that the test was necessary to monitor improvement, he agreed to a final one at the end of his six weeks of therapy.

Since his recent setbacks, his family has asked to take him home to pursue ethnic treatments (application of leaves and lotions to his skin; taking of homemade herbal mixture by mouth), believing that hospital treatment has failed to cure him. They have not been antagonistic. Part of their cultural beliefs is that spirits of deceased relatives cause illness and/or failure to respond to conventional therapy. They also put faith in dreams, and the family reports that some dreams about this patient and his course of illness have come true.

Psychiatric consultation has confirmed that the patient does not now have **decision-making capacity**. The infectious disease consultant states that he will surely die if he leaves the hospital, and may die even with continued treatment. The most recent neurology note states that his prognosis is guarded, even with treatment, since he is not responding to current therapy, presumably on the basis of immunosuppression. His vision will not improve, and his cognitive recovery is questionable. On exam, he is somnolent and appears to be in no distress.

DISCUSSION

We traditionally allow competent patients to refuse treatment, even life-saving treatment, as long as they understand the consequences of their decision. We are more reluctant to honor such requests from **surrogates**. When working with surrogate decision-makers, the primary questions are: (1) Is the proxy making the decision the patient would make? and (2) Is the proxy acting in the patient's **best interests**? It is often helpful to articulate the goals of therapy before judging a particular decision about a particular modality.

These matters become even more complex when dealing with patients from another culture. Requests for unorthodox therapies can sometimes be accommodated without compromising conventional therapy; at other times this is not possible.

This patient (and his family) apparently chose a goal of cure and accepted conventional medical therapy. Now that he has worsened in spite of therapy and has lost decision-making capacity, his caring family still want to pursue that goal of cure through other means. At the same time, the care team believes that the possibility of cure (restoration of previous level of impaired function) with continued therapy is fading.

RECOMMENDATIONS

1. If the proposed ethnic interventions are not recognized as toxic and can be administered in hospital in conjunction with continuation of conventional therapy, this option should be offered to the family. If this is acceptable to them even for a few days, his prognosis may become even more clear.

2. In light of his poor prognosis for recovery (and for survival) even with continued therapy, if (1) is not possible, or if his family insist on his discharge, a nonadversarial meeting with them should be held in an effort to determine whether the patient would choose this move. They must clearly realize that it is the care team's understanding that he will die if they take him home. If the care team is convinced that the family is making a truly informed **substituted judgment**, it would be ethically permissible to allow them to take him home **AMA**.

3. If this cannot be determined, or if the responsible physicians are not willing to do this, the only alternative would be an adversarial court proceeding.

FOLLOW-UP

The patient's **neurologist** permitted the family to apply the topical therapies but could not be convinced by the family or the nurses to allow the internal herbal mixture. The patient initially seemed to show some improvement and was a bit more alert. However, his fever continued and his kidney function deteriorated, probably from the prolonged use of amphotericin. The spinal fluid tests monitoring his progress initially improved, then bounced up and down. His mental capacity also fluctuated considerably. Phone consultation with a nationally known expert in cryptococcal infections offered no other options. The patient's family considered flying him back to Samoa, but the cost was prohibitive. Nearly four months after the consultation (over five months after admission), he was found unresponsive in bed. No resuscitation was attempted.

COMMENT

Would it have been better to allow his family to take him home, or at least to allow the administration of the herbal mixture in hospital? It is difficult to know. The administration of unknown chemicals might have adversely affected the antibiotics, worsened his failing renal function, or caused other unexpected side effects. The chemicals might have had no effect at all. Could they possibly have helped? While this seems unlikely, in a patient with a very poor prognosis it might have been helpful to the family as they looked back on the sequence of events to be able to think they had fulfilled their duty to the patient.

Case 9.05

QUESTION

Must we continue painful therapies in this dying Muslim child at the insistence of her father?

STORY

Basha'ir is a six-year-old girl in an intact, devout Muslim family. She was found to have an incurable malignancy of her spinal cord (ependymoma) twenty months ago and had noncurative surgery to alleviate some of her symptoms. When the tumor recurred eight months ago, she again had surgery to reduce the bulk of the tumor in another attempt to reduce her symptoms, realizing that she was terminally ill.

Her parents have cared for her at home, managing her pain, paralysis, incontinence, and seizures with help from visiting nurses. Two months ago she developed respiratory problems requiring home oxygen. Her condition gradually deteriorated, and two weeks ago she was readmitted because of increasing respiratory distress and diminishing awareness. She initially received palliative therapy,[5] but her father insisted she be transferred to the

---

5. Palliative therapy has a goal of patient comfort and dignity rather than patient survival.

intensive care unit for maximal therapy, even though he recognized no more therapy was available to slow the tumor. She was **intubated** and given **ventilator** support, but her pulmonary status has progressed to **adult respiratory distress syndrome**, which, in her situation, is irreversible. Her nurses feel she is suffering needlessly and are suggesting that her life support be withdrawn.

Her physicians are convinced she will never awaken or be able to breathe on her own. Her oncologist, **pulmonologist**, and intensive care specialist have all asked her father to allow withdrawal of life support, which they believe is merely postponing her inevitable and imminent death and prolonging her suffering. He maintains that "Only Allah can take a life," and as her father, he feels it is his responsibility to do everything possible to postpone death. He is also concerned that increasing her doses of morphine to treat her suffering may shorten her life.

I met with the patient's father, the intensive care physician, and a Muslim pediatrician who understood both the religious tenets and the therapeutic limitations. After prolonged discussion her father recognized that she was already on maximal ventilator settings, and that when her heart stopped, it would be because of insufficient oxygen, and that could not be reversed with **cardiopulmonary resuscitation. Limitation of treatment** orders were agreed upon as outlined in the recommendations below.

DISCUSSION

Vitalism is the belief in the moral imperative to continue biological life as long as it is physically possible, regardless of the quality of that life. When based on religious belief, it is often called theological vitalism, and usually comes from a focus on the sanctity of human life and the sovereignty of the Divine. Theological vitalism may be held by some, but not all, individuals in fundamentalist sects of Judaism, Christianity, and Islam. When a patient or **surrogate** holds this stance, failure to give maximal life-prolonging therapy incurs moral culpability.

Health-care professionals have a professional obligation to preserve human life and postpone death when that is possible and desired by the patient or surrogate. Recognition of the inevitability of death, however, allows decisions to limit death-postponing therapies when desired by patient or surrogate. In addition, professionals have a concurrent obligation to reduce suffering. Occasionally, as in this case, these two obligations conflict. In general, health-care professionals recommend treatment to reduce suffering over treatment to postpone inevitable and imminent death.

In this case the professionals were able to convince the patient's father of the moral necessity of trying to maximize her comfort. They were, in turn, convinced by her father of the moral necessity of postponing her death as long as was possible, somewhat diminishing their frustration.

RECOMMENDATIONS

1. It is ethically permissible to continue to provide full death-postponing measures; however, a **do-not-resuscitate order** may be written.
2. Efforts to maximize the patient's comfort should be used. Since she is on full ventilatory support, there should be no concern about hastening her death from the generous use of opiates.
3. Her parents should continue to receive support from the chaplaincy and social service department.

FOLLOW-UP

The patient received increased dosing with morphine and appeared to her nurses to be less uncomfortable. She progressed to cardiac arrest eleven days after the ethics consultation. Her parents and professional caregivers felt satisfied with the sequence of events.

COMMENT

When confronted with a patient or surrogate who stakes a vitalistic claim, it is important for professionals to focus on the goals of therapy rather than on the specific modality of therapy in question. When the vitalism comes from religious belief, it is imperative for the professionals to clearly understand the tenets of the faith. This may often be enhanced by having a religious interpreter. In addition, the presence of someone from the same faith tradition as the patient may defuse some adversarial situations.

Occasionally, it may be possible to discuss other tenets of the patient's faith that may balance the one under focus. For example, when the focus is on the sanctity of human life, a discussion of the finitude of life may help clarify the situation. Then again, it may not. This could be perceived as coercive, so must be used judiciously if at all.

Case 9.06

QUESTION

Must we continue the ventilator in this young woman who is dying if her parents continue to insist upon it, anticipating miraculous intervention?

STORY

Adina is a nineteen-year-old Hispanic female who was found to have an incurable brain tumor *(posterior fossa medulloblastoma)* seven months ago. She had noncurative surgery to remove the bulk of the tumor, surgical placement of a shunt to reduce **intracranial pressure**, insertion of a permanent feeding tube, radiation therapy, and chemotherapy. Although she had several medical complications, she was able to go home.

She was admitted from clinic two weeks ago because of weakness and weight loss. She has had further chemotherapy and aggressive therapy of her medical problems. Plans were being made for discharge home when she developed continuous seizures *(status epilepticus)*, and she had a respiratory arrest five days ago. The seizures were controlled with some difficulty, but she has had no spontaneous efforts at breathing, so has remained on the **ventilator** since then. Repeat **MRI** showed diffuse cerebral involvement with tumor and **herniation of the brain stem**. She has remained comatose, but she does not meet the criteria for declaration of brain death.

We do not know the patient's desires about aggressiveness of therapy. Her parents have been very attentive and have been informed that she is imminently dying. They were at first insistent on all possible treatment, but one week ago they agreed to a **do-not-resuscitate order**. She has continued on the ventilator, antibiotics, seizure meds, antihypertensives, and nutrition. Dr. Shuck, the neurosurgeon, reports that the family's reluctance to withdraw the ventilator is "because we are Christians." They are convinced that God is able to perform a miracle that will allow their daughter to live, even though the doctors are convinced she is dying. They are devout Roman Catholics and have been ministered to by both the hospital chaplain and their own priest. The parents are also grieving the death of the patient's paternal aunt, which occurred several weeks ago.

DISCUSSION

Whether to continue therapy deemed inappropriate by the physician but requested by a patient's **surrogate** depends on two primary factors: whether use of that therapy will add to the patient's burden, and whether nonuse of that therapy will add to the surrogate's burden. Since the patient's **best interests** are preeminent, if there was consensus on the care team that continued ventilation and support were causing Adina further pain and suffering that could not be relieved, it would be appropriate to make a unilateral clinical decision to withdraw therapy. Since it seems unlikely that she is sensate, this is probably not justified.

If the patient's best interests are not being violated by continued treatment, the burden to the family brought on by withdrawal of therapy must be considered. If they believe that it would be immoral to stop, therapy should be continued until they come to understand that this is not so because of the inevitability and imminence of death. If they are hoping for a miracle, they should be gently confronted with the reality that we must use reasonable medical judgment in making clinical decisions. Further, although God is able to intervene supernaturally when he chooses, he does not require our cooperation to produce miracles; he can perform them even after biologic death.

Other factors that might come into play if prolonged support were a possibility include the effect on the morale of the care team and the cost to society of continued care.

RECOMMENDATIONS

1. If the team in the intensive care unit (ICU), neurology, and oncology all agree that further therapy is inappropriate, that she is suffering because of it, and that this suffering cannot be relieved, the family should be told firmly, but compassionately, that her therapy will be discontinued at a specified time.
2. If the ICU team, neurology, and oncology agree that further therapy is inappropriate but that her suffering can be controlled, the family should be given a firm recommendation that therapy be discontinued (versus asking permission to do it). If they are insistent that the ventilator not be stopped, their specific reasons should be ascertained. (a) If they believe it would be immoral to stop, their own priest should be asked to join a management conference. (b) If they are awaiting a

miracle, the above reasoning may help them to better understand the ICU team's position.

3. If there is agreement about limitation of therapy to comfort measures, everything may be stopped except good nursing care and seizure and pain medication.

FOLLOW-UP

Three days after the consultation, the patient made some respiratory effort. She was gradually **weaned** from the ventilator over the next forty-eight hours. However, she slipped back into respiratory failure and was **intubated** again fewer than twenty-four hours later. One week later her blood pressure dropped and did not respond to standard treatment. The following day her heart stopped.

COMMENT

The belief in miracles is common in all three monotheistic faith traditions, and is based on a belief in divine sovereignty and omnipotence. Some believe that God performed miracles in antiquity but does not now. Others believe in and often see miracles all around them.

A belief in God's ability to miraculously intervene in seemingly hopeless human situations should not, however, translate directly into an expectation of a miracle in a given situation. Miracles are rare, by definition. A conversation about this is infinitely more difficult if the believer also believes that God's performance of the miracle is contingent on his or her faith and actions, as will be seen in the next case.

Case 9.07

QUESTION

Is it ethically permissible to limit therapy for this infant over the objection of his parents, who insist God told them he will survive?

STORY

Joshua is a four-month-old boy who was admitted to the intensive care unit soon after birth with diagnoses of **Down syndrome** and congenital heart disease. At six weeks of age, because of **congestive heart failure** and failure to thrive, he had his first surgery.[6] He has had two subsequent surgeries for septic breakdown of this original repair. In addition, he has had repeated bouts of **sepsis** with organisms resistant to most antibiotics and progressive multiple organ system failure. He has been on a **ventilator** for several weeks and is also on peritoneal dialysis, drugs to sustain his blood pressure, **total parenteral nutrition**, and multiple antibiotics. At present his white blood count is markedly elevated (118,000)[7] without an obvious source of infection. He receives frequent sedation because the oxygen content of his blood falls when he is agitated.

On examination, his abdomen is distended (from dialysis), he is on a ventilator, and he has multiple intravenous and arterial lines. He responds to stimulation but is sedated. His nurse reports that he responds to and withdraws from painful procedures.

Dr. Laska reports that the family is devoted and has consistently requested that "everything" be done, but when recently informed that Joshua's prognosis for survival is very poor and that it will be impossible to **wean** him from the ventilator, they have begun to consider limitation of therapy.

I met with his mother. She is a special-education teacher, has two other children, and has a strong Pentecostal faith (shared by her husband and parents). She is grateful for Joshua's care. He was named for an Old Testament leader, and his mother believes that many Scripture references to Joshua now apply to her son. She says God has told her that he will get better, and she believes that he has survived this long because of her unwavering faith. She does not expect indefinite life support for him, but she is at present unwilling to put a time limit on continued efforts to prolong his life. She says God will tell her if and when it is time to limit therapy. While she believes that prolonged ventilation would be an unacceptable quality of life for him, she does not feel that this will be necessary. She does say she would want treatment stopped if he were to be declared brain dead. She also does not desire any further surgery.

6. Repair of a persistent atrioventricular canal and ligation of a patent ductus arteriosis.

7. Normally the white blood count is below 10,000; most serious infections elevate it to 20,000-40,000.

DISCUSSION

In a patient with a very poor prognosis for survival, it is appropriate to discuss **limitation of treatment**. This is especially so when the patient is capable of suffering and continued life support is prolonging that suffering.

Limitation of treatment decisions for children should generally be made jointly by the care team and a caring family. The family's preferences should generally be followed. Rarely may it be permissible to override a request for continued therapy if the team believes the family is not acting in the patient's **best interests**, for example, by insisting on treatment that causes unrelievable pain and cannot benefit the patient.

In the face of unprecedented survival, there is no consensus on how long to continue life support while awaiting supernatural intervention.

RECOMMENDATIONS

1. It seems appropriate to continue Joshua's present level of support and to search for correctable causes of his instability and **multi-organ system failure** (MOSF).
2. It would also seem appropriate for the care team to establish some time-limited goals (*x* degree of improvement in *y* period of time) beyond which they are unwilling to continue aggressive life support that is causing this child continued suffering.
3. It is ethically imperative to make every effort to bring him comfort, even if this should have the unintended secondary effect of shortening his life.

FOLLOW-UP

Full therapy for his MOSF was continued for the next four days. He then suddenly deteriorated and had a cardiac arrest, which did not respond to intensive efforts at resuscitation.

COMMENT

I felt particularly pained for Joshua's mother. I was unable to reach her Pentecostal pastor to learn if her understanding that God's performance of a miracle was dependent on her continued faith was part of his teaching. She felt a huge burden. She clearly loved Joshua and did not want to cause him unnecessary suffering, but she felt morally constrained to continue treatment that his professional caregivers felt was inappropriate. I was also unable to speak with her after his death to learn whether the sequence of events would have a detrimental effect on her faith.

Case 9.08

QUESTION

Is it permissible to continue treatment the patient seems clearly not to want at the request of his sister who believes he is not spiritually ready to die?

STORY

Mr. Patterson is a sixty-six-year-old widower who was admitted nine days ago with severe chest pain. The pain has continued intermittently, and he has developed other problems including poor circulation to his brain and his kidneys. It has been determined that he has a large, previously undiagnosed aneurysm of the aorta in his chest, and it developed a rupture partway through its wall nine days ago (called a dissecting aortic aneurysm). When diagnosed, it was far too extensive to be surgically repaired. The tear has progressed both directions along the aorta. The resulting diminished flow of blood to his brain has somewhat compromised his ability to communicate, and diminished flow in the other direction has now totally stopped his kidney function. A **do-not-resuscitate order** has been written. His physician in the intensive care unit (ICU) has asked his two adult children whether dialysis should be started, though he recommends against it since Mr. Patterson will almost certainly die from this condition within several days. The children have spoken with him and think he has said no, though it is not clear that he fully understands. His children believe this refusal of temporary postponement of his death would be consistent with his previous life choices.

The patient's younger sister, Genevieve, a devout Southern Baptist from out of state, has been at his bedside since shortly after admission. She says, "He's not ready to die!" She reports that the patient is not a believer, but he has seemed receptive to Genevieve's witnessing over the past week.

She thinks the patient is about ready to accept Jesus, and she pleads for the use of dialysis to allow him time to make this eternal decision.

DISCUSSION

When a patient loses the capacity to participate in treatment decisions and has left no written instructions, those decisions should be made by an appropriate **surrogate**. In many jurisdictions there is statutory hierarchical designation of surrogacy; in others this has not been codified into law. From an ethics perspective, the appropriate surrogate is the person or persons who best know the individual, his or her wishes and values. This may or may not be the person who appears at the top of the hierarchy in law. This state has no statutory surrogacy law, so by tradition we look to "next of kin" for assistance with surrogacy decisions. Generally, adult children are given priority of surrogacy over the patient's siblings, though this is subject to some flexibility depending on individual circumstances.

Once a surrogate is determined, that person should make decisions using **substituted judgment**, that is, an understanding of the patient's wishes or values, rather than making the choice the surrogate would make in a similar situation or making a choice based on the surrogate's values. In this case the request for continuation of treatment felt to be inappropriate by the professionals has been based on the wishes of the patient's sister, rather than on the presumed wishes of the patient.

RECOMMENDATIONS

1. It would not be appropriate to institute dialysis for this patient if his children and professional caregivers are sufficiently convinced that he would decline it if he were able.
2. His sister may continue to witness to the patient if he seems able to understand, as long as this is not perceived as badgering by the ICU staff or the patient's children.

FOLLOW-UP

Moments after the consultation was completed, the aneurysm ruptured into the patient's stomach causing massive hemorrhage. He died very quickly. Genevieve was present and appeared to be devastated. Counseling from the hospital chaplain was arranged for her.

COMMENT

I spoke with Genevieve at length immediately after her brother's death. She was overwhelmed with grief. She voiced a feeling of personal failure and anger at God for not allowing her more time. Having some understanding of her perspective, I tried to talk with her about individual choice for or against an acceptance of God's offer of salvation, the differing role of the Holy Spirit and the human witness. She did not seem assuaged. It was my hope that subsequent counseling could bring her a sense of peace.

Case 9.09

QUESTION

May we accept the refusal of a blood transfusion by this adolescent Jehovah's Witness?

STORY

Debbi is thirteen and a half years old and was well until two weeks ago when she developed knee pain without obvious trauma. She subsequently developed a fever and was admitted to the hospital with an infected knee joint found to be caused by staphylococcus aureus. She was started on appropriate antibiotics, but developed toxic shock[8] and has subsequently been found to have staph **sepsis**, osteomyelitis[9] of the femur, and bilateral staph pneumonia with large pleural effusions.[10] Her osteomyelitis has been surgically drained. Her sepsis has come under control with the use of two antibiotics (vancomycin and cefotaxime). She is on supplemental oxygen and **total parenteral nutrition.**

Debbi's pneumonia is improving, but it has not been possible to relieve the pleural effusions with either needle aspiration or placement of

8. Toxic shock is a life-threatening but treatable condition caused by a few types of bacteria, including the staphlyococcus. It consists of high fever, low blood pressure, rash, and multi-organ system failure.

9. Localized infection of a bone, often caused by spread of the bacteria through the blood stream.

10. Collection of fluid in the pleural space, between the lungs and the chest wall; it may compress the lungs and cause difficulty breathing; it often needs to be removed by needle aspiration or continuous drainage through a chest tube.

chest tubes, and surgery was proposed for this afternoon.[11] Her red blood cell count has dropped from normal level on admission (hemoglobin = 11.5) to a very low 6.1. She was begun on erythropoietin (an enzyme to stimulate her bone marrow) several days ago.

Debbi is the oldest of six children in an intact family. The family has a long and strong Jehovah's Witness tradition. Her parents were accepted into full membership as adolescents; her maternal grandfather and uncle are Jehovah's Witness elders. The patient is an excellent student in the eighth grade. She was accepted as a full member of the Jehovah's Witness community five months ago after examination by the elders found her to be of sufficient understanding.

I spoke with the patient (parents, uncle, and grandfather present), and she clearly articulated the Jehovah's Witness position on receiving blood or blood products. She quoted Scripture and explained her understanding of Jehovah's prohibition and did not "want it on [her] conscience" to accept blood. She asked that blood not be used, "if possible." When gently challenged on this last point, she clearly stated that she did not want blood even if it meant that she might die as a result. She repeated this sentiment on rediscussion without her family present and after being told that I would accept her statement as her true desire rather than assume she wanted us to override her refusal.

Her physicians believe they must proceed with more aggressive intervention because of her pulmonary condition. I spoke with the pediatric thoracic surgeon, and he reported that decortication is likely to involve significant blood loss. Because her anemia makes surgery risky, repeat chest tube placement under fluoroscopy will be attempted today while waiting a few more days for a response to erythropoietin.

DISCUSSION

The Jehovah's Witness belief about blood transfusion is a deeply held rational belief based on their interpretation of Scripture. There is strong ethical precedent for honoring such a request from an adequately informed patient with **decision-making capacity**, even if nonuse of blood will lead to death. Some suggest that many Jehovah's Witnesses will state the de-

---

11. When the fluid is collected into multiple small cavities, it is necessary to do a procedure called "decortication," a peeling away of this thick infected layer. This is a large and bloody operation since innumerable small blood vessels have grown between the lung and the abnormal tissue.

nomination's position but secretly hope that medical or legal professionals will override their refusal in order to save their lives. It is my belief that health-care professionals should not engage in this charade, but should honestly accept their statement as their desire.

There is legal precedent to obtain a court order to transfuse children of Jehovah's Witnesses over the objection of their parents if the nonuse of blood is likely to lead to death or disability. There is growing sentiment, however, that it is not the legal age of majority that is morally relevant, but the child's level of understanding, so that the refusal of a mature minor should be honored as if he or she were an adult. (See chapter 11 for discussion of consent for adolescents.)

In this case, I believe this adolescent is making an informed, non-coerced choice against potentially lifesaving blood transfusion.

RECOMMENDATIONS

1. It is my recommendation that this patient's physicians and the hospital should respect her refusal of blood products and should continue to do everything possible short of using blood products to improve her condition. Should she deteriorate to the point where she will surely die without blood, I believe we should reluctantly accept that tragic outcome.

2. If her physicians wish to honor her refusal, they should make it clear to her that her words of refusal will be accepted as her true desire; it will not be assumed that she wants to be rescued by seeking a court order over her objection.

3. Because of the legal precedent of overriding the refusal of Jehovah's Witness parents, her physicians should initiate a report of this situation to child protective services. If her physicians agree with my stance, the purpose of the report would be to seek judicial relief from the precedent. If her physicians disagree with my stance, the purpose of the report would be to seek the court order authorizing transfusion.

FOLLOW-UP

Child protective services and subsequently the juvenile court were notified of the situation. A hearing was held three days later, with testimony from pediatrician, surgeon, and ethicist. By this time the patient was slightly better (no fever, some drainage from the new chest tubes). The judge said she would issue an order for transfusion over parental objection if the patient's condition deteriorated. When the tube drainage slowed and her fever returned several days later, her parents chose to transfer her to a hospital where surgeons said they would operate without giving additional blood. This transfer was accomplished with the judge's approval. It is not known whether surgery was in fact done, but it is known that the patient survived the illness.

COMMENT

Three of the most difficult ethics consultations I have done have been on adolescents in Jehovah's Witness families. Each was handled a bit differently, varying with the circumstances.

In this case, I felt the patient was very mature and was making a truly informed decision based on the views she adopted when she became a Jehovah's Witness several months earlier. Her answers to my questions seemed a bit rote, but this probably reflected her recent teaching. At the same time, they seemed sincere and informed.

It has been my observation that physicians coming from a strong faith perspective usually take one of two positions in relation to transfusion of patients from the Jehovah's Witness tradition. The majority, relying on the importance they place on the tenets of their own faith, reluctantly accept the refusal of blood products. A minority, believing their own faith is correct on this issue and that the Jehovah's Witness teaching is in error, are often more willing to ignore the patient and transfuse over his or her objection, believing their professional mandate is to save lives when possible.

Case 9.10 ───

QUESTION

"Please write something in the chart so that the doctors will not give blood transfusions to my daughter."

STORY

Jesse is a thirteen-year-old girl who was admitted to the hospital seven days ago, a few hours after she apparently attempted suicide by swallowing a large amount of someone else's prescription medication, which led to seizures and **aspiration** of stomach contents into her airway. Her family has requested full treatment except that no blood or blood products be given because of their long-standing Jehovah's Witness faith.

She has remained critically ill with **adult respiratory distress syndrome, sepsis, congestive heart failure**, acidosis, and progressive anemia, and recently has developed kidney failure. She is currently supported with a **ventilator, total parenteral nutrition**, two drugs to sustain her low blood pressure, two antibiotics, and two sedatives for agitation. I see nothing in the chart to suggest that she has suffered any neurological damage. Her team feels that her condition is worsening, but none of her clinical problems is clearly irreversible. The ICU (intensive care unit) team has respected the family's request until this time and has made efforts to improve her profound anemia without the use of blood products. However, her blood count has dropped to a dangerously low level (hemoglobin = 5.2 grams; normal = 11-14 grams), and the team believes she cannot survive without being given blood, and may die even with transfusion.

Her mother reports that Jesse has been exhibiting "mood swings" for several months, and her teacher has complained about her mood and attitude. They were suspicious of illicit drug use but were not certain until drug screens done on admission were positive for opiates, cocaine, and marijuana. The patient's older sister says significant intrafamily stresses have been present for several years.

Her parents have been Jehovah's Witnesses for eleven years and have raised their children in that faith. Her mother reports that they have taught their children the restriction about blood and they faithfully attend services at Kingdom Hall. She reports that children are accepted as full members of the faith when they reach the "age of accountability" sufficient to understand the implications. They had begun to talk with Jesse about membership, but no steps had been taken. Her mother says she is willing to accept the possibility of the patient's death, but is unwilling to accept blood or blood products, and she wants the chart to clearly reflect her strong opposition to this treatment. The ICU team has notified child protective services of this patient's medical need for blood, and a hearing is scheduled for today on this issue. Her mother paged me with the above request.

DISCUSSION

There is a strong and growing ethical consensus that even life-prolonging treatment should not be given involuntarily to a patient with **decision-making capacity** who gives a rational reason for refusal. This clearly applies to lifesaving blood transfusions in adult Jehovah's Witnesses. Their refusal is based on belief in a divine command that carries eternal consequences for disobedience.

The consensus is nearly as strong that it is ethically permissible to override parental refusal of lifesaving transfusions for children of Jehovah's Witnesses who have not yet adopted the tenets of the faith. The reasoning is that the child's right to life has greater moral weight than parental discretion or parental religious liberty. The ethical decision about whether to override parental refusal in a particular case hinges on the likely benefit of transfusion. In some cases, if the benefits of transfusion are minimal, it may be justifiable to respect parental wishes against transfusion.

In this case, if it is probable that transfusion will significantly improve Jesse's chances of survival, it would appear to be justifiable to proceed with transfusion. The history of intrafamily stress and her suicide attempt are extra factors that would make it problematic to withhold transfusion in this case even if the likely benefits are minimal.

RECOMMENDATIONS

1. If this patient's professional caregivers are convinced that transfusion has a significant chance of increasing the patient's survival, it would be ethically permissible to seek a court order to transfuse her over parental objection.
2. If, on the other hand, it is highly likely that the patient will not survive even with transfusion, it would be permissible to honor the parental refusal of blood products.

FOLLOW-UP

A court order was obtained and six units of packed red blood cells were transfused over the subsequent forty-eight hours. The patient improved immediately (improved urine output, improved blood pressure), reversing a progressive downward trend. Her mother felt she was not involved in the decision, so she felt no guilt.

The patient continued to improve over the next several weeks, had a **tracheostomy**, was **weaned** from the ventilator, and was transferred to the rehabilitation service. Child protective services remained involved, providing a counselor who saw the patient frequently to discuss family relationships.

COMMENT

In general, it is appropriate to honor parental wishes about avoiding blood products when this can be done without significant risk to life or limb of the child. This may involve prolonged hospitalization, increased risk of infection, or other nonlethal outcomes detrimental to the patient. However, when the patient is in danger of dying or being disabled, it is generally held to be ethically permissible to override the parents' refusal in order to protect the child. As difficult as this decision is for a health-care professional, I try to frame it personally: How would I feel if persons in authority said my religious beliefs were irrelevant, and they were going to treat my child over my objection as they saw fit?

The patient in Case 9.09 was the same age as this patient. The major difference in recommendations is that patient 9.09 had already made a faith commitment to the Jehovah's Witness tradition. Patient 9.10 had not, thus it did not seem permissible to allow her to die for a religious tenet she had not personally accepted.

It is important for health-care professionals to remember that all Jehovah's Witnesses (at least in my experience) refuse whole blood, packed red blood cells, white blood cells, platelets, and plasma. The use or nonuse of other blood products is a matter of conscience; some Jehovah's Witnesses may accept albumin, coagulation factors, erythropoietin, or specific blood-saving techniques ("Cell Saver," hemodilution).[12]

12. The Cell Saver is an instrument that sucks up the patient's blood lost during a procedure, passes it through a filter, and reinfuses it into the patient's circulation. Hemodilution is a procedure that removes one or more units of blood from a patient just before a procedure that is expected to entail significant blood loss, leaving it in place in bags still attached to the patient, then giving the patient an infusion of nonblood fluid like saline, doing the bloody procedure, and then reinfusing the patient's own blood when the procedure is completed.

Case 9.11 ────────────────────────────────

QUESTION

Is it permissible to withhold aggressive treatment from this child in the persistent vegetative state, treatment that her parents request based on their Orthodox Jewish beliefs?

STORY

Miriam is a six-year-old girl who was born with microcephaly.[13] She was cared for at home by her parents for eighteen months, then admitted to a high-quality pediatric long-term care facility. She has previously had two or three brief hospitalizations for treatment of pneumonia. She was transferred here eight days ago with respiratory distress and was found to have pulmonary congestion caused by renal failure not previously recognized. She has been treated aggressively (including assisted ventilation) and has been found to have end-stage kidney disease from glomerulonephritis.[14] She does not currently need dialysis but may at some undetermined time in the future if she becomes unable to make urine. She is being **weaned** from the **ventilator** and is on **total parenteral nutrition** (decreasing as tube feedings through her nose are tolerated), antibiotics, and a diuretic to encourage urine output. A **neurologist** has stated that she is in a **persistent vegetative state** (PVS), although her nurses report that she is given occasional doses of sedation for seemingly agitated head motion. Her ICU (intensive care unit) physicians believe it is inappropriate to use invasive or aggressive measures such as dialysis or long-term assisted ventilation to prolong the life of a child in a PVS. In addition, the dialysis acceptance committee of the hospital has unanimously voted against dialysis for this patient.

Her parents have requested full treatment for Miriam. They are Orthodox Jews and have conversed with their rabbi. While they understand that she is, and will continue to be, incapable of any human interaction, and they believe she will have a better existence after her death, they state

---

13. Microcephaly is a condition of significant underdevelopment of the brain and skull with varying degrees of functional impairment.

14. Glomerulonephritis is a group of inflammatory conditions that affect the small filtering blood vessels in the kidneys. There are several causes, but in many cases no cause can be found.

that they are obligated to do everything humanly possible to prevent her death.

DISCUSSION

Caring parents are given considerable discretion regarding treatment for children who have profound neurological impairment in that they are often allowed to accept or decline treatments recommended by their child's physicians. It is an unsettled question whether this discretion extends to their requests for treatments deemed "inappropriate" by the child's physicians.

Physicians might believe a particular treatment is inappropriate for a particular child because (a) it won't work, (b) it would cause the child disproportionate suffering, (c) it is too expensive, (d) it is scarce and another patient has a greater need or will achieve a greater benefit, or (e) it is outside the professional standard of care. Such "standards of care" may be articulated in the medical literature or in policy statements of institutions or professional bodies, or they may merely be personal practice patterns. Physicians consider dialysis or artificial ventilation to be obligatory for some children, optional for some children, and inappropriate for others. These professional value judgments are usually based on the child's overall condition.

Since this request from Miriam's parents is based on a long-standing and firm religious belief shared with their faith tradition (as opposed to an idiosyncratic or irrational belief or an unrealistic expectation of benefit), any reason for denial would have to be weighty.

In this child, dialysis and long-term ventilation: (a) would work in that they could postpone death; (b) would not cause the child disproportionate suffering since she is in the PVS and is incapable of awareness; (c) are expensive but would likely be covered by Medicaid; and (d) are not sufficiently scarce in our setting to consider rationing on that basis. Thus the only ethically justifiable reason to withhold these modalities from this patient would be that they are outside the standard of care.

Policies adopted by professional organizations, authoritative statements in the literature, or local institutional policies that preclude or recommend against dialysis or long-term ventilation for children in the PVS could be used as justification for declining to provide these modalities for this patient.

A literature review on the issue found five references that clearly state that dialysis is inappropriate for permanently unconscious patients (two personal opinions offered by **nephrologists**, one institutional recommendation, one from the End-Stage Renal Disease Advisory Committee of the U.S. Department of Health and Human Services, and one from the National Kidney Foundation) and none suggesting otherwise. This suggests a developing consensus.

RECOMMENDATIONS

1. If this child should deteriorate so that either of these modalities is indicated, it would be permissible for her physicians to make a strong recommendation against their use and to try to dissuade her parents from their request. The cited literature may be used to demonstrate a developing consensus. Since, however, there is as yet no definitive uniform professional stance, it would be ethically problematic to deny their persistent request.

2. Physicians who feel very strongly that these treatments are wrong for this patient should not be forced to provide them if transfer of responsibility to a willing physician is possible.

FOLLOW-UP

After reading the cited literature, the parents and rabbi agreed that dialysis would be outside the standard of care for Miriam. The physicians recommended transfer back to her long-term care facility with hospice care. However, when her kidney function rapidly deteriorated over the next few days, the rabbi insisted that she remain in the hospital, even that she be transferred back to the ICU, and that she receive all possible treatments short of dialysis to postpone her death. Her deteriorating kidney function would inevitably lead to disturbance of her fluid and salt balance and to cardiac arrest. When asked about **cardiopulmonary resuscitation** (CPR), he said, "We are not doctors. The doctors should do what they think best." In light of that, I wrote this follow-up note in her chart: "In a patient with renal failure who is not a candidate for dialysis, aggressive management of fluid and electrolytes may postpone death, but death is inevitable from electrolyte problems. CPR will not be effective in restoring circulation when the arrest is from uncorrectable electrolyte abnormalities. Therefore CPR is futile for this patient, but aggressive management of her fluids and electrolytes would still be appropriate given the parents' expectation of all treatments to postpone death. It is thus ethically permissible to write a **do-not-resuscitate order** for this patient based on **futility**." Three days later Miriam's heart stopped. Her body was released for immediate burial.

COMMENT

This case is a good example of a situation where close involvement of a spiritual adviser to the patient's family was very helpful to the clinical team. Once the tenets of faith were clearly outlined, it was possible to work within them to honor the family's religious beliefs with only moderate compromise of the standards of the medical profession.

Case 9.12

QUESTION

Should we continue treatment in this Hindu man who is imminently dying when his family is still hopeful for recovery?

STORY

Chintan is a fifty-four-year-old man from India with a complicated medical history of diabetes, coronary artery disease, and arterial disease of his legs. He was admitted nearly one month ago with severe **congestive heart failure**. He consented to high-risk coronary artery bypass grafting since it appeared to offer the only hope for improvement. He has done poorly since surgery. He has had respiratory failure, kidney failure requiring dialysis, gastrointestinal hemorrhage, liver failure, repeated episodes of **sepsis**, seizures, and he has not awakened since surgery, presumably because of multiple small strokes that occurred during surgery. It is reported that the patient is minimally responsive when addressed in Hindi, although he also spoke English before this illness. He has had continued aggressive treatment, but several consulting physicians are suggesting to the primary ICU (intensive care unit) team that further treatment is not warranted. The team has scheduled a conference with the family for this afternoon to discuss **limitation of treatment**.

The team reports that the patient's brother appears to be the family spokesperson and decision-maker, although the patient's wife is present and involved.

DISCUSSION

In most circumstances, families of critically ill patients who have a poor prognosis are given adequate information and may be asked to consent to withdrawal of life-prolonging treatment. This is particularly so when survival is unprecedented and the patient is capable of suffering. When patients are from other cultures, we try to be sensitive to their different approaches to revealing a prognosis and to decision making.

It is my understanding that in this culture, patients and families are unable to make a decision to limit life-prolonging treatment because they are expected to remain optimistic. If it is clearly felt that this patient's condition is incompatible with survival, it might be culturally sensitive for the team to make a unilateral decision against continuing the current level of treatment on the basis of medical **futility**.

In addition, my reading suggests that in this culture the physician's words are felt to have power, so that it would be considered inappropriate to predict death since that might make it happen. It might be more culturally appropriate to state that everything possible has been done; whether the patient survives is out of the doctors' hands. It would likely be appropriate to recommend that all family be encouraged to come to the bedside because of the severity of the patient's illness.

If the team does make a unilateral decision to limit treatment, it should be done in such a way that it does not appear to be a life-terminating event; for example, withholding new antibiotics might be more acceptable than discontinuing the **ventilator**. Or the team could say that dialysis was instituted for kidney failure and it is time to stop the dialysis to see if the kidneys have recovered.

RECOMMENDATIONS

1. A unilateral decision by the care team to limit treatment may be appropriate in this case based on medical futility.
2. If such a decision is made, it should be instituted in a culturally sensitive way.

FOLLOW-UP

The ICU team met with the patient's wife and brother using the above suggestions. There was agreement to write a **do-not-resuscitate order** and to stop dialysis. The patient died two days later. I spoke with his brother, who is grieving but understands that the accumulation of organ problems was not survivable.

COMMENT

In this case, brief research into cultural and religious beliefs revealed a differing perspective on appropriate communication about end-of-life issues rather than differing beliefs about the accompanying natural or supernatural events. This understanding allowed a more cooperative approach to a very difficult situation.

Case 9.13

QUESTION

Please help establish an end point of treatment for this dying woman whose husband insists that everything be done.

STORY

Virginia is a forty-five-year-old woman who has had scleroderma[15] for about four years that has involved many organ systems (skin, lungs, gastrointestinal tract, kidneys) as well as depression and osteoporosis with compression fractures. She was admitted with a pulmonary embolus (blood clot that had formed in her leg and traveled to her lungs) two months ago and has been in the intensive care unit (ICU) nearly constantly. She has had a **tracheostomy** and insertion of a permanent feeding tube. Her condition has worsened in the past two weeks, and she is now described as having end-stage scleroderma with overwhelming infection,

---

15. Scleroderma is a chronic condition of unknown cause that consists of tissue changes in multiple organs. It generally leads to death from failure of the heart, lungs, and kidneys.

skin breakdown, and massive swelling of her entire body. Her ICU care team is certain that her condition is irreversible and she is imminently dying, and would like to limit treatment, but her husband believes she will survive and insists that all treatment be continued.

The nursing staff describe her husband as very devoted. They believe that he hears only the good news and does not absorb information of a negative nature. He spends many hours each day at her bedside, either reading the Bible or being involved in her care. He is a retired electrician and is somewhat older than she. Each has children from previous marriages. It is reported that they met over the phone through their church affiliation, and she moved from out of state to marry him four years ago.

On admission the patient signed the general "consent to treatment" document and penciled in "no tracheostomy" and "CPR [**cardiopulmonary resuscitation**] yes." A durable power of attorney for health care in her chart names her husband as her **agent**; however, the page with the date and her signature is missing. In the space for a statement of desires concerning life-prolonging treatment is written, "Once I am brain dead, my husband has full authorization to make the final decision as to when to disconnect me from any and all life support machines, but all medication including pain treatment is to continue."

DISCUSSION

Decisions about **limitation of treatment** for an imminently dying patient should ideally be made jointly by the patient (or more likely the **surrogate**) and the professionals involved in the patient's care. When these two parties disagree about goals or about the use or nonuse of specific modalities, this can sometimes be resolved by further discussion, listening, and explanation, or through compromise. Sometimes, however, no consensus or compromise can be reached. The reason underlying such irresolvable conflicts is often a clash between medical facts and predictions and the religious or cultural beliefs of the patient.

In almost all situations of irresolvable conflict, further management decisions should be guided by the patient's values and beliefs. A medical professional is not, however, required to offer or use a treatment that clearly will not work (physiologic **futility**) or violates his or her own personal or professional conscience, such as causing unrelievable pain without clear benefit.

In this case we have a fairly clear statement (missing date and signature) of the patient's vitalistic beliefs, and her appointed surrogate is trying to accomplish her goal of postponing death for as long as possible. It is not clear why he consented to her tracheostomy, since she had declined this. If we are convinced that this document truly represents her wishes, aggressive treatment should continue until it clearly will not work, as long as her suffering can be controlled.

RECOMMENDATIONS

1. A conference with her husband and pastor might help to clarify the husband's understanding of the clinical situation, and our understanding of their theological beliefs. Even though it may be uncomfortable for him, it is important that he be made to acknowledge the reality of the medical facts and the degree of certainty of the prognosis.

2. Unless this conference leads to a different understanding of her wishes, all treatments that have a reasonable chance of forestalling death should be continued. There is, however, no obligation to start or continue treatments that will not work or are not working, nor is there a requirement to continue treatment "until she is brain dead."

3. The patient should probably remain in a **full code status**, so that any reversible events can be treated. This does not, however, mean that full resuscitative attempts must be continued for a prolonged period. If such attempts are not working after a reasonable effort has been made, they may be stopped. This might even mean stopping after only a few minutes of effort if the clinical situation is such that reversibility is unprecedented.

FOLLOW-UP

A management conference was held with the ICU attending physician, the patient's ICU nurse, the patient's husband, his pastor, and the clinical ethics consultant. We discussed the patient's current situation and very poor prognosis; talked of her values and our responsibility to pursue them as long as it was feasible; and also talked of changing goals to comfort care when there seemed little and diminishing potential for survival.

With support from his pastor, her husband seemed to understand, agreed to a **do-not-resuscitate order**, and agreed to call her children to see if they wanted to come from out of state before he further contemplated the possibility of withdrawal of life support. They were unable to travel quickly, so he requested that the medication to sustain her blood pressure be stopped. She died in about four hours.

COMMENT

This was not a case of differing religious beliefs, but one where personal devotion and intense religious beliefs led the patient's husband to deny the reality of her imminent death. His trusted pastor was able to be somewhat more objective and was able to help him see the reality of the situation.

*   *   *

Other Cases Involving Cultural/Religious Beliefs

Cases 4.10, 4.12, 10.05, 10.08, 11.07, 13.09, 14.04, 14.08

References on Ethical Issues Involving Cultural and/or Religious Beliefs

Fadiman, A. *The Spirit Catches You and You Fall Down*. New York: Farrar, Straus and Giroux, 1997.

Health and Medicine in the [Anabaptist, Anglican, Catholic, Christian Science, Eastern Orthodox, Evangelical, Hindu, Islamic, Jewish, Latter-Day Saint, Lutheran, Methodist, Reformed, Shamanic] Tradition. This series of fourteen books was published by Crossroad Publishing Company (New York) in the 1980s and 1990s and focused on various denominational traditions.

Marty, M. E., and K. L. Vaux, eds. *Health/Medicine and the Faith Traditions*. Philadelphia: Fortress, 1982.

Pellegrino, E., P. Mazzarella, and P. Corsi, eds. *Transcultural Dimensions in Medical Ethics*. Frederick, Md.: University Publishing Group, 1992.

PART IV

CHAPTER 10

Ethical Issues in the Neonatal Period

Assisting with treatment decisions for newborns in distress, whether from prematurity, birth injury, or congenital anomalies, can present among the most challenging ethical dilemmas. A combination of appropriate attitude (especially sensitivity), skills (e.g., mediation), and knowledge of ethical and judicial precedents, plus some basic knowledge of clinical neonatology, is essential and will well serve individuals who enter the neonatal intensive care unit (NICU).

For at least a generation there has been a presumption in North America in favor of vigorous treatment of newborns, perhaps even more so than for adults. This presumption is primarily based on the newborn's heightened potential for recovery, survival, development, and adaptation, but likely has an emotional component as well. However, all these favorable aspects of the neonate are often shrouded in a cloud of uncertainty.

The 1963 filming at the Johns Hopkins hospital of a decision to withhold corrective surgery from a newborn with **Down syndrome** and congenital blockage of the small intestine started a public debate on the issues.[1] When a 1973 article appeared in a major medical journal suggesting it was sometimes permissible for parents and **neonatologists** to decide to provide less than maximal therapy,[2] there was considerable skepticism and criticism — amplified in light of the 1973 Supreme Court decision on

1. J. A. Gustafson, "Mongolism, Parental Desires, and the Right to Life," *Perspectives in Biological Medicine* 16, no. 4 (1973): 524, 529-33.

2. R. S. Duff and A. G. Campbell, "Moral and Ethical Dilemmas in the Special-Care Nursery," *New England Journal of Medicine* 289, no. 17 (1973): 890-94.

abortion. Concerns were raised about discriminatory decisions leading to the deaths of newborns with handicaps based on a prediction of diminished quality of life.

Over the ensuing decade the public and professional conversation became quite heated. A 1983 publication by the Stinson family of their pleadings with NICU staff to withdraw support from their infant was both insightful and evocative.[3] The President's Commission report in 1983 lent support to the prevailing pediatric position that allowed some parental discretion when there was significant clinical uncertainty.[4] Things came to a head after public discussion of the case of Baby Doe in Bloomington, Indiana, who was also born with Down syndrome and a correctable gastrointestinal problem (tracheoesophageal fistula, an abnormal opening between the esophagus and the airway). That case was taken to court rather than becoming the subject of a documentary. The court allowed her parents to refuse corrective surgery, and she died a public death from dehydration. The federal government responded to this case with rigid rules disallowing such quality-of-life decisions, and the controversy became even more contentious. The resulting compromise, called the "Baby Doe Regulations,"[5] has been in place for over twenty years. These regulations, passed as an amendment to the Child Abuse Law, retain a presumption in favor of treatment but articulate exceptions where full treatment is not legally mandatory: (a) if the infant is irreversibly comatose (e.g., an infant with **anencephaly**, which is failure of development of the upper portion of the brain); (b) if treatment would be futile in terms of survival; or (c) if the treatment would be virtually futile and inhumane.

Some physicians, philosophers, and ethicists maintain that the Baby Doe Regulations are too restrictive,[6] that some conditions do not fall within these strict parameters when parents should have some discretion about continuation of life-sustaining measures. Most are willing to live within the constraints of the regulations, relying on some interpretation of the terms "reasonable medical judgment," "effective," and "appropriate" to

---

3. R. Stinson and P. Stinson, *The Long Dying of Baby Andrew* (Boston: Little, Brown, 1983).

4. President's Commission for the Study of Ethical Problems in Medicine and Biomedical and Behavioral Research, *Deciding to Forgo Life-Sustaining Treatment* (Washington, D.C.: U.S. Government Printing Office, 1983).

5. *Child Abuse Amendments of 1984*, 42 USCA §5102 (1984).

6. L. M. Kopelman, T. G. Irons, and A. E. Kopelman, "Neonatologists Judge the 'Baby Doe' Regulations," *New England Journal of Medicine* 318, no. 11 (1988): 677-83.

allow a bit of discretion.[7] However, when cases with conflict have been taken to court, judges have varied in their decisions.

In 1992 Stephanie Keene (known then as Baby K) was born in Virginia with anencephaly. Her mother was informed of the diagnosis before birth, and based on her strong religious faith and her belief in the right to life, she insisted that the baby receive full treatment when she was born, including **ventilator** support if needed. The standard of care in the delivery room for a newborn with anencephaly is comfort measures, without efforts to sustain life. Her mother's wishes were followed; Stephanie was resuscitated in the delivery room and subsequently given respiratory assistance with a ventilator. She eventually was **weaned** from ventilator support and later transferred to a long-term care facility. She had several readmissions to the hospital with respiratory problems, and the hospital physicians felt it was inappropriate to continue to use vigorous measures on this infant who would never have any awareness. The hospital went to federal court seeking a ruling that it was not obligated to provide inappropriate treatment that was outside the standard of care. The federal district court, and subsequently the U.S. Court of Appeals,[8] decided in the mother's favor, based not on a right to life or on the Baby Doe Regulations, but on federal law that requires emergency rooms to provide lifesaving treatment to patients in need rather than transferring them. Stephanie lived two years and four months.

A more recent Texas case again highlights the struggle over who holds the trump card in decisions about how aggressively or how long to treat a neonate.[9] Mrs. Miller was admitted to the hospital in 1990 at twenty-three weeks' **gestation** in premature labor. The fetus was felt to be at the lower limit of viability. When it was determined that her baby was very small and had a dismal prognosis, she and her husband requested that the baby girl receive only comfort care. A hospital administrator said (incorrectly, it turns out) that the hospital system had a policy requiring resuscitative efforts if the baby weighed more than 500 grams (1 pound 2 ounces), so she was resuscitated. She survived, but with major neurological disabilities, and her parents sued the hospital (HCA). They won a multimillion-dollar judgment, but this was overturned by the Texas Supreme Court. The final

---

7. "Bioethical Review Committees in Perinatology," *Clinical Perinatology* 14, no. 2 (June 1987): 379-93.

8. *In the Matter of Baby K,* 16 F. 3d 590 (4th Cir. 1994).

9. *Miller v. HCA,* 47 Tex. Sup. J. 12, 118 S.W.3d 758 (2003).

court decision returns the authority to make split-second delivery room decisions about whether to resuscitate premature newborns to the physician, allowing him or her to proceed over the objections of the parents. However, the court also stated that parents generally have the right to request **limitation of treatment** in the NICU as long as their decision is within a reasonable range of acceptable options.

Because emotions can run high in difficult NICU situations, it is vitally important to recall the adage "good ethics begins with good facts." It is important to have input from neonatologists (usually two or more), nurses, and pediatric subspecialists in the area of interest (e.g., neurology, cardiology, gastrointestinal) as well as consultation with pediatric radiologists. Support for parents from social workers and chaplains or family clergy is almost always needed. I find that I recommend a multidisciplinary conference in the process of ethics consultations in the NICU even more often than I do in the adult setting. Some hospitals have established an infant care review committee process for such discussions, usually with input from clinical ethicists and hospital legal counsel.

NICUs tend to be staffed by tightly knit professional teams. When a decision is made to withdraw support from a neonate, especially one who has been in the unit for some time, I often suggest someone (nurse manager, social worker) do an informal poll of all staff on all shifts to see if there are any concerns or any significant dissent. Not infrequently I will meet with a group of nurses to address such concerns, preferably before, but sometimes after, such a decision is implemented.

Do-not-resuscitate orders are perhaps of lesser importance in the NICU than in the adult setting because the strong newborn heart often continues to function well, with some other organ or system being the tipping point.

Another difference from adult consultations lies in the assessment of the newborn brain. There is not a mathematical correlation between structure and function, but then, this is true in adults too. What is different is the newborn's potential for development and adaptation; the newborn brain is more plastic than the adult brain (see Case 10.05).

Neonatologists tend to be very good at keeping records and documenting outcomes. Using many years' data on survival, recent studies have equally emphasized "intact survival" and functional outcomes. Measuring this outcome requires long-term follow-up, and is still often difficult to interpret and apply in the NICU crisis (see Case 10.06).

As a point of reference, when a baby is born, he or she is given an **Apgar score** as a measure of how well he or she is doing with the transition from the protective environment of the uterus to the outside world. This universally accepted scoring system assigns 0, 1, or 2 points to each of five parameters: heart rate, breathing, color, muscle tone, and reflex irritability. Thus the score ranges from 10 (ideal) to 0 (stillborn). The scoring is done at one minute after delivery and repeated at five minutes. The typical healthy newborn has Apgar scores of 8-9 at one minute and 9-10 at five minutes. If the five-minute score is less than 7 or 8, the scoring is generally repeated at five-minute intervals. Thus, for a compromised newborn, you may see Apgar scores of 4/6/8/9 (one minute, five minutes, ten minutes, and fifteen minutes).

Let's now look at some cases in the NICU that raised significant ethical dilemmas, a few involving premature infants (see Cases 10.01 and 10.02), but most at or near full term, and most of those with severe illnesses or anomalies.

Case 10.01

QUESTION

Is it ethically permissible to honor the request of this pregnant woman that no treatment be given her premature newborn in a situation where full treatment is ordinarily used?

STORY

Melinda is thirty-eight years old and at twenty-one weeks' **gestation** in her second pregnancy. She is not in labor, but she is thinking ahead. Her first child was born seven years ago at twenty-five weeks' gestation, is blind, and has significant developmental delay. Given the nature of her first child's prolonged stay in the neonatal intensive care unit (NICU) and current impairments, Melinda is requesting no resuscitation for this child if it is born prior to twenty-eight weeks' gestation.

The neonatology service met with Melinda and her husband to review the limits of viability and to discuss treatment options. The parents were informed that prior to twenty-five weeks the physicians and nurses were willing to defer to parental preferences by providing no resuscitation. During the twenty-fifth week they would take parental wishes into account, but their decision about resuscitation would be based on the clinical condition of the child. And after twenty-six weeks, full resuscitation would have to be provided to the infant. Given the patient's reservations about this proposed course of action, the obstetrical service offered her the possibility of termination of the pregnancy, as her fetus had not yet reached the point of viability. She declined.

The patient has also requested that the medical team abide by her current request that a premature infant not be resuscitated, even if (as she anticipates) immediately after delivery she expresses a change of heart and requests vigorous resuscitation. The patient feels that such a natural, parental response would be irrational and would not reflect her considered decision on this matter.

Melinda had a career in interior design, but has stayed at home to provide care for her handicapped daughter for the past seven years. Her husband, Ivan, works part time as a pharmacist and spends many hours per week assisting in home care. They have no current religious affiliation, but consider themselves to be quite spiritual.

DISCUSSION

This case raises a number of important issues. The first is the limitation of parental authority in terms of neonatal treatment decisions. Parents are the presumed guardians of their children, but their authority is not unlimited. Thus the American Academy of Pediatrics (AAP) states: "The rights of parents in decision making must be respected. However, physicians should not be forced to undertreat or overtreat an infant if, in their best medical judgment, the treatment is not in compliance with the standard care for that infant."[10] This has direct application to this case, for providing only comfort care (as requested) to a twenty-seven-week-plus fetus, for example, would constitute inappropriate undertreatment. The treatment plans set forth by the neonatology staff are well within the standard of care.

From a legal standpoint, a physician who resuscitates a child of twenty-six or more weeks — even over parental objections — is on firm

10. "The Initiation or Withdrawal of Treatment for High-Risk Newborns," *Pediatrics* 96 (1995): 362.

ground. The Texas Supreme Court decision stated that "a physician, who is confronted with emergent circumstances and provides life-sustaining treatment to a minor child, is not liable for not first obtaining consent from the parents."

Withholding life-sustaining treatment from a child of fewer than twenty-five weeks' gestation (or perhaps twenty-five to twenty-six weeks, depending on the child's clinical appearance) is less clear. The Baby Doe Regulations, mandated by the federal government in 1984, state that the only indications for limitation of life-sustaining treatment for newborns are (1) if the child were to be permanently unconscious, or if the treatment were (2) futile or (3) virtually futile and inhumane. In light of these rules, the AAP position statement, and the arguable definition of "virtually futile and inhumane," the plan proposed by neonatology is ethically acceptable.

As for the patient's request that the medical team disregard any authorization she gives after delivery to resuscitate a child of fewer than twenty-six weeks, this is not ethically permissible. To do so would force the medical team to make an immediate judgment of her **decision-making capacity**, and even if she was found to lack capacity, most would argue that her authorization would still be binding. Her request is an example of a "Ulysses clause,"[11] whereby patients request that treatment be withheld at a later time over their incapacitated consent. There is no precedent for such a course of action in this context.

It is impossible at this time to predict the neonate's specific condition in the NICU, and thus to do any concrete advance planning for situations in which treatment can be limited. The most that can be said is that the parents should be fully informed of their child's condition, and that their latitude is increased in a nonemergent setting.

---

11. The name is derived from Homer's *Odyssey*, which speaks of female Sirens who sang with voices so seductive that no captain could resist steering toward their island, and then crashing on the rocks. However, Ulysses very much wanted to hear the voice of the Sirens, and he devised a plan to do so without jeopardizing the safety of his ship. He instructed his crew to follow a course he charted for them, a course that would take them near enough to the Sirens so he could hear them but not so close as to cause the ship's demise. He further ordered his crew to lash him to the mast and to plug their ears with beeswax. He instructed them not to obey him until they reached a location out of range of the Sirens' voices.

RECOMMENDATIONS

1. It is ethically permissible to withhold life-sustaining treatment at the parents' request for a newborn of fewer than twenty-five weeks' gestation, as well as to take the parents' wishes into account for a child between twenty-five and twenty-six weeks. It is ethically obligatory to pursue vigorous resuscitation for any otherwise healthy newborn of twenty-six or more weeks.
2. If the parents in the delivery room were to authorize resuscitation of a child at fewer than twenty-five weeks' gestation, and this was felt to be within the standard of care by the medical team, it is ethically permissible to pursue resuscitation, regardless of the parents' previously stated wishes.

FOLLOW-UP

No follow-up information is available.

COMMENT

It is ironic that the physicians caring for this pregnant woman and her baby would offer to terminate her pregnancy at twenty-one weeks but would insist on full treatment if the baby were born after twenty-six weeks. At least it is reassuring that they uphold the sanctity of human life after the point of viability.

Most people of faith have a high regard for individuals with disabilities, and a protective stance for handicapped newborns who are vulnerable to decisions made by others. Some might be judgmental of parents who seem willing to sacrifice their child to prevent its life with disabilities. I think, instead, that we should come alongside these parents who have followed a difficult course for the past seven years, try to understand their needs and limits, and offer to help in any way we can. Ethics and law require that we protect this infant, but we also have an obligation to these parents. If their child should have significant disabilities, we should offer to help them with placement in a loving foster home so they can continue to focus on the needs and gifts of their first child without additional burden.

Case 10.02 ⸻⸻⸻⸻⸻⸻⸻⸻⸻⸻⸻⸻⸻⸻

QUESTION

What are the ethically permissible treatment options for this eleven-day-old, critically ill premature infant (born at twenty-six weeks' gestation)?

STORY

This eleven-day-old infant girl was born at an estimated twenty-six weeks' **gestation** to Betsy, who has three prior children, after medication failed to stop her premature labor. Her **Apgar scores** were 2, 4, and 7. She was admitted to the neonatal intensive care unit (NICU) with severe respiratory distress, low blood pressure, and acidosis[12] with a clinical diagnosis of **sepsis**. She has been treated vigorously but, in addition to her respiratory failure, has had the following complications: kidney failure (slowly improving), a grade III-IV **intracranial hemorrhage**,[13] and seizures. She has unexplained **cyanosis** of her trunk and legs indicating a lack of oxygen. An **electroencephalogram** done today because of her worsening clinical condition shows no electrical activity. This finding is unprecedented in preemies, and therefore is not a clear prognostic guide; however, it is suggestive of an even more dismal neurologic outcome. With the passage of time and the worsening clinical condition, the NICU staff is becoming increasingly pessimistic about survival in general, but specifically about intact survival.

The infant is currently on high-frequency ventilation,[14] antibiotics, **total parenteral nutrition**, medication to sustain her blood pressure, and two drugs for seizures. On examination she is flaccid and cyanotic.

Her mother, Betsy, has a history of drug abuse and is currently in jail on an assault charge. Her father's whereabouts are not known. Her mother has been in daily telephone contact with the NICU staff, and has signed an authorization for her brother, Rudolph, to make routine treatment decisions. It is reported that he is leaning toward **limitation of treatment**.

---

12. Acidosis is an abnormal chemical condition of the body in which the blood takes on an acidic quality with consequent disturbance of many chemical processes. It can be caused by a deficiency of oxygen or by several other mechanisms.

13. Intracranial hemorrhages in neonates are described on a scale from grade I (small, with no or minimal consequence) to grade IV (large, indicating significant brain damage).

14. A form of assisted ventilation with rapid breaths, used when conventional ventilatory assistance is not effective.

However, a maternal aunt (a social worker who has not seen the infant) is pushing for increased treatment aimed at survival. Betsy has not seen the baby since admission. She has told the **neonatologist** that she would like treatment used, but she does not want her daughter to suffer needlessly.

The NICU social worker has checked with child protective services and learned that Betsy does not automatically forfeit her maternal rights to her children because she is incarcerated.

DISCUSSION

Treatment decisions for a critically ill premature infant should be guided by the **best interests** of the baby. If parents decline treatments that are deemed clearly beneficial by the infant's physicians, those treatments should be used until the decision can be reviewed by others (e.g., a hospital Infant Care Review Committee or the court). If, conversely, parents request treatments that the infant's physicians deem clearly futile, these too should probably be continued, pending review, unless they would also entail unrelievable suffering. In those intermediate situations where specific treatments are of uncertain efficacy (i.e., neither clearly beneficial nor clearly futile), parental discretion is ethically appropriate, and physicians should almost always honor their decision. However, legal constraints may sometimes require treatment that parents would prefer to forgo. As a patient's prognosis becomes increasingly dismal, the patient's physicians have an increasing obligation to recommend limitation of treatment to prevent needless suffering of the infant.

In this case, the patient's unique social situation should not significantly change decision-making methods or treatment options. Her precarious but uncertain situation would make either continuation or withdrawal of treatment ethically permissible. Her treatment team should continue to try to facilitate a bedside visit by and discussion with her mother. While further discussion with other family members is appropriate, and family consensus would be ideal, it is the patient's mother who has ultimate decision-making authority. Her physicians should also continue to reshape their recommendations based on the patient's changing condition.

RECOMMENDATIONS

1. Efforts should be continued to facilitate a bedside visit by the mother at the earliest possible time. She should not be required to make a life-

or-death decision for her daughter over the telephone without having the opportunity to see her.

2. Conventional bedside decision-making methods should be used by attempting to balance potential benefits and burdens.

3. If the infant's physicians come to believe that she cannot survive in spite of continued vigorous treatment, and that treatment is causing her to suffer, they should strongly recommend that life-sustaining treatments be stopped and only comfort measures be continued.

FOLLOW-UP

The warden refused to release the mother from prison for even a few hours. A request to the prison chaplain was also unproductive. The infant's condition continued to slowly deteriorate; her kidney failure grew worse and she developed gangrene of her fingers. At about one month of age, the NICU nurses were preparing to make a video of the infant to send to her mom, but at that same time the neonatologist informed the mother by phone that further increases in level of treatment were futile and would not be used. She accepted this, but her (social worker) sister was upset that the doctors were "giving up." The baby died on full support thirty-four days after her premature birth.

COMMENT

At the time of the ethics consultation, this premature infant's condition was very poor. Though the prognosis was not necessarily uniformly fatal, it was nearly certain that she would have some neurologic compromise if she did survive. Her condition slowly deteriorated after that. A decision to withdraw treatment could probably have been justified earlier, but this was hampered by her mother's incarceration.

Complicated social situations often slow medical decision making. This is often acceptable, and perhaps even preferable, but may not be if the infant is experiencing suffering that cannot be adequately relieved.

Case 10.03

QUESTION

Is it ethically permissible to stop the ventilator in this six-week-old baby who was born at thirty-one weeks' gestation and has a congenital condition (myotonic dystrophy) with a poor prognosis?

STORY

This six-week-old girl was born prematurely (at thirty-one weeks' **gestation**) and was noted in the delivery room to have some dysmorphic features (e.g., club feet, underdevelopment of the jaw) as well as markedly reduced muscle tone. Because of poor respiratory effort, it was necessary to **intubate** her airway and assist her ventilation in the delivery room before she was transferred to the neonatal intensive care unit (NICU). Her lung function remains poor so that she has not been able to be **weaned** from the **ventilator** during these six weeks. Her **electroencephalogram** is abnormal. The right side of her muscular diaphragm between her chest and abdomen is weak. Workup has now shown that she has myotonic dystrophy, an inherited progressive weakness of voluntary and involuntary muscles.

She is currently stable, on tube feedings, conventional ventilator settings, and maintenance medications. She is on no sedation. Several reports in the medical literature have found that infants with congenital myotonic dystrophy severe enough to require assisted ventilation at birth all remain ventilator-dependent and all die in the first year from pulmonary complications. Her NICU care team believe that, because of her poor prognosis, continued aggressive treatment would be inhumane. If such vigorous treatment is chosen for this child, she will need a permanent **tracheostomy** and surgical placement of a permanent feeding tube.

Her mother, Jesse, is twenty-one years old and is significantly mentally delayed. She may in fact suffer from a milder case of dystonia herself. She is minimally verbal and unable to care for herself. Her living situation has been unstable. She currently is staying in a motel with her mother, who has a history of drug abuse. It is reported that her mother may have hired Jesse out as a prostitute to obtain money for her own drug habit. Because of this unstable social situation, the infant has been made a ward of the county court, and an attorney has been appointed to represent her. The father of the child has not been identified.

DISCUSSION

When a newborn is critically ill, medical professionals generally recommend the use of all treatment that will be of benefit to the patient, but they may occasionally recommend against such treatment if it is felt to be disproportionately burdensome. Generally, professionals caring for an infant with handicaps look to the baby's parents for guidance about such decisions. They have an obligation, however, to challenge any parental request they believe is clearly not in the child's **best interests**.

In addition to this professional advocacy for handicapped newborns, society and the courts have a bias toward life support. This has been codified in the 1984 "Baby Doe Regulations," which mandate use of full treatment for handicapped newborns except: (a) when the infant is irreversibly comatose; (b) when treatment would be futile; or (c) when treatment would be virtually futile in terms of survival and would be inhumane.

In this case, the infant's mother is mentally unable to participate in decisions about goals of therapy or about the use or nonuse of specific modalities, and she is socially unable to provide infant care even if the baby could leave the hospital. Her professional caregivers believe that continued invasive treatment would be disproportionately burdensome for her. In addition, continuation of vigorous life support will require additional surgical measures that will further add to her treatment burden. Their recommendation for discontinuation of her death-postponing treatment is based on the burdens to her, not on her developmental potential or lack of social support.

RECOMMENDATIONS

1. It is ethically permissible for this infant's caregivers to seek consent from her court-appointed **surrogate** to change treatment goals from survival to comfort care, including the withdrawal of measures currently being used to postpone her death.
2. It is my opinion that this infant's condition falls within exception (c) of the Baby Doe Regulations, that is, continued aggressive treatment is virtually futile and would be inhumane.

FOLLOW-UP

A petition was filed with the county court with the recommendations of several professionals that life support be withdrawn. The court hearing one month after the consultation focused only on the issue of surrogacy (who could make decisions for her). Consent was given by the court for surgical placement of a feeding tube and tracheostomy. A second hearing was scheduled for one month later. By this time the patient had stabilized and shown some signs of awareness (tracking with her eyes, occasional smile). The court overruled the recommendation about **limitation of treatment**, and the patient was transferred to a long-term pediatric facility on the ventilator.

COMMENT

The social situation of this infant was overwhelmingly sad. Clinicians confronted with situations like this must guard against allowing the psychological factors to move them either in the direction of premature limitation of treatment or toward an overprotective stance that might lead to inappropriate overtreatment. While withdrawal of support from this infant seemed justified at the time of consultation, delays secondary to legal proceedings allowed her condition to slightly improve such that the initial conclusion might be questioned. Her long-term prognosis remained very poor, but we do not have any follow-up information beyond her date of discharge.

Is life for a few months on a ventilator requiring frequent blood tests better than death in the newborn period? I don't know.

Case 10.04 ───────────────────────────────────

QUESTION

Should this child with a poor prognosis for intellectual development (CHARGE syndrome) have lifesaving surgical interventions?

STORY

This six-week-old male was born at thirty-four weeks' **gestation** weighing three pounds and two ounces, and he was noted to have a heart murmur.

He was admitted to the neonatal intensive care unit (NICU) with diagnoses of respiratory distress syndrome and complex congenital heart disease. Staff have determined that he has the CHARGE association of anomalies,[15] multiple structural abnormalities that happen at a specific time in early development. All affected infants also have developmental delay, varying from minimal to severe. Those with sensory deficits are more severely delayed.

This child has been found to be blind in the right eye, but may have some central vision in the left. He has a heart abnormality that required a minor intervention and will require further procedures that cannot be done until he gains considerable weight. He has undeveloped nasal passages, which interfere with his ability to breathe (newborns can breathe only through their noses, not through their mouths). Though kidney problems are common in this syndrome, his kidneys appear to be functioning adequately. His genitalia are immature and underdeveloped. He has had poor growth. His ears are low-set, and results of hearing tests are pending. He is currently on a **ventilator** with minimal settings. Since he is unable to breathe through his mouth, he will require a **tracheostomy** until his nasal passages are surgically repaired, and that cannot be done until he is larger. He is being fed through a tube in his nose.

He has two parents, Tom and Theresa, and a healthy three-year-old sister. The **neonatologist** feels they have not bonded well with him and do not appear to be vigorous advocates for him. Even before the CHARGE diagnosis was made, his parents were suggesting that either his heart should be fixed so he could go home and be normal, or his therapy should be stopped.

DISCUSSION

Therapies that have the potential for physiologic benefit to an infant should be offered to parents. They then make a value assessment of whether the anticipated physiologic benefit sufficiently outweighs the burdens of the therapy and the burdens of the disease to warrant pursuing that therapy.

If parents choose to accept the proposed therapy, it is generally done, whether the treatment team feels the potential benefit is clear or marginal.

---

15. This developmental condition has been given an alliterative name based on the medical names of the constellation of symptoms.

Parents are generally allowed to decline proposed therapy that is of questionable or marginal benefit to their infant if they appear to be acting in the child's **best interests**. If parents decline proposed interventions that are not merely of marginal benefit but, in the treating team's estimate, would be clearly beneficial to the infant, there is strong ethical consensus and significant legal precedent to request judicial imposition of that treatment over the objection of the parents.

Mental retardation in and of itself is not sufficient justification for withholding lifesaving therapy from an infant. The motivation behind this precept is the feeling that mentally handicapped life is generally perceived to be better than no life. This assessment is often tempered, however, if the infant also has unrelievable suffering.

It is also generally felt that factors such as family integrity, degree of bonding, cost, and societal impact should not be determinative in making decisions for handicapped infants.

RECOMMENDATIONS

1. The proposed interventions all appear to have some potential for benefit to the infant. Thus they should all be offered, and if accepted by the parents, should be done.
2. If the parents decline any of the proposed interventions, the response of the team will depend on whether they feel the potential benefits to the infant are marginal or clear, and whether they feel the parents are acting in the infant's best interests. (a) If the parents decline therapy that the team feels is clearly beneficial to the infant, they should try to persuade the parents to accept it, and failing that, they should be willing to go to court to seek judicial intervention. (b) If the parents decline therapy that the team feels is of marginal benefit to the infant, it may be forgone as long as the team feels the parents are considering the infant's best interests over their own. If they appear to be making the decision for their own relief, it should be questioned and might need to have further review, either within the institution (e.g., by an ethics committee or an infant care review committee) or in court.

FOLLOW-UP

The baby's mother was reported to be unduly pessimistic from the outset, and the day after the consultation she requested that all treatment stop.

She was informed that the hospital staff was legally and ethically obliged to pursue beneficial treatment. When the parents were still declining consent for surgery one month later, the case was reported to child protective services. An attorney was appointed to represent the interests of the infant. At a subsequent hearing, the judge declined to remove custody from the parents. The infant's attorney appealed to the state appellate court and subsequently to the state supreme court. Both higher courts declined to hear it. Four months later this infant's ventilator was stopped at the insistence of his parents, and he died.

COMMENT

Courts are often supportive of parental rights, but even more often take very seriously their mandate to protect vulnerable infants from premature or inappropriate decisions to limit therapy. In this unusual court decision, judges held parental rights to be a higher standard than this protective mandate.

Most people of faith place a very high regard both on family integrity and on protection of vulnerable individuals. When these two elements conflict, as they did in this case, some may come down on one side of the issue and others on the other side. The wisdom of Solomon may be needed to reach a conclusion, and even after the fact, we may not always be sure we did "the right thing."

Case 10.05

QUESTION

Is it ethically permissible to continue painful treatments on this infant who has little, if any, potential for cognitive development because of holoprosencephaly?

STORY

This one-month-old infant boy was born at another hospital at thirty-six weeks' **gestation**. It was known from prenatal ultrasound studies that he had clefts of his lip and palate, but soon after birth he was transferred to the neonatal intensive care unit (NICU) because he also had severe anomalies of the brain, now diagnosed as semilobar holoprosencephaly[16] with diabetes insipidus.[17] He is deaf and blind, he responds to painful procedures (needle sticks, suctioning), and he even reacts poorly to diaper changing. He receives small doses of narcotics for discomfort and distress. He sucks reasonably well, and it is possible to comfort him with soothing. He was initially able to sustain spontaneous breathing, but he subsequently required **intubation** (and later a **tracheostomy**) for treatment of pneumonia and to protect his airway. It is not clear yet if he can be **weaned** from the **ventilator**. He is still receiving **total parenteral nutrition**, but it is anticipated that his stomach and intestines will work at some time in the future. His cognitive potential is also unclear, but is almost certainly very poor. With continued vigorous treatment he may survive for months or years.

His parents, Ron and Louise, are loving and visit for an hour or two daily, though they live some distance away. They have no other children. Louise is twenty-nine and a part-time college student; Ron is forty-one and works as a cable TV installer. They are reported to be of strong nondenominational Christian faith, but have little or no family support and do not belong to a church. The NICU staff believe they have not fully accepted the poor prognosis and are praying for miraculous intervention.

Some of his bedside nurses are becoming increasingly uncomfortable giving him fully vigorous treatment, fearing that they are inflicting pain with very little prospect of benefit to him.

DISCUSSION

Treatment decisions for handicapped newborns are ideally made jointly by parents and professionals. Parents are generally allowed some discretion in such matters and may choose a treatment plan that is not the first recommendation of the professional caregivers. They sometimes even choose treatment that the professionals believe is not in the child's **best interests**. Still, the parents' choice generally prevails. The professionals may be justified in refusing to provide a requested treatment (a) if that treatment is

16. Holoprosencephaly is the name given to a group of developmental anomalies of the brain and face with a spectrum of severity. The semilobar form of holoprosencephaly is intermediate in severity. However, all forms result in moderate to severe mental retardation.

17. An inability to concentrate urine resulting from lack of a hormone made in the brain (not related to diabetes mellitus). In this case, it indicates a rather severe malformation of the brain.

truly physiologically futile, or (b) if they believe the parents' choice is causing the child unrelieved suffering. In such cases, a challenge to parental surrogacy in court may be justified. At the same time, there is a societal and judicial bias toward using treatments for handicapped newborns. Thus parents are usually supported by the courts in their choice for "inappropriate" treatment, though usually not for truly futile treatment.

Current treatment of this child is not futile in that it is working to prolong his life. Some of his caregivers may feel it is inappropriate and not in his best interests. However, there remains some uncertainty about his future, and it is possible that currently burdensome treatments may be short term so that his burden/benefit ratio may change with time.

RECOMMENDATIONS

1. It is ethically permissible to continue his current treatment plan.
2. It is also ethically permissible to continue to educate his parents about his condition and to periodically recommend some limits to treatment if his professional caregivers agree strongly that it is not in his best interests. However, such recommendations should not be frequent or harsh so as to be perceived as badgering. A second opinion from outside the institution might encourage parental acceptance of his condition and prognosis.
3. Continued efforts at supporting the parents in their belief system are also appropriate. If there is concern that their beliefs may be significantly different from others in their faith tradition, it may be beneficial to ask a pastor with a similar perspective to sit in on discussions.
4. His bedside nurses should continue to focus their efforts on his comfort as well as his survival, and they should encourage and relieve each other if they feel stress from providing treatment they deem inappropriate.

FOLLOW-UP

The parents continued to be optimistic, searching the Internet for other options and requesting consultation at pediatric specialty centers. Three months later he weaned off the ventilator, had abdominal surgery to reduce reflux, and was switched to tube feedings. He was discharged home at ten months of age. Six months later his physician reported no significant change in his condition.

COMMENT

Nursing concerns that the parents were "too loving" or "unrealistically optimistic" or "hoping for a miracle" in this case may have been a response to their religious fervor. Or they may have been based purely on compassion for this infant for whom the nurses were continually being asked to provide treatments that clearly made him uncomfortable.

Continued treatment of this neonate in the face of a poor prognosis was ethically justified, some would even say ethically obligatory, because the treatment itself entailed little burden to the infant. Treatment was neither "futile" nor "virtually futile and inhumane."

Case 10.06 ──────────────────────────

QUESTION

Is it ethically permissible to limit diagnostic or therapeutic interventions for this infant with multiple anomalies when there is some uncertainty of prognosis?

STORY

This one-week-old male infant was born to Nancy after thirty-six weeks' **gestation**, weighing four and a half pounds, with **Apgar scores** of 4 (one minute) and 7 (five minutes). He was small for his gestational age, required **intubation** in the delivery room, and soon required ventilatory assistance. He was transferred to the medical center neonatal intensive care unit (NICU) for evaluation of multiple anomalies.

Three weeks prior to delivery an ultrasound had been done because of large uterine size, and it showed an excess of **amniotic fluid** and limb deformities. Although chromosomal anomaly was suspected (perhaps trisomy-13 or -18, syndromes resulting from an extra chromosome #13 or #18), his chromosome studies were found to be normal.

Evaluation of the infant and workup to date have shown microcephaly (small head), frontal bossing (prominent forehead), underdevelopment of his face, small eyes, flat and rotated ears, right-sided stomach, diminished growth of the left side of the body, and multiple limb anomalies (lack of flexion of arms; short, tapered, and clenched fingers; dislocated hips and left knee; clubbed feet; underdeveloped left toes). His heart and lungs appear to be normal, but he did not tolerate accidental **extubation** and had to be quickly reintubated, probably because of underdevelopment of the cartilage in his airway. Head ultrasound is normal except for the obvious smallness of the brain, and **MRI** imaging of the brain shows nonspecific abnormality on the surface of the cortex (the upper surface of the brain where centers are located that involve much sensation and voluntary motion). The ear-nose-throat consultant recommends **bronchoscopy** to assess the airway, and he would prefer to do a **tracheostomy** first, feeling this would be safer due to his fragile respiratory status. The neurology consultant says his neurologic prognosis is "difficult to ascertain, but most likely to be poor with decreased purposeful activity and limited intellectual capacity."

Specialists believe this represents Larsen's syndrome. In this condition the musculoskeletal problems tend to dominate, but some are reported to have mental retardation. There is a less common lethal form where infants die of underdevelopment of the lungs.

This infant's current treatment consists of tube feeding, serial casting of his legs to try to straighten his clubbed feet, and intubation to maintain his airway; he is on minimal **ventilator** settings and could probably breathe unaided if he had a tracheostomy.

His parents are very loving and concerned for his well-being. Nancy is a stay-at-home mom, and her husband works in human resources for a large corporation. They attend a Presbyterian church two or three times a year. They are both concerned about this baby's quality of life and his suffering. They are comfortable raising a child who is "slow," but they want to avoid having him "propped up in a corner in an institution." In addition, they have raised the issue of the impact of a severely disabled child on their family (three healthy children) and the question of who would care for him if he should outlive them. At the time that the consultation was requested, they were reluctant to consent to either bronchoscopy or tracheostomy (surgery to allow attachment of the ventilator to his neck rather then going through his mouth).

DISCUSSION

There exists in our culture a professional inclination toward treatment of handicapped newborns. In addition, we have an even stronger societal (legal) mandate to not withhold lifesaving therapy from vulnerable newborns. This infant does not fit any of the three exceptions for mandatory treatment.

From an ethics perspective, it is important to have the best possible prognostic information before making any irreversible decisions. When there is a high degree of certainty that an infant will have minimal cognitive development, it is ethically permissible to weigh the benefits against the burdens for each treatment used. For example, there is generally felt to be no moral obligation to use burdensome life-extending technology to prevent death in a child who will not be able to engage in relationships.

In this case, there is sufficient uncertainty about his prognosis that there appears to be an ethical (as well as a legal) obligation to use standard therapy. If, as time passes, it becomes clear that he will have very limited cognitive potential, it would then be ethically permissible to withhold or withdraw any therapy for which the burdens appear to outweigh the benefits. It might even be permissible to withhold antibiotics for a life-threatening infection if he appeared to be suffering from treatments needed to sustain his life.

RECOMMENDATION

Evaluation of this patient's airway is both legally and ethically obligatory. (a) If only the upper airway is underdeveloped and he can achieve independent respiration with merely a tracheostomy, this and other standard therapy should be continued until his developmental potential is better understood. (b) If, however, his lower airway is also significantly underdeveloped and he requires some form of mechanical ventilatory support, it would be permissible to reassess the benefits-and-burdens equation for him.

FOLLOW-UP

After the consultation his parents consented to a tracheostomy. Further evaluation showed an "immature" **electroencephalogram**, and an ophthalmologist determined that he is blind in one eye and has a cataract in the other. Soon after the tracheostomy, he was removed from the ventilator, began moving his extremities and started sucking. His parents learned how to give tube feedings and how to care for his tracheostomy, and he was discharged home at five weeks of age.

COMMENT

While we give considerable discretion to parents regarding such decisions, our primary responsibility as health-care professionals is to seek the **best interests** of the infant. It is understandable that parents would look to the future (e.g., their concerns about ongoing care if he should outlive them), but we must protect vulnerable newborns from parental decisions that focus on their (parental) needs or concerns.

Case 10.07

QUESTION

Is it ethically permissible to suggest withdrawal of life support from this infant who has a very poor prognosis for survival and is suffering from his current therapy?

STORY

This three-month-old boy was a full-term baby who was healthy until admitted at one month of age with pneumonia caused by a virus known to cause extensive pulmonary tissue destruction. He has been critically ill since admission, and received nearly five weeks of extracorporeal membrane oxygenation (ECMO).[18] After he failed to respond adequately to this prolonged course, his professional caregivers and his parents made a difficult decision to stop the ECMO with the expectation that he would not survive on a lower level of ventilatory support. However, he did not die. He has since been on high-frequency ventilation (rather than standard ventilation) with 100 percent oxygen and high pressure settings, but has had repeated pulmonary complications including repeated lung collapses requiring insertion of new chest drainage tubes nearly every day. His chest X-ray shows progressive scarring and very little functional lung tissue. He continues to be infected with resistant bacteria and has received multiple

18. ECMO is a complicated invasive form of treatment that can be used for the short-term (several days) replacement of function of the lungs plus or minus the heart; available at a few pediatric centers around the United States.

transfusions for anemia. He has had seizures, and his liver is enlarged and functions poorly, but the cause of the latter is unknown.

At an infant care committee meeting today, with several current bedside caregivers and multiple other neonatal intensive care unit (NICU) staff who know him well, there was unanimity that (a) this child will never be free of his need for ventilatory support, (b) he cannot survive more than a few days or weeks even with continued support, and (c) he is suffering from current therapies. Everyone present wanted to make a strong professional recommendation to his family to withdraw life support so that he can be released from his suffering.

His mother has likewise expressed concern about his suffering. She agreed with the stopping of ECMO after some discussion and was prepared for him to die, but has again become hopeful since he did not die. She has one other child who is healthy. Her husband travels on overseas business much of the time, but he was able to come home for a short time to participate in discussions about discontinuation of the ECMO.

DISCUSSION

It is ethically and legally permissible to withdraw support from a critically ill newborn with the expectation that the child will not survive if: (a) the child is irreversibly comatose, (b) further treatment is futile for survival, or (c) further treatment is virtually futile and is inhumane. Parents are the appropriate **surrogates** for seriously ill children and, after being adequately informed of the options and likely outcomes, should most often make decisions about goals of therapy and about the use or nonuse of specific treatment modalities. In some cases, however, as when a child is experiencing irremediable suffering from the interventions used, it is professionally appropriate for the child's caregivers to make a strong recommendation for withdrawal of support, and to try to persuade reluctant parents to consent to this course of action. In some rare circumstances, it may be ethically appropriate to even seek judicial permission to withdraw painful interventions over the objection of parents who remain insistent on continued treatment.

In this case, continued treatment is not clearly futile in that it could temporarily postpone the child's death, as it has for the past several weeks. However, as time has passed, and with continued deterioration, it seems that treatment is quickly approaching physiologic **futility**. Even if continued vigorous therapy is not yet physiologically futile, it is "virtually futile and inhumane." Thus it is not only ethically permissible to recommend withdrawal of support, it is ethically obligatory to do so if his caregivers believe his suffering cannot otherwise be relieved.

RECOMMENDATIONS

1. It is ethically permissible to withdraw support from this infant with the expectation that he will not survive.
2. If his caregivers believe that continued vigorous treatment cannot reverse his underlying condition so that he can survive, they should make a recommendation to his mother that his support be stopped.
3. If his caregivers believe that continued aggressive treatment cannot reverse his underlying condition, and they further believe that continued treatment is causing him unrelievable suffering, they should make this recommendation to his mother very strongly, and on his behalf they should try to persuade her if she is reluctant. Though she may need some time to again accept his imminent death, this time of reflection and consideration should not be allowed to be prolonged because of his continued suffering.

FOLLOW-UP

The **neonatologist** made a strong recommendation from the entire NICU team to stop life support. The baby's mother consented, her husband agreed, support was stopped, and the patient died quickly.

COMMENT

On the basis of a belief in family integrity, it is most often appropriate to support parental decisions and to try to meet their goals. However, in those rare instances when a parental decision to continue treatment causes the infant suffering that cannot be relieved, and the chosen treatment has virtually no prospect of benefiting the infant, professionals have an obligation to advocate for relief of the infant's suffering.

In retrospect, it may have been better when the decision was made to stop ECMO to remove all respiratory support rather than putting the infant on conventional and, later, high-frequency ventilatory support. This decision may have been considered a compromise acceptable to the parents who were reluctant to limit treatment.

A professional recommendation to withdraw life support is a major turn of events and should never be done lightly. These decisions should remain difficult, especially when parents demonstrate an understandable natural inclination to continue treatment. Determining the proper timing for such a recommendation may likewise be difficult; different individuals often reach this conclusion at different times. Developing unanimity of the NICU team is often a good indicator that the time has been reached.

Case 10.08 ─────────────────────────────

QUESTION

Should we continue to provide the life-sustaining treatment requested by the parents of this infant with a lethal condition (thanatophoric dwarfism)?

STORY

This seven-day-old girl is in the neonatal intensive care unit (NICU). Her mother, Maria, is a twenty-six-year-old Italian woman, and this is her first baby. The father, also Italian, is fifty-three and has four older children from a previous relationship. It is reported that Maria took prenatal vitamins but received no prenatal care during this pregnancy. She gave birth one week ago at another hospital, approximately at term, by Cesarean section because of obstructed labor.

At birth the baby was noted to have short limbs and a large head and to be in respiratory distress. She was **intubated**, given ventilatory support, and transported to the medical center NICU. A geneticist and a dysmorphologist (a specialist in congenital anomalies) have seen her, and made a diagnosis of thanatophoric dwarfism.

Thanatophoric dwarfism is a uniformly lethal condition that occurs sporadically, without a familial or genetic pattern. Its manifestations include multiple characteristic skeletal anomalies, and it is differentiable from other nonlethal forms of dwarfism. Its lethality stems from the presence of a small bony chest cage and consequent underdevelopment of the lungs. Since this condition is always lethal, the standard of care is to give infants with this diagnosis comfort care, and most die within a few days.

Her parents were informed of the diagnosis and prognosis, and they requested a few days of intensive treatment. Attempts at **weaning** from the **ventilator** have been unsuccessful, and she now in fact requires increased ventilatory support. Her parents, especially her father, have become increasingly resistant to the NICU staff's recommendation to withdraw support. The father has now taken the position that "we are obligated to treat her because she needs help," and he has requested six weeks of treatment to see if she will grow and improve. She was baptized yesterday by the Catholic chaplain at the request of her mother. Characteristic of the Italian culture, Dad is clearly the dominant person in the marriage; Mom is quiet and defers to him during discussions.

On exam the patient is severely dysmorphic (multiple unusual physical structures and features) but does not appear to be uncomfortable. She is on a ventilator, which is usually considered moderately burdensome. In addition, she requires suctioning every three hours, receives intravenous fluids, and has punctures for blood gases every day, or more frequently.

DISCUSSION

The goal of treatment for a seriously handicapped newborn is generally chosen jointly by the parents and professional caregivers of the child. Some parental discretion is allowed in that parents may sometimes choose a goal that would not be the first recommendation of the professionals but is still within the bounds of accepted medical practice. Occasionally, however, the parents choose a goal that is either not achievable or outside the bounds of accepted medical practice.

In this case, the dad's request for continued support "so that she can grow" indicates the parents have chosen a goal of survival. The neonatal literature confirms that this is not an achievable goal; all infants born with this condition die. The current treatment is not technically "futile" because it is postponing her death, but her caregivers consider it "inappropriate" because it is *merely* postponing her inevitable death and it is burdensome to the patient and causing her to suffer without receiving the commensurate benefit of long-term survival. At the current time, her burden is not felt by her caregivers to be sufficiently great to warrant unilateral withdrawal as a matter of conscience.

RECOMMENDATIONS

1. The current treatment should be continued while efforts are made to persuade the child's parents to consent to withdrawal of support. It should be repeated to them that this is a clearly lethal condition, and that continued support will not change that but does cause her to suffer needlessly. This message should be reinforced by physicians, nurses, social workers, chaplains. Other educational efforts (pictures, written descriptions) may help.

2. A second opinion from **neonatologists** at another institution might help the parents understand that the recommendations are the current standard of care.

3. If, in the estimation of her caregivers, her suffering becomes uncontrollable, they would be justified to take the position that they cannot in good conscience continue to provide the requested treatment. If her parents are still unwilling to accept the recommendation to withdraw support, they should be given assistance in seeking another institution willing to give the support. If none is found after a short time, it would then be ethically justifiable to inform them that the treatment will be stopped at a specified time. Their only option then would be to seek a court injunction to prevent withdrawal of support.

FOLLOW-UP

Mom slowly came to an acceptance of the child's inevitable death. However, Dad became increasingly resistant, hostile, and threatening. Staff perceived that his resistance was based on his understanding of their Roman Catholic belief that stopping treatment would be murder. Counseling with a Catholic chaplain made no apparent difference. After further pulmonary deterioration (two weeks after the consultation), including several episodes when both parents were present, they said they could accept her death "if it is God's will." They consented to a **do-not-resuscitate order** but were unwilling to consent to removal of the ventilator. At six weeks of age, she had a cardiac arrest while still on the ventilator, and she was not resuscitated.

COMMENT

When parents think medical recommendations are inconsistent with their values or wishes, they frequently become angry or even hostile. This tension may increase the difference of opinion. If the basis for their opinion is their understanding of a religious tenet, it may be helpful to encourage them to speak with a hospital chaplain, or preferably with their own clergyperson. Sometimes, however, they are so focused on one particular belief (e.g., the sanctity of life or their parental obligation) that they may be unable to fully understand complementary beliefs (e.g., the finitude of life, compassion, relief of suffering). Because of this dad's dominance and this mom's reticence, the difference of opinion in this case did not become evident until late in the course of events.

Case 10.09

QUESTION

Is it ethically permissible to withdraw intravenous fluids from this neonate with severe brain damage?

STORY

This twelve-day-old girl was born at term to Laura, age twenty-nine, after an uncomplicated pregnancy. Delivery was slowed when the baby's shoulders became wedged in the birth canal, and the baby was floppy and had poor color at birth (**Apgar scores** of 3, 6, and 6). She had early seizures. She was transferred to the neonatal intensive care unit (NICU) and required minimal ventilatory assistance for forty-eight hours. She has a rudimentary suck, but cannot swallow and has had some difficulty handling her secretions. She shows little motion and occasional seizures. She has opened her eyes at least once. She is currently receiving intravenous (IV) fluids and no medications. After consultation with her parents, orders were written for no resuscitation or **intubation** if she should deteriorate. Serial exams and an **MRI** of her head have led the neurology consultant to say with confidence that she has suffered severe brain damage from lack of oxygen. His best prediction is that she will demonstrate marked developmental delay and very limited function or ability to communicate or eat.

Her caring parents have been aware of her situation and supportive of investigations and treatments. They have said from the beginning that they can handle a lot and are willing to care for a disabled child. Both have had personal experience with relatives who had significant disabilities. They own and operate a bakery, but have sufficient employee help that they could devote considerable time to caring for a child with special needs. However, when the severity of her compromised future became clear, they asked that her IV fluids be stopped with the expectation that she would not survive. All members of the NICU team (several physicians and nurses, a social worker, a chaplain) support this request.

DISCUSSION

In caring for infants with disabilities, there is a professional and societal presumption that life is inherently good and even compromised life is to be preferred to death. However, in some situations the prospect is for such severely compromised quality of life that the burdens of treatment necessary to maintain life are disproportionate to the benefits of that life. In those situations, most believe it is permissible to provide less than maximal treatment.

From an ethics perspective, parents are recognized as the appropriate **surrogates** for their children. Health-care professionals have an obligation to ensure that parents are not making premature or inappropriate decisions to limit treatment for children who might enjoy a reasonable quality of life with adequate care and support. With the recognition that not all parents will reach the same decisions in similar cases, the ethics question becomes whether a given parental decision is within a reasonable construal of parental discretion.

From a legal perspective, however, our court system has put in place a higher standard. Federal "Baby Doe Regulations" (1984) require that all disabled infants receive standard treatment, including fluids and nutrition, unless (a) they are permanently unconscious; (b) treatment would be futile in terms of survival; or (c) treatment would be virtually futile in terms of survival and the treatment needed for survival would be inhumane.

In this case, the fact that all the many professionals caring for this infant support the parental request to discontinue fluids and nutrition suggests that their decision is probably within a reasonable construal of parental discretion. However, the patient's prognosis does not clearly fit within the Baby Doe exemptions from the requirement for full treatment. This state enforces these regulations through the agency for child protective services (CPS).

RECOMMENDATIONS

1. If the prognostic certainty about this infant's developmental potential is high, it is ethically permissible to honor this parental request to withdraw artificially administered fluids and nutrition.
2. Because the legal constraints may be tighter than ethical standards, CPS should be consulted before this decision is implemented.
3. If there will be any significant delay in implementing a decision to stop IV fluids, consideration should be given to supplemental nutrition in order to avoid further neurologic compromise from incomplete nutrition.

FOLLOW-UP

The CPS pediatric consultant and the CPS commissioner supported the parents' decision the day after the ethics consultation. IV fluids were withdrawn. The parents continued to hold the infant and grieved appropriately. They were initially hesitant to allow morphine for facial grimacing, concerned that they do nothing to hasten death. The NICU staff agreed to use a half dose, which appeared to keep her comfortable. She died in her mother's arms several days after the IV fluids were stopped.

COMMENT

The parents' familiarity with caring for children with handicaps and their willingness to raise a handicapped child of their own suggested that they were caring and giving. Thus their request to limit treatment raised few questions about selfish motivation, which might have been a consideration if other parents made a similar request based on their own needs.

The fact that all the NICU team supported the parents' decision should not by itself be determinative. It is possible that the team were merely charmed by the parents' attitude, or even that the professionals in this particular NICU had less respect for the value of disabled life than average. The latter seems very unlikely because NICU clinicians as a group are among the most optimistic and hardworking of all clinicians, almost always reluctant to "give up" on their appointed task of pursuing survival of their charges. And it has been my experience that individuals within that team are very willing to stand up and voice a minority opinion. So when such a team offers unanimous support for withdrawal of life support from a severely compromised neonate, it usually does indicate that the decision has ethical merit.

Case 10.10 ————————————————————————————————

QUESTION

Is it ethically permissible to withdraw support from this infant with congenital infection at the request of his parents?

STORY

This two-week-old boy was delivered by Cesarean section (due to slowing of the baby's heart during labor) at thirty-nine weeks' **gestation**. At birth he was noted to have respiratory distress, rash, enlarged liver and spleen, and an abnormal blood count. He was transferred to the neonatal intensive care unit (NICU) for evaluation and treatment of presumed congenital infection. Congenital cytomegalovirus (CMV) disease was recently confirmed. This infection occurs during pregnancy.

He has been treated vigorously with high-frequency ventilation, repeated platelet transfusions, an antiviral agent, and antibiotics. His pulmonary status has improved somewhat in the past few days, but he still requires high-frequency ventilation and his blood platelets remain dangerously low, putting him at serious risk of bleeding into his brain. Head ultrasound shows brain swelling and cysts; no brain calcifications are present, which suggests his CMV infection occurred late in gestation. Ophthalmology consultation says he has "poor visual function" without specific evidence of CMV infection in the eye. Neurology consultation shows normal head circumference at birth and subsequent growth, and the consultant says the prognosis is guarded, with normal development unlikely.

The literature states that there is no effective therapy for symptomatic congenital CMV disease, which carries a 30 percent mortality rate. In addition, the neurological prognosis for the survivors is difficult to quantify, but is known to be worse with the presence of microcephaly, eye infection, and brain calcifications.

One of the NICU staff suggested to the parents that they might want to consider withdrawal of life support. The NICU care team and consultants are supportive of this, but requested ethics consultation before proceeding. The infant's parents are married and have a healthy four-year-old girl. While this was an unplanned pregnancy, they had adjusted and were looking forward to the birth. They are both observant Roman Catholics. They are anguished over a decision to stop life support, and are asking questions that indicate they are clearly seeking the **best interests** of the infant.

DISCUSSION

Parents are the presumed **surrogates** for their children. Medical professionals generally honor the treatment requests of parents unless they are clearly not acting in the child's best interests. When parents of a critically ill newborn request the withdrawal of life support, it is important to consider the overall prognosis of the child, both for survival and for subsequent developmental potential. Federal regulations, while very protective of vulnerable handicapped newborns, recognize the appropriateness of withdrawal of treatment in those situations when treatment would not be effective in ameliorating or correcting all the life-threatening conditions, so that continued treatment is merely prolonging the dying process.

In this case, there is no effective therapy for this infant's underlying condition. He has received vigorous supportive treatment, but his abnormal blood condition is still life-threatening and his neurological prognosis is poor.

RECOMMENDATION

If all his professional caregivers agree that further aggressive treatment will not correct his condition so it is clear that he will die in spite of continued treatment, it is ethically and legally permissible to change goals to comfort care and to discontinue life support.

FOLLOW-UP

After talking with the pediatric **neurologist**, both parents requested that life support be stopped. The baby was baptized. The **ventilator** was stopped, and he died in his mother's arms about one hour later.

COMMENT

The fundamental medical problem in the baby, the CMV infection, carried a 30 percent mortality rate, that is, a 70 percent chance of survival. It would seem prudent, perhaps even ethically mandatory, to continue treatment in light of this. However, his uncorrectable blood problem (low platelets) made his particular prognosis much worse than that stated in the textbooks. This unquantifiable information tilted the scale here so that withdrawal of support was deemed ethically permissible.

Case 10.11

QUESTION

Is it ethically permissible for this infant's mother to decline standard surgical procedures?

STORY

This three-and-one-half-week-old girl was the product of a full-term normal second pregnancy in a thirty-four-year-old woman named Elizabeth. She was born vaginally at an outlying community hospital weighing just under six pounds, and she looked healthy at birth. She was soon noted to have a high-pitched cry, some unusual physical features, and a right-left transposition of her internal organs. At eighteen hours of age she was transferred to the medical center neonatal intensive care unit (NICU) with respiratory distress that had started after vomiting and choking. She has been found to have "*cri du chat* syndrome" (French, cry of the cat), caused by a chromosomal abnormality. Hers is an unusually large chromosomal defect. She is awake and fussy, has a poor suck reflex, produces a lot of respiratory mucus, coughs and chokes frequently, and is tube-fed in the prone position with her head elevated. At times she temporarily stops breathing.

Some babies survive this syndrome with severe mental retardation (average IQ = 20), but most succumb to respiratory infections from **aspiration**. Nearly 90 percent of survivors display self-injury or mutilating behavior. This baby has severe gastroesophogeal reflux,[19] which is part of this syndrome. Because of this she will probably not be able to avoid repeated respiratory infections. Two surgeries have been proposed: a minor procedure to insert a feeding tube through her abdominal wall and a major operation to reduce her risk of aspiration. Her mother has declined both.

---

19. Reverse flow of stomach contents up the esophagus, with the potential for aspirating said material into the lungs.

Her mother is a business executive. She describes herself as basically optimistic and says her life is otherwise good; she is financially secure. She is divorced from the father of her healthy nine-year-old daughter, but in close contact. The father of this child is not involved. She has researched these diagnoses extensively, is well informed, and has discussed matters with her Seventh-Day Adventist pastor. In light of the baby's poor long-term prognosis, she has consented to orders for no resuscitation and no ventilatory assistance. The reason she gives for declining the proposed surgeries is, "I love her too much to do that to her." Her plan is to take her daughter home for comfort care. She volunteers that she would give up working to care for her if she had a chance for a decent quality of life, which she describes as breathing, eating, and experiencing some joy. She is personally comfortable with the chosen treatment plan, but she requested ethics consultation because she wanted to make sure she was within ethical bounds as well.

DISCUSSION

Neonatology operates under a professional and societal mandate to protect infants with physical or mental disabilities from premature or inappropriate **limitation of treatment** decisions. The federal "Baby Doe Regulations" clearly define when it is legally permissible to withhold or withdraw therapy from handicapped newborns. States, hospitals, and individuals interpret these regulations with varying degrees of latitude, some allowing more parental discretion than others. The primary ethical imperative is that the decision-makers, both professional and family, seek the **best interests** of the infant; survival in a compromised but comfortable condition should ordinarily be sought if it is feasible.

In this case, the two offered surgeries are standard procedures that would be used for this infant if she had severe reflux without the chromosomal anomaly. However, her short-term ability to appreciate her environment is very limited. And in both the short and long term, she will experience the burdens of her compromised life (aspiration, choking, shortness of breath, self-injury). Even if surgeries were done to reduce reflux, she would still have respiratory distress from her heavy secretions. Both her professional caregivers and her mother appear to be seeking her best interests.

RECOMMENDATIONS

1. It is ethically permissible to withhold vigorous lifesaving therapies if this infant should deteriorate.
2. It would be ethically permissible to provide the two recommended standard surgical procedures.
3. It is also ethically permissible to forgo these invasive procedures that might temporarily forestall death but would do nothing to enhance her poor quality of current or future life.
4. The permissibility of withholding other nonburdensome modalities (feeding, antibiotics) is less clear. Most would maintain that these are morally obligatory; others would say they are required only if needed for patient comfort.
5. It might be worthwhile to discuss these matters with all NICU staff involved in her care to ensure understanding and to determine if any of her caregivers have significant dissenting opinions.

FOLLOW-UP

The baby did not have the proposed surgeries. She was discharged home on hospice care at four weeks of age.

COMMENT

Some people of faith oppose any decisions to limit treatment that are based on the infant's current or future quality of life. This resistance is often warranted since some parents are more concerned about their own quality of life than they are about the child's. Had this been an average case of *cri du chat* syndrome, this would have to be considered. However, the fact that her particular chromosomal defect was larger than the average for this syndrome suggested that her abnormalities would be of the more severe type. In addition, the mom's extended research and her willingness to sacrificially care for this infant lent support to her request.

Case 10.12

QUESTION

Should lifesaving cardiac surgery be done on this infant with severe brain damage?

STORY

This eleven-day-old girl was born by Cesarean section at thirty-eight weeks' **gestation** with **Apgar scores** of 8 and 9. Her mother is twenty-two years old and has no other children; she has had two induced abortions. She had little prenatal care during this pregnancy.

At about forty-eight hours of age the patient was noted to be breathing rapidly and not feeding. Evaluation showed she had congenital heart disease (type B interrupted aortic arch with ventricular septal defect, atrial septal defect, and patent ductus arteriosis). During cardiac catheterization she suffered a prolonged period of low blood pressure. She was transferred to the neonatal intensive care unit (NICU) and has been treated aggressively. Her cardiovascular status is now stable, and corrective surgery is planned when she is cleared neurologically. Surgery for this condition is standard therapy and has less than 15 percent mortality. Since she is stable, it would be possible to delay surgery for a few weeks, but this would increase her risk of developing other problems.

She was noted to have seizures soon after admission to the NICU. In addition, a **CT scan** has shown thrombosis of multiple veins (cause uncertain; not from **ischemia**, possibly from sludging), swelling of both sides of her brain, and mild hemorrhage into her brain. In spite of this, her cerebral blood flow appears to be adequate. Her neurological diagnosis is significant hypoxic-ischemic **encephalopathy**, i.e., brain damage from lack of oxygen. This condition has been stable for the past several days, but the long-term prognosis is uncertain and will not be totally clear for several months. It is certain that she will not be neurologically normal, and there is a significant likelihood that she will be severely impaired, quite possibly in a **persistent vegetative state** (PVS). Without the neurologic problem, standard therapy would be cardiac surgery as soon as feasible. Without the cardiac problem, standard therapy would be supportive care and watchful waiting.

The baby's mother is single and has some support from her own mother. She has a history of substance abuse (marijuana, amphetamines, alcohol). Her wishes about surgery or other aggressive intervention have not yet been explored. The baby's father has little involvement.

DISCUSSION

Parental decisions about treatment of severely handicapped newborns should be followed unless they refuse standard therapy that is clearly in the infant's **best interests**. The second applicable standard here is that negative effects of the child's continued existence on other individuals and on society should be excluded from the calculus.

Determining what is in the infant's best interests is very difficult in this case where it is certain that the child will be neurologically handicapped but uncertain to what extent. The generally accepted standard in these situations is that permanent handicaps justify withholding life-sustaining treatment only when they are so severe that continued existence would not be of net benefit to the infant. Net benefit is absent if the burdens imposed on the patient by the disability or its treatment would lead a competent person to choose to forgo treatment. This standard is unfortunately subjective and imprecise.

We could visualize cardiac surgery for this infant as we would supportive therapy for an infant with similar neurological problems but a normal heart. In other words, cardiac surgery should be provided if the brain problem would lead us to do supportive therapy. If the benefits to the infant of continued life are sufficiently ambiguous that we would either not offer supportive therapy or allow the mother to reject it, then it would be justifiable to not offer cardiac surgery or to allow the mother to reject it.

RECOMMENDATIONS

1. Cardiac surgery should be recommended to this infant's mother. There does not appear to be sufficient certainty of a PVS to recommend against surgery.
2. If her mother declines consent for the recommended surgery, the NICU team must decide if they feel strongly enough about this advocacy position to go to court to impose surgery over her refusal. Since there is significant doubt about this child's future quality of life, some **neonatologists** would be uncomfortable going to court and would reluctantly accept maternal refusal of surgery.

FOLLOW-UP

Corrective cardiac surgery was recommended to this patient's mother, though nonsurgery was discussed. Mom consented to surgery, which was done successfully four days after the ethics consultation.

COMMENT

Cardiac surgery for this compromised newborn seems very appropriate in light of the uncertainty about her cognitive potential from the severe brain damage she received during catheterization. However, if her mother had declined consent for surgery, many neonatologists would have been reluctant to request a court order for it, based on the high likelihood she would have a poor neurological outcome and would thus be unable to appreciate the benefits of painful surgery.

*   *   *

Other Neonatal Cases

Case 9.07

Reference about Neonatal Issues

Lantos, J. D., and W. L. Meadow. *Neonatal Bioethics: The Moral Challenges of Medical Innovation.* Baltimore: Johns Hopkins University Press, 2006.

CHAPTER 11

Ethical Issues in Children

Early in medical school I was taught that "Kids are not small adults," leading on to the assertion that they are different not only anatomically but
also physiologically and psychologically. I would now hasten to add — and
ethically. The primary ethical differences between adults and children are
(a) a different locus of decision making and (b) a different standard for decision making.

Locus of Decision Making

Treatment decisions in pediatrics are almost always made by a **surrogate**,
and that surrogate is almost always one or two (or sometimes more) parents. Sometimes, however, foster parents or state agencies are responsible
for treatment decisions for children (see Case 11.02). As a child matures, the
locus of decision making gradually shifts from the parents to the child. The
legal authority for medical decision making in the United States is determined by each state, and it shifts at midnight on the child's eighteenth
birthday in most states. Everyone realizes that this arbitrary line does not
recognize either the variation between children or the gradual development
of moral authority. The policy statement on consent, permission, and assent by the American Academy of Pediatrics Committee on Bioethics explores this ethical transition and provides practical applications.[1]

---

1. Committee on Bioethics, American Academy of Pediatrics, "Informed Consent, Parental Permission, and Assent in Pediatric Practice," *Pediatrics* 95 (1995): 314-17.

Standard of Decision Making

The child has not previously had **decision-making capacity**, so we cannot search for a **substituted judgment** but are always making **best interest** decisions. In addition, of course, the child does not get to choose his or her surrogate, as an adult is able to do. Parents and physicians almost always agree on what is in a particular child's best interests. So those situations rarely present ethical dilemmas.

Ethical problems arise when there is a difference of opinion about what is in a child's best interests. Most often such disagreements are between the physician on one side and both parents on the other. The disagreements may involve either a lack of parental consent for something recommended by the physician (see Case 11.08) or a parental request for an intervention that the physician believes to be inappropriate (see Case 11.05). These can most often be managed by discussion or negotiation, or in some instances by compromise. In other instances the problem is that two parents disagree (see Case 11.06). This can make resolution more difficult. And sometimes, of course, two or more health-care professionals may not agree on what should be done for the child (see Case 11.03).

Requests for inappropriate treatment can be managed relatively easily, at least from a physician's perspective. If a parent requests antibiotics for a viral infection, the physician can merely decline.[2] If parents want a child of average or slightly below average height to receive growth hormone injections so he or she will be the tallest child on the basketball team, a physician may easily say, "No, that is outside the standard of care and I am unwilling to do that." The parents are free to look elsewhere, but the ethical issue from the physician's perspective is over and done with. It is, however, more difficult for physicians to convince parents to discontinue a treatment the doctors believe is no longer working when the parents think it is still beneficial (see Case 11.05).

Refusal of recommended treatment, on the other hand, is not so easy to manage. The state has given physicians who care for children the responsibility to report to child protective services (CPS) instances of what they consider medical neglect. Sounds straightforward, but it isn't always

---

2. Unfortunately, physicians not infrequently relent, rationalizing that if it is perchance a more serious bacterial infection, the child may get worse or even die, and in addition, the parents would then have a legitimate claim for negligence and might sue. Thus antibiotics are often misused for minor or viral infections, and this leads to a rapid rise in bacterial resistance. But the ethical issue is that the physician has the option to decline.

so. If parents allow a child to eat junk food and watch violence on TV, is that neglect? If a parent doesn't bring a child back for a recheck after treatment for an ear infection, is that neglect? What about missed appointments for well-child care? Or even more specifically, what if the parent brings the child in for routine checks but refuses to allow immunization, believing that the risk of side effects from the vaccine is greater than the risk of infection with what are now rare diseases in North America?[3]

At least part of the physician's assessment when trying to make a decision about possible parental medical neglect is based on the parents' reason for refusal. Some reasons are easier to accept than others. If the failure is because of inattention or overbusyness, that is handled one way. If it is a financial problem, other options are explored. The most troubling refusals are those based on differing values. Some may be idiosyncratic, some may be philosophical (e.g., dietary restrictions or excesses). Others may be based on religious beliefs.

Religiously based treatment refusals[4] are fairly common and often lead to requests for ethics consultation. Parents who forgo all formal medical treatments (e.g., Christian Science adherents and several others), including those who rely instead on prayer for divine healing, are not encountered too often since they don't typically bring their children to clinics or hospitals for medical care. Stories of tragic deaths often make headlines and sometimes result in legal charges against the parents.

Much more common are situations where parents want good treatment for their children but have specific beliefs about specific treatments. The paradigm here is the Jehovah's Witness tradition where transfusion of most blood products is believed to cause eternal separation from Jehovah.

A 1988 report on 172 children known to have died over a twenty-year period from such religiously based "medical neglect" speculated that most of them would probably have survived had they received timely appropri-

---

3. This dilemma arises more frequently than one might imagine. The parents are statistically correct, but their refusal is really a matter of them riding on the coattails of others. The concept of disease prevention through immunization requires maintenance of "herd immunity," that is, a certain percentage of susceptible individuals must have protective antibodies to prevent epidemics. Since most childhood immunizations are effective in only 80-90 percent of children, if a significant number of parents refuse immunization of their children, the entire population will be at risk, especially the 10-20 percent in whom the immunization was not effective.

4. See also chapter 9.

ate care.[5] As a health-care professional, one is tempted to get angry at these parents and to encourage courts to remove parental rights. However, family integrity and religious freedom are also important societal values and must be seriously considered.

I think a better response is to understand that these are generally good people who have a different value system or different worldview. They want what is best for their children, but they have come to a different conclusion than I have. I encourage health-care professionals to try to understand the parents' values, their limits, and their reasons, and then to try to work within that value system to give as good care as they will accept. This may involve extended discussions, a longer hospital stay, prolonged recovery, increased risk of infection, etc. But protecting family integrity may be worth it in some circumstances. However, when the parental limits raise a serious threat to life or limb, then, as a professional, I am both legally and morally obligated to be the child's advocate by reporting the situation to CPS.

Adolescents

Parental values that pose a potential threat to child welfare, whether based on religious values or idiosyncratic beliefs, become especially challenging when the child becomes an adolescent. Three of the most challenging ethics consultations I have done have been on girls twelve or thirteen years old in three different families who followed the Jehovah's Witness teachings, all of whom had life-threatening situations that could be treated with blood products. Each situation was unique, and each was handled a bit differently.

Caring for adolescents can raise ethical issues, even without religious or personal value differences. Issues of confidentiality and disclosure (see Case 11.08), access to care, capacity to make decisions (see Case 11.10), fear of threatening or abusive parents, noncompliance with treatment (see Case 11.12), and lifestyle choices can all present challenges. In addition to declaring an age of majority, each state also provides statutory guidance to physicians about when they may treat adolescents without parental permission. Most of the exclusions have to do with sexual activity, reproductive choices, substance abuse, or mental health. Physicians (and others involved in these discussions) must be aware of state laws that govern such

---

5. Swan Asser, "Child Fatalities from Religion-Motivated Medical Neglect," *Pediatrics* 101, no. 4 (1988): 625-29.

matters. In addition to the law, however, we must bring to bear precepts of ethics: capacity, consent, best interests, patient advocacy, access to care, and many more.

Caring for *children with chronic illness* can also present ethical challenges. Some chronically ill children become "prematurely mature" in making treatment decisions (see Case 5.04) because they have been through the intensive care unit, **ventilator** support, etc., or because they have seen friends from their clinic go through difficult times or even die. For others, part of the chronic illness is a cognitive disability that requires ongoing surrogacy by parents or by some societal agency. I coauthored an article in 1994 that highlights some of the issues found in doing consultations on critically and chronically ill children.[6]

Among the first journal articles that I clipped and saved in my ethics files were several on ethical issues in pediatrics. Pediatric issues have been, continue to be, and will likely always be prominent in our discussions in clinical ethics.

Let's now look at some ethical dilemmas encountered in the care of children, presented in the order of increasing age.

Case 11.01

QUESTION

Is it ethically permissible to withdraw support from this seven-month-old infant with an undiagnosed progressive neurologic condition at her parents' request?

STORY

Hilary is now seven months old. She appeared normal at birth, developed appropriately, and appeared to be healthy until about five months of age when she demonstrated some regression in developmental milestones. This quickly progressed to episodes when she temporarily stopped breathing, which prompted hospital admission nine weeks ago, and subsequent

6. R. D. Orr and R. M. Perkin, "Clinical Ethics Consultations with Children," *Journal of Clinical Ethics* 5, no. 4 (1994): 323-28.

respiratory failure requiring full-time **ventilator** support in the pediatric intensive care unit (ICU).

She has had innumerable tests looking for a neurologic or metabolic diagnosis, but without success. Her condition has been discussed with specialists at three large pediatric hospitals, and she was sent to a fourth for further evaluation. She returned from this evaluation three weeks ago; at that time plans were discussed for long-term care (either at home or in the nearest long-term ventilator facility, which happens to be out of state) while the group awaited final results from the consultation. She has had a **tracheostomy** and surgery to prevent reflux of stomach contents.

Hilary is currently on full-time ventilator support with only an occasional spontaneous breath. She is blind; her hearing status is uncertain. She exhibits spontaneous movement, occasionally smiles, and grimaces during uncomfortable procedures. In the past two weeks she has demonstrated cardiopulmonary instability (major fluctuations in blood pressure and pulse), recently with increasing frequency. The consultation report has now been received from the referral center, and her condition is deemed undiagnosable, but it seems to be progressing toward inevitable death. On the basis of this prognosis, her parents two days ago agreed on the phone to a **do-not-resuscitate order** and also asked about the possibility of "ending her life."

Her father is a plumber and her mother does not work outside the home; she cares for their other children, ages five and three, and she does not drive. They live in a small community over an hour away. During the early part of Hilary's hospitalization, both parents were at the bedside constantly, but in recent weeks they have visited infrequently and now do not even call every day. Hilary's nurses report that they seem appropriately bonded to her and suspect their withdrawal is partly for social or financial reasons, and may also represent anticipatory grief.

Dr. Rudd, the pediatric ICU physician caring for Hilary, is comfortable with a change to comfort care and withdrawal of support, but he is uncomfortable with the wording of the father's last request and with the fact that it was made by phone rather than in person. He asked both parents to come in to discuss the decision and the process.

FAMILY MEETING

Dr. Rudd, Hilary's nurse, and I met with both parents. The parents asked appropriate questions, appeared to be grieving appropriately, and asked the doctor's recommendation. He recommended withdrawal of support with the expectation that Hilary would die in hours or days. They concurred. They reported that other family will visit tomorrow and have asked that her ventilator be withdrawn the following day. They are Roman Catholic; Hilary has been baptized, and her parents would like a priest present when support is withdrawn. Their choice of words ("ending her life") appears to be from lack of understanding of their significance rather than from malevolence.

DISCUSSION

When a child has a progressive illness and appears to be headed toward death, it is obligatory to use all reasonable measures to find the cause in order to determine if any therapy might alter the course of the illness. When it becomes clear that the child will die, whether because the diagnosis is known and is clearly fatal or the condition is undiagnosable but all reasonable measures have been taken and the clinical course is clearly progressing toward death, it is ethically permissible to change goals from survival to comfort care, including the withdrawal of death-postponing measures that are in use.

Such decisions are based on serving the child's **best interests**, and are generally made jointly by health-care professionals and caring parents. In situations where the parents are absent or uninvolved, or even appear to be uncaring or neglectful, it is still ethically permissible to withdraw support if all involved professionals strongly agree that death is inevitable and imminent. If parents are uninvolved and there is not unanimity among the professionals, it may be necessary to seek judicial involvement (via guardianship) before an irreversible decision is made.

In this case, there is professional unanimity that withdrawal of support is not only permissible but also recommended, based on the patient's inevitable and imminent death. Hilary's parents, though somewhat withdrawn from the clinical setting, are actively involved in decision making and agree that withdrawal of life support is the best course of action.

RECOMMENDATIONS

1. It is ethically permissible to change goals to comfort care and to withdraw support from this infant with the expectation that she will not survive. It is not permissible to do anything to intentionally hasten

death, but unintentional hastening of death secondary to needed comfort measures is ethically justifiable.

2. The timing of withdrawal of support may be negotiated to meet the convenience of her family.

FOLLOW-UP

On the evening of the day of the ethics consultation, Hilary's parents decided it would be too difficult to wait, and they asked that her ventilator be discontinued that evening. The staff of the pediatric ICU agreed to this. She died in her mother's arms two hours after the ventilator was discontinued.

COMMENT

Rarely parents will ask professionals to do something to intentionally hasten death, usually as a result of their perception that the child is suffering. More often, as in this case, parental requests that might sound like requests for euthanasia merely reflect an acceptance of a child's inevitable death leading to a request for the professionals to stop whatever measures are postponing death so that the inevitable can happen. However, it is wise for professionals to thoroughly evaluate such requests to ensure that the meaning and motivation are ethically and legally acceptable.

Case 11.02

QUESTION

Is it ethically permissible to honor a mother's request for no further treatment for this ten-month-old child who is a temporary ward of the state?

STORY

Beatrice ("Bea") is a ten-month-old infant who was born at term with **Apgar scores** of 7 (one minute) and 8 (five minutes), but she was found to be small for her age of **gestation** (2.7 kilograms, a little under six pounds). She was subsequently found to have complex **cyanotic** congenital heart disease. She also has hypothyroidism and no spleen. She underwent emergency surgery at three weeks of age to revise the vascular connections; this was a temporizing lifesaving measure, not a cure. At three months she was operated on again for pulmonary vein narrowing; at six months she had subsequent nonsurgical redilation of this same obstruction. In recent weeks she has been eating less and requiring more oxygen, suggesting recurrence of the narrowing, though this has not yet been found on ultrasound. If her deterioration progresses, the therapeutic options under consideration are: (1) heart-lung transplantation, (2) repeat dilation of the narrowed pulmonary vein, or (3) comfort care.

The patient spent the first four months of her life in hospital, and since discharge has been in the temporary custody of Mr. and Mrs. Green, who are foster parents for medically fragile children. Her biologic mother has been diagnosed as "mildly mentally retarded" and has led a life described as "chaotic." It was determined that she had insufficient insight and resources to care for Bea. The patient's father has not been identified.

If a decision is made to pursue heart-lung transplantation, the patient would have to relocate to be near a large pediatric medical center six hours away from the Greens' home. With the current shortage of organs for double transplant in a child this size, it is anticipated that 75 percent of children will die on the waiting list. If this transplant becomes available, it usually offers a 75 percent five-year survival and a 25 percent ten-year survival. The surgery itself is quite burdensome to the patient, and follow-up requires meticulous care and medication plus frequent professional follow-up.

Repeat pulmonary vein dilation could be done locally. While much less burdensome to the patient, it is only a temporizing measure. In addition, it is uncertain whether it would be successful a second time, and if it were, how long before the narrowing would recur.

Nonintervention and comfort care, with the expectation of death within a relatively short time, is another option offered to parents in these situations. Some parents choose this route if they believe the child has a very poor quality of life, has suffered enough, and that the burdens of further interventions outweigh the potential for benefit of continued life. At least one consulting cardiologist has said this is not an unreasonable option for this patient. The patient's primary cardiologist, however, evaluates her as "sick, but not dying," and recommends repeat dilation if a repeat narrowing is identified.

Mrs. Green describes Bea as joyful, social, communicative, and oblivious to her condition. She is felt to be developmentally normal.

State child protective services reports that the birth mother is unwilling to relinquish parental rights, is asking the court to authorize increased visitation, and is requesting no further interventions because she believes the patient has suffered enough.

DISCUSSION

When treatment decisions must be made for an ill or disabled child, medical professionals generally discuss available options with the child's parents and may recommend the option they believe to be the preferred approach. Parents are allowed some discretion in making these decisions. But our society has mandated that children, because of their vulnerability, be protected from parental decisions that are clearly not in their **best interests**. Determining what is the "preferred approach" and what is in the child's best interests, however, are value-laden assessments and are rarely objective. There is professional, societal, and judicial consensus that low-burden, low-risk, highly effective interventions should be provided for a child, even if they must be imposed by the court over the objections of the parents. There is less consensus on the use of interventions felt to be high-burden, high-risk, or low-efficacy, and parents are often allowed to bypass interventions that others might choose for their own children.

The situation becomes even less clear when a child has been removed from the custody of parents who are unable to provide either ordinary care or the extraordinary care required by chronic illness or disability. In these situations, state agencies and courts assume decision-making authority, usually in consultation with both biological and foster parents.

RECOMMENDATIONS

1. Though nonintervention and comfort care is a not unreasonable option for this patient, based on the recommendations of her cardiologist and the report from her foster mother of her current vitality, it would be ethically problematic. Another attempt at dilation of her pulmonary vein narrowing would seem to be ethically obligatory because her caregivers believe it to be in her best interests. This recommendation is based on an assessment that it is relatively low burden and low risk, and it has a reasonable expectation of efficacy. If further assessment led to a conclusion that this was not the case, this recommendation would change.
2. Pursuing heart-lung transplantation is not ethically obligatory for this

patient, but remains optional. It has a less than 20 percent chance of working (25 percent chance of happening, 75 percent chance of five-year survival if it does happen), is high risk (significant perioperative mortality) and high burden (trips of many miles for evaluation; relocation if listed for transplant; probable transfer of custody to CPS in a different state, and introduction to a new foster home; significant pain from surgery and post-op care). The low chance of success combined with the high burden of an attempt does not justify the social disruption that would be required — a disruption likely to be detrimental to this child in what would probably be her last weeks or months of life.

3. On the basis of the inherent goodness of life and the current good quality of Bea's life, some would encourage her decision-makers to pursue every available option to prolong her life. A decision for or against pursuit of this option could be influenced by the best available prognostic data, which might require a preliminary visit to the transplant center for evaluation of her unique situation. If the prediction is worse than the above figures, that would lend weight to the choice against transplantatiom. If better, it would lend support for this option. However, her outlook seems sufficiently poor, even with pursuit of transplantation, that there is no ethical obligation to even pursue further evaluation.

FOLLOW-UP

Repeat dilation was done successfully about one month after the consultation. There was discussion of using chemotherapy to try to prevent renarrowing, but because of her absent spleen, which elevates her risk of infection, this was not done. She was legally adopted by her foster family two years later, and they describe her as "one of God's precious miracles." Consideration was still being given to future transplantation or other cardiac surgery because she had done so well in spite of seriously compromised heart-lung function. However, unexpectedly and inexplicably, restenosis of her pulmonary artery did not occur. Six years after the consultation she was growing and thriving.

COMMENT

Foster parents who are willing to provide the level of care needed by this child and who are also willing to advocate for seriously handicapped children are few and far between. They should be provided as much support and guidance as they need and, as in this case, should be encouraged to advocate for the child. Bea's biologic mother, herself somewhat compromised, was removed from the intimacy of the situation. She may have felt that she was seeking her daughter's best interests, or she may have been seeking to reestablish some degree of control over the situation. Bea was very fortunate to have foster parents, professionals, and CPS workers who protected her from an unwarranted **limitation of treatment**.

Case 11.03

QUESTION

Is it ethical to continue aggressive treatment that is causing this boy to suffer when the treatment has almost no chance of saving his life?

STORY

Christopher is twenty-two months old. He was admitted to the emergency department three weeks ago with blunt trauma to his abdomen from "falling off the bed," but the injury is now felt to be nonaccidental. He was in extremis and was immediately taken to the operating room where it was found that his duodenum (first part of the small intestine) was ruptured, his liver was lacerated, traumatic pancreatitis (inflammation of the pancreas caused by injury) was present, and the peritoneal cavity was contaminated from duodenal spillage. A portion of the duodenum was removed and the two ends of the small intestine were connected. He was transferred to the pediatric intensive care unit (ICU) for further management.

In the ensuing three weeks his condition has been precarious with **ventilator** dependence and worsening pulmonary function, three cardiac arrests, repeated bleeding with hemorrhagic shock, seizures, and **sepsis** (life-threatening, widespread infection). In addition, he has had to be taken back to the operating room twice for breakdown of the original repair, and removal of his pancreas and spleen. All his abdominal contents have suffered significant damage. It has been impossible to close his abdomen, so this is being cared for as an open wound.

Christopher's nurses have requested an ethics consultation because they feel he is suffering immensely from the current treatment, they believe he cannot survive, and they further believe he has suffered brain damage from his turbulent clinical course. In addition, they point out that his care is very expensive, and with no chance of survival, future expenses represent poor stewardship of medical resources. His surgeons remain of the opinion that he has a small, but real (perhaps 5 percent), chance of survival. His parents want treatment to continue.

Chris's injury has been deemed "nonaccidental" because, in addition to the injury being inconsistent with the story given, he was found to have multiple other bruises of varying ages as well as cigarette burns on his skin. The alleged perpetrator of the injury is a teenage relative who babysat for him on several occasions.

DISCUSSION

When children are clearly dying, it is appropriate for their professional caregivers and family to reject futile therapies and even to consider withdrawal of life-sustaining treatment to shorten their time of suffering. However, when the outcome is uncertain, it is more appropriate to continue therapy while seeking to maximize pain control. As the degree of uncertainty increases, the obligation increases.

Parents generally want all treatment felt to be beneficial for their child. Legal consequences for themselves or for relatives may sway their position; however, those legal consequences should not be allowed to be determinative. If the professional caregivers believe requested treatment is truly futile, especially if the treatment is causing the patient unrelievable suffering, it is permissible to consider withdrawal of support, even if this might lead to legal consequences.

In this case, professional caregivers differ regarding the degree of uncertainty about the patient's outcome.

RECOMMENDATIONS

1. Current therapy should continue pending (2) and (3).
2. Neurology consultation might help to determine if he has suffered significant brain damage.
3. A multidisciplinary management conference to include physicians and nurses as well as others involved in Chris's care may help to clarify his current situation and his future.

4. Increased efforts at pain control may help the patient and also help to reduce the nurses' discomfort.

FOLLOW-UP

Against the odds, Chris survived. He was hospitalized for seven months, during which he had a rocky course but his health progressed steadily upward. He eventually was able to eat, began to speak a few words, and was able to stand. He was discharged to foster care. Cost of his hospitalization was over $2,000,000.

COMMENT

What can one say? When I first saw this patient, I seriously doubted he could survive. But when confronted by an unusual constellation of injuries that offer no good data on which to base a prediction, one is forced to err on the side of life until evidence of nonsurvival is overwhelming.

Was it worth the cost? If Chris were able to weigh in, I suspect he would say that life is worth both the pain and the financial cost. Some, thinking of other patients who are unable to afford even basic health care, might challenge this huge expenditure for a patient with a very small chance of survival. Fortunately, such questions should not be addressed to patients, families, or bedside caregivers, but must be looked at by those expert in health policy.

Case 11.04

QUESTION

How vigorous should we be investigating and treating a bronchial obstruction in this two-and-one-half-year-old child with multiple anomalies (Schwachman's syndrome)?

STORY

This two-and-one-half-year-old girl was born with incomplete closure of her abdominal cavity, which was surgically repaired in the neonatal period.

At two months of age she was diagnosed with probable Schwachman's syndrome (a recessively inherited condition with pancreatic insufficiency, elevated blood sugar, malabsorption, and low white blood count). She has had repeated hospitalizations with respiratory infections and **sepsis**, and her overall function has deteriorated progressively, specifically her cognitive function. Between her frequent hospitalizations she has been cared for at home. She had a **tracheostomy** placed six months ago, and she is fed via a gastrostomy tube.

She was admitted this time six weeks ago with pneumonia and septic shock after a short stay at home. She is currently dependent on a **ventilator** and one of her main airways is obstructed. The cause of this obstruction has not been adequately defined by two **bronchoscopies** or by **MRI**, but it appears to be from an unknown mass pressing on the outside of her airway. Further evaluation would require invasive testing.

On examination, the patient is sedated but moves when stimulated. Her care team reports that she becomes agitated when sedation is reduced but does appear to be calmed when her mother holds her. She is on moderate ventilator settings, tube feedings, and intravenous antibiotics. There is a **do-not-resuscitate order** in place.

Her social worker reports that the parents are caring and concerned about her continued deterioration. She believes they are ready to consider further limitation of therapy, and she also believes they will follow whatever recommendation the care team makes about further care.

DISCUSSION

When a child is predictably dying of a disease process, it is appropriate to evaluate all diagnostic and therapeutic options to see whether the potential benefits to the child outweigh the burdens to the child. Using this calculation, it is ethically permissible for the child's **surrogate** to decide against specific options when the burdens of therapy outweigh its benefits. It is also ethically permissible not to employ options when the burden of the disease outweighs the benefits of continued life.

In a chronically ill child, it is important (and sometimes difficult) to make these burden/benefit calculations from the child's perspective, rather than on the basis of burdens to the family or to the care team. In a situation where a surrogate may be easily influenced by the recommendations of the care team, it is tempting to make only the recommendation the team wants to carry out. While it is permissible to make a professional recommendation, in a situation like the present where decisions will significantly affect the duration and quality of life, it is very important to let the parents know of other options that would be considered acceptable or conventional therapy.

RECOMMENDATIONS

1. If consensus on the care team holds that the minimal benefit of continued life in her severely compromised state is outweighed by the burdens of continued ventilation, or by the invasive testing needed to further evaluate her bronchial mass, it would be permissible for the team to recommend to her parents that she be **weaned** from the ventilator and not reconnected to it should she deteriorate. It would likewise be permissible to withdraw or withhold antibiotics or other antidisease medications. However, since this is a value judgment by the team, the parents should be apprised of the option of continued ventilation in an institutional setting. If they seem to have the patient's **best interests** in mind and choose a more aggressive plan, that should be honored as well.

2. If a **limitation of treatment** recommendation is made and that plan is followed, it would be appropriate to decide what setting would be best for her continued care once she is off the ventilator. She might be cared for in the hospital pediatrics ward (as opposed to the pediatric ICU), in a hospital nearer the parents' home, or at home if they can receive adequate hospice support.

FOLLOW-UP

The pediatric intensive care team met with the patient's parents several times over the next few days. Her parents were reluctant to "stop treatment," so slow weaning attempts were made with the understanding that her pulmonary treatment would not be increased again if she should deteriorate. After two weeks without significant progress, her parents agreed to stop the ventilator, and she was given some mild sedation. She died about ten hours later.

COMMENT

The clinical recommendations of health-care professionals are very important. Some professionals, recognizing this, merely give the facts and allow the patient or family to make their own decision based on their own values. Sometimes this is appropriate, for example, when two or more treatment plans are equally acceptable and equally efficacious. Sometimes, however, this "delicatessen approach" represents failure by the professionals to shoulder their responsibility. If one treatment plan clearly offers benefits to a patient, the professional has an obligation to point that out and to recommend its acceptance. Of course, the patient or surrogate may choose to ignore this recommendation and choose another acceptable option.

In other situations, professionals may not adequately recognize the weight patients and families give their recommendations. In these cases it is important for the professionals to ensure that the decision-maker is aware of all treatment options rather than accepting the recommendation as the only option.

Some people of faith believe it is morally obligatory to continue life if this can be done. Most, however, recognize the need to consider the balancing effect of patient suffering and the caregivers' obligation of compassion. Prognostic uncertainty, of course, muddies this calculation in many instances.

Case 11.05

QUESTION

Is it ethically permissible to stop the off-label use of an expensive drug in this two-and-one-half-year-old girl with Gaucher's disease who may be suffering because of its continued use?

STORY

Bonnie is a two-and-one-half-year-old girl who was evaluated at seven months of age for failure to thrive and enlargement of her liver and spleen. She was found to have Gaucher's disease, a genetic (recessive) lipid storage disease, the manifestations of which are due to the absence of an enzyme. She was seen in consultation at the National Institutes of Health (NIH), and because it was not known which of three types of this disease she had, she was begun several months ago on a six-month trial of a replacement enzyme approved for and effective in preventing the manifestations of the disease in two of the three types. The family was unable to return to Washington for the six-month follow-up visit. The treatment has been continued, and, at her parents' urging, the dosage has been increased to higher than normal. She has had frequent long admissions (for infectious and neurologic complications), and she has developed problems that suggest progressive disease (including respiratory failure — she has been on a **ventilator** at home for several months), strongly suggesting that she has the one type of this disease that does not benefit from enzyme replacement.

On the other hand, her liver and spleen have decreased in size, she has survived longer than the average for patients with the more severe type (death before age two), and her parents point out that she has grown some and they are convinced that she shows signs of neurologic development while at home. However, during her frequent hospitalizations she has shown minimal awareness; at best she smiles, responds to her parents, and follows simple commands. She is currently at home and receives **total parenteral nutrition**, home mechanical ventilation, a morphine drip (for bone pain), and the intravenous enzyme every fourteen days.

Her overall therapy is very expensive (to date over $1,000,000); the enzyme alone costs several thousand dollars per month. Both Dr. Burgess, Bonnie's primary pediatrician, and the NIH consultant believe the enzyme is no longer indicated. The medical director of her managed care organization is denying payment for the enzyme until she is convinced of a valid medical indication to continue. In addition, Dr. Burgess is concerned that progressive disease and invasive treatments are causing Bonnie sufficient suffering and that continued treatment may be inappropriate if it is merely postponing her inevitable death.

Her parents are her caregivers at home, and they have declined assistance from home nursing. Her mother is at home full time, and her father has reduced his work as an accountant to part time in order to help.

DISCUSSION

When a child is felt to be suffering because of burdensome treatments that are merely postponing inevitable death, it is appropriate to consider **limitation of treatment**. However, since it is very difficult to assess a child's quality of life or degree of suffering, we usually look to parents and other bedside caregivers for guidance about both how much analgesia or sedation to use and when it is appropriate to withdraw life support because of suffering. When a physician is clearly convinced that a child is suffering needlessly because parents insist on continued therapy, it may be appropriate to challenge the parents' surrogacy in court.

In this case, the patient's parents and professional caregivers do not agree on her quality of life or her degree of suffering.

It is generally accepted in our system of health-care finance that an insurer is obligated to pay for contracted services that are medically indicated. Insurers may be legally justified in denying payment for not-indicated or nonefficacious therapies, but their moral obligation to a patient who is already receiving an off-label[7] therapy is less clear. The morally relevant feature is whether that therapy is effective and beneficial. The determination of effect and benefit is the responsibility of the physician and should be based on objective observations.

In this case, opinion differs about the effect and benefit of the enzyme. This difference of opinion should be resolved using objective evidence of either (a) disease stability or progression or (b) presence or absence of neurologic development (or presence of neurologic deterioration). This may require professional observation of the patient in her home environment when she is not acutely ill.

RECOMMENDATIONS

1. If there is objective evidence over time of neurologic deterioration in spite of continued therapy, withholding enzyme therapy over the objection of her parents might be ethically justified. If, however, it appears to the physicians that the enzyme has been or continues to be effective in slowing the natural course of her disease, it would be ethically problematic to withhold it based on cost alone.
2. Since her physicians are concerned about her suffering, it may be appropriate to increase analgesia or increase home surveillance to ensure her comfort. But, absent evidence of her irremediable suffering, it is not ethically justifiable to seek court-ordered withdrawal of the enzyme or the life support based on patient suffering.

FOLLOW-UP

Four months later Dr. Burgess reported that the patient was still receiving the enzyme. Her mother had become more realistic about the outcome. And

---

7. Use of a drug for a condition for which it has not been approved by the Food and Drug Administration.

her professional caregivers were more convinced that she had actually improved (videos of her motor function at home showed considerably better function than they had observed at the hospital). There was no further discussion about discontinuing the enzyme. Nine months after the consultation, Bonnie developed uncontrollable seizures, and her parents consented to a **do-not-resuscitate order** and to withdrawal of the ventilator.

COMMENT

It is not infrequent that parents and professional caregivers disagree about a child's level of awareness or function. Sometimes this is because the parents have an understandable bias in favor of their child. Often, however, it is because the parents see the child when the child is at maximal level of function, while the professional caregivers see the child only when hospitalized, ill, and in an unfamiliar environment.

As soon as the cost of care enters the discussion, the focus shifts from clinical ethics (i.e., what is best for this patient) to health policy or social ethics (i.e., what is best for other patients). This is a totally different endeavor. For decades in North America, it has been assumed that we should always do what is best for the individual patient. Very slowly our society has come to accept what had been realized earlier in other societies, that with the astronomical increases in cost of care, some priorities and limits must be set. We have not yet sorted out how to do this, but it is clear that rationing must be done at a policy level rather than at the bedside.

Case 11.06

QUESTION

Is it ethically permissible to withdraw support from this disabled six-year-old child with cerebral palsy who has a potentially reversible condition (pancreatitis) when her parents disagree?

STORY

Jenny is a six-year-old girl who developed sluggishly and had several critical illnesses in the early months of her life. After extensive workup, she was diagnosed just before one year of age with cerebral palsy and developmental delay (of unknown cause) and possible autism. Her parents continued to be hopeful that she would improve, but when she was about two-and-one-half they acknowledged that she would have little further development and would need ongoing total care. They felt unable to provide long-term care for her at home and believed their marriage in jeopardy from the stress of caring for her. They made arrangements for foster care, though they retain custody. For the past three years she has remained in the foster home without further hospitalization, though her condition remains fragile. Her parents see her two times per week. They have three older children.

Jenny was admitted four days ago with dehydration and possible **sepsis**, has been found to have acute pancreatitis, and has now developed **adult respiratory distress syndrome**. Her acute condition has stabilized, and her caregivers in the intensive care unit (ICU) believe she has more than 95 percent chance of surviving this crisis and returning to her baseline condition, though she will likely need ICU support for two to three more weeks.

Jenny's mother says she has come to terms with her poor prognosis, and she believes Jenny is suffering pointlessly even at her baseline status. She is no longer comfortable with vigorous life-prolonging treatment. However, her husband, both foster parents, and her professional caregivers believe it is premature to make this decision because her baseline condition, in their estimation, is satisfactory and her short-term prognosis is good. She is now on a **ventilator** at moderate settings, she is medically paralyzed and sedated, and she is receiving **total parenteral nutrition** (TPN) and antibiotics.

Both foster parents and Dad describe her as joyful when she is healthy, which they report is about 50 percent of the time. She is bothered with frequent respiratory and urinary infections, as well as significant gastrointestinal problems (reflux, constipation, abdominal pain). She smiles, snuggles, vocalizes (no words), loves music, and recognizes individuals. She rarely cries.

Her parents are both concerned and thoughtful. Dad works regular hours as an architect. Mom reports that her views of disability and quality of life are significantly affected by providing care for her father for many years as he died slowly from cancer. She participated in **limitation of treatment** decisions for him. She has been in therapy for some time for anxiety and depression. Foster Mom is a licensed respite care provider who cares for three disabled children and her own two healthy children.

Foster Dad works part time as a financial planner and helps with child care at home.

DISCUSSION

Parents are generally the appropriate **surrogate** decision-makers for their children. However, society expects medical professionals who care for children to advocate for their patients and to intervene to protect them from any treatment decisions that may harm them. Professional guidelines are a bit more lenient, allowing some parental discretion, primarily when the outcome of a proposed treatment is uncertain.

Societal guidelines that mandate care for disabled children cannot, however, stipulate where that care is to be provided. If parents are unable to provide care that society says is obligatory, society then has a concomitant obligation to provide an appropriate place of care.

In this case the patient's underlying condition is of uncertain etiology, with some uncertainty of long-term outcome, though it seems unlikely she will develop significantly beyond her current condition. Her acute problem is life-threatening but is almost certainly reversible. Her parents have felt unable to provide long-term total care and have made arrangements to have that care provided. Her mother now questions the wisdom of continuing standard care, but the patient does not meet the criteria society has set to allow parental discretion for withholding or withdrawing standard treatment.

RECOMMENDATIONS

1. It would be ethically problematic to withdraw life support from this child at this time. If any of her family insists on this course of action, this should not be done until the situation is reviewed by child protective services or the court.
2. It is appropriate to discuss goals of therapy and possible limitations of treatment. (a) For example, if the agreed-upon goal is to return this patient to her baseline condition, it would be ethically permissible to agree that, should her condition change (e.g., additional hypoxic brain damage) or should this goal no longer be medically reasonable (e.g., worsening pulmonary situation, other organ failure), a decision could be made to change goals to comfort care and to withdraw life-prolonging measures. (b) It would also be ethically permissible to

agree to withhold new modalities that would either be unlikely to work or disproportionately burdensome to her (e.g., dialysis, long-term TPN).

FOLLOW-UP

Mom became quite upset with the consultation recommendations and left town for several days. When she returned, another planning meeting was held, and the following treatment guidelines were agreed upon: (a) all want what is best for Jenny; (b) because of her compromised baseline condition, some aggressive interventions that might be technically feasible are not appropriate (e.g., organ transplantation, long-term vent support or dialysis); (c) because her current condition is reversible and improving, continued treatment and support are appropriate; (d) she will likely come to a point when continued standard interventions are no longer appropriate because they have become disproportionately burdensome, for example, with deterioration of her baseline function or with the need for repeated and frequent hospital admissions or other burdensome treatments; (e) until (d) is reached, when urgent decisions must be made, the default will be to provide the treatment; (f) treatments started may be withdrawn if it becomes clear that they are not working or are no longer appropriate; and (g) her parents and foster parents will continue to discuss their perceptions of the patient's level of pleasure and suffering and will reevaluate treatment goals and the use or nonuse of specific modalities as her condition changes.

Jenny was discharged back to her foster home about five weeks after admission.

COMMENT

These parents must be commended for recognizing they were becoming overwhelmed with caring for this handicapped child, for making alternative arrangements, and for their willingness to remain involved in decisions about her care. Her mom was particularly distressed by the current situation, perhaps influenced by the stress she experienced in caring for her own father when he became disabled. However, stepping back from the situation a bit, she saw more clearly that Jenny's baseline condition was satisfactory, and the prospect of returning to that condition was good. This led to the conclusion that a decision to limit treatment at this point would be premature and ethically troublesome.

Case 11.07

QUESTION

Is it permissible to follow the parents' request to withhold information from their ten-year-old son regarding the scheduled surgery to amputate several gangrenous extremities?

STORY

Juan is a ten-year-old Hispanic boy admitted to the pediatrics intensive care unit (ICU) three weeks ago with a life-threatening meningococcal infection.[8] He has been treated vigorously but developed fulminant **sepsis** (positive cultures of both blood and cerebrospinal fluid); kidney failure that required temporary dialysis; disseminated intravascular coagulation,[9] which ultimately resulted in multiple sites of gangrene of his extremities. He continues to require mechanical ventilation and he receives **total parenteral nutrition.**

The plastic surgery consultant has recommended the following amputations: the right leg below the knee, the right fingers, and the left hand. There had been some question of how much the patient can comprehend since he may have suffered some brain damage as well; his **electroencephalogram** is severely abnormal. The true mental status of the patient has been difficult to establish because of the heavy sedation needed to control his agitation and pain.

Juan's parents have consented to the amputations, but his father asked that Juan not be told before surgery what was going to happen. The pediatric ICU nurses believe this child has a right to know and are very uncomfortable with this failure of disclosure.

On examination, the patient is sedated, **intubated,** and has multiple areas of blackened skin over several areas of his extremities, trunk, and abdomen. He is able to shake his head yes or no appropriately to simple questions, and is able to move all extremities.

---

8. A bacterial infection, primarily involving the surface of the brain, which may also affect many other tissues, including causing gangrene.

9. Disseminated intravascular coagulation is a disorder of the blood in which the blood clots abnormally within the blood vessels so there are insufficient clotting factors remaining to prevent hemorrhage. It has several causes, including severe infection.

DISCUSSION

In most situations, the preferences of parents regarding treatment decisions for their child should be followed. Parents usually best understand what is in the **best interest** of their child. When the parental preference is in conflict with what the treatment team believes is in the patient's best interest, then the parents' rationale should be sought. Most often, when parents are educated about the risks and benefits involved with certain treatment options, they are eager to follow whatever course is most beneficial to their child.

In some cases, if parents insist on withholding information from the patient and the treatment team believes this failure to disclose imposes more harm than disclosing, it may be ethically permissible to override the parents' wishes.

Removal of limbs is a permanent, irreversible surgery with lifelong implications. Failure to disclose this to the patient could result in significant loss of trust, making future treatment more difficult. Thus, it would be difficult in this case to justify not informing the patient of the amputations. At the same time, the Hispanic culture is more paternalistic than ours, and children are often not given important information about decisions made by parents.

Deciding whether or not to inform the patient about the surgery may be a moot point if he does not have the capacity to understand the information. However, in light of this uncertainty, it would seem reasonable to attempt to convey this information on a level he would likely understand.

RECOMMENDATIONS

1. There should be further discussion with Juan's parents about disclosure. The physicians and nurses should tell them why they feel strongly that the patient be informed. The primary physician should encourage Juan's father to inform Juan of the scheduled amputations and the ramifications of the surgery.
2. While the patient's ability to understand may be impaired by his current condition, the explanation given him should be made in terms appropriate for his level of understanding in the event he is able to process the information.

FOLLOW-UP

After further discussion, Juan's father agreed to tell him that surgery would be done "to remove all the dead tissue so [he] could get better," without specifying the extent of amputation. When this was done, he nodded.

COMMENT

It is not always easy to determine when cultural beliefs trump contemporary ethical standards. This case was marginal. Thus the compromise reached seemed quite satisfactory.

Case 11.08

QUESTION

Is it ethically permissible for this eleven-year-old child's parents to refuse potentially lifesaving treatment for his malignancy?

STORY

Joel, age eleven, was found six months ago to have a bone cancer in his femur that was felt to have a 75 percent chance of cure with vigorous therapy. He was referred to a children's hospital and evaluated there. Upon recommendation of pediatric cancer specialists, he received and tolerated six weeks of preliminary chemotherapy given by Dr. Martin, a pediatrician in this community. Though his parents initially preferred amputation, they were persuaded to return to the children's hospital two months ago for more elaborate surgery that would remove the tumor but preserve the leg. This surgery is much more difficult than amputation, but it has a much better functional result. Unfortunately, the pathology report showed the tumor to be more advanced than originally suspected, reducing Joel's prognosis for cure to 40-50 percent. Standard therapy calls for six months of follow-up chemotherapy. The drug to be used has a low incidence of brain toxicity; however, this side effect is seen only when the drug is used in higher doses than he would get.

His parents are considering no further chemotherapy based on their belief that he is dying and the chemotherapy is too toxic. They openly talk about his death in front of him. All his professional caregivers here and at the children's hospital believe it is clearly in the child's **best interests** to have the chemotherapy since his prognosis for long-term survival without it is near zero. Though his parents have not made a definitive refusal of further therapy, they have been postponing meetings, discussions, and a decision, and his prognosis worsens with such delays.

Joel's parents are concerned that he has a baseline defect in cognitive function, and they fear the chemotherapy may cause further brain damage. They are well intentioned and well read. They have sought counseling for him for over four years and have requested sedating medication that he has used both at home and at school.

DISCUSSION

Parents have the right to make treatment decisions for their child and the responsibility to act in his or her best interests. Since a child's "best interest" is not easily defined, and since not all parents will come to identical decisions in similar situations, our society allows parents some ill-defined degree of discretion in making treatment decisions.

Physicians have the responsibility to recommend to parents what they believe to be in a child's best interests. That recommendation should be based on the best available data, and in cases of doubt, should include consultation and second opinion. Physicians likewise have the responsibility to oversee the scope of parental discretion. They are expected to notify child protective services (CPS) if parents are making a choice that is clearly outside a "reasonable construal of the child's best interests."

In this case, there is strong professional agreement on what treatment is in this child's best interests. His parents are postponing a semi-urgent treatment decision, and their behavior raises questions about their understanding of his best interests.

RECOMMENDATIONS

1. Dr. Martin should document the joint recommendation for further treatment, and inform the parents again, in person or via registered mail, of this joint recommendation and the urgency of beginning therapy.
2. If the parents do not agree to begin therapy within a clearly specified

time, CPS should be notified of the medical staff's concerns about medical neglect.

FOLLOW-UP

Dr. Martin sent a certified letter to Joel's parents saying chemotherapy should begin within seven days, and failure to do so would necessitate a report to CPS. After another short delay, Joel was admitted for the chemotherapy. Unfortunately, a chest X-ray done at that time showed that the cancer had spread to his lungs, making cure impossible. The new tumors had probably been present for several weeks, so earlier initiation of chemotherapy would not likely have made an ultimate difference.

COMMENT

Respect for family integrity and protection of vulnerable children are both important societal values. When they appear to conflict, it is often very difficult to know when is the appropriate time to use the agencies of society to intervene. Such was the case here. The pediatrician tried to work with the parents to find a reasonable approach that would meet their goals and protect the child's best interests. What eventually became clear was that Joel's parents seemed to be preparing themselves (and him) for his death before it was clear that he would not survive. Once this became clear, there was no option except to marshal external forces to make them move forward quickly. Unfortunately, even this did not allow him to reach the hoped-for outcome.

Case 11.09

QUESTION

Is it ethically permissible to do less than optimal therapy for this eight-year-old developmentally delayed child with malignancy?

STORY

Johanna, age eight, was taken to her pediatrician about one month ago with weakness and was found to have acute lymphoblastic leukemia

(ALL). It was subsequently determined that she has an uncommon variant of ALL that carries the worst prognosis (25-30 percent overall survival). Standard therapy for ALL includes four weeks of induction chemotherapy followed by continuation therapy. Because of the poor prognosis for this variant of ALL, standard chemotherapy is not an option for continuation. Aggressive chemotherapy is still used at some centers, but has not yet been standardized. Recent data indicate that bone marrow transplant (BMT) gives better survival rates — in the range of 30-40 percent five-year survival at experienced centers. However, the small numbers of patients with this diagnosis make such data less reliable than one would like, and make the specific patient's prognosis even less certain.

Johanna has finished her induction therapy, which she has tolerated well in spite of its significant side effects. Her local pediatric oncologist and consultants at a referral center have recommended BMT. After two discussions, her well-informed parents remain pessimistic and are inclined toward **palliative care** (focused on patient comfort rather than on fighting the disease) only, or possibly aggressive chemotherapy rather than BMT, though they are still considering all options. Tissue typing is pending to determine whether a parent or sibling would be a compatible tissue donor. Johanna's oncologist believes that aggressive chemotherapy carries about the same burden and risk as BMT with slightly lower survival rates, though this difference is difficult to quantify.

The patient is the oldest of three children in an intact, caring family. Her father owns a telecommunications company and her mother is at home. Johanna has a history of dysmorphic features (abnormal appearance) and developmental delay without a specific diagnosis. Though she "gets sicker than other kids," she had never been hospitalized prior to this diagnosis of ALL. She displayed some behavioral problems as a preschooler, but her family and school have worked hard to develop a nurturing and protective environment for her. She does not recognize that she is different from the other kids. Her parents are concerned about not only the physical burden of the proposed treatment (e.g., would the total body irradiation given prior to BMT, even if it would lead to cure, cause her additional neurologic problems?), but also the social and psychological burdens (e.g., she does not develop rapport easily with strangers; she has never "slept over").

DISCUSSION

Treatment decisions for a child should be made jointly by the parents and health-care professionals after each has had the opportunity to consult with others (extended family, referral specialists, families of other patients, etc.). Treatment decisions should be based on the best available data and an assessment of what will be in the child's **best interests**, taking into consideration not only the physical well-being of the child but also the child's emotional, social, and spiritual well-being. When parents and professionals disagree on a treatment decision, generally the parents' wishes should prevail. Parents are allowed some discretion in making decisions, but professionals are obligated to challenge parental choices that are clearly not in the child's best interests, even going to court if necessary.

Health-care professionals have a particular obligation to scrutinize parental decisions for less than optimal therapy for a child who is physically or mentally disabled. This special scrutiny is needed because some individuals or families undervalue handicapped life and others may make poor decisions because they are overwhelmed by fatigue or burden.

In this case, the patient has a very caring and well-informed nuclear and extended family who are searching for what they believe to be in her (whole-person) best interests. In addition, she has professionals who have searched out the best available data from around the country, though that data is limited because of the rarity of her precise condition.

RECOMMENDATIONS

1. It would be ethically permissible to use aggressive chemotherapy rather than BMT for this patient if her parents are convinced that the physical risks, social disruption, or psychological burden of the latter would be too great, or if BMT would preclude the home-based palliative care they desire.
2. It is important that her parents are fully aware of the option of beginning chemotherapy and switching to home-based palliative care if certain milestones should arise indicating a worsening prognosis.

FOLLOW-UP

There were no tissue matches for BMT found in Johanna's nuclear family. Aggressive chemotherapy was begun. Her parents took her to a large medical center to discuss BMT using an unmatched donor. The parents were somewhat divided, Dad wanting no BMT, and Mom ambivalent.

COMMENT

As advocates for vulnerable patients, pediatricians and family physicians are expected to encourage parents to accept therapy that has the best chance of helping their child. Their recommendations should consider not only the disease process but also an assessment of the whole person, including psychological, social, and spiritual dimensions. They are especially expected to prevent parents from making unwarranted or premature decisions to withhold or withdraw therapy from a child with handicaps. Assessing parental motivation is sometimes difficult. (Is it because of parental fatigue from the burden of caring for this disabled child or a lack of assistance or social support? Is it based on a poor regard for disabled life? Is it something else?) This case was easier to assess than some due to the obvious good motivation of the parents.

Case 11.10

QUESTION

Is it ethically permissible to restrain this fifteen-year-old adolescent to treat his severe constipation against his will?

STORY

Charles is a fifteen-year-old boy who has a history of significant constipation since childhood and has required four or five hospitalizations for evacuation of his bowels. It is recorded in his chart that he has not been consistently compliant with medication and has been resistant to seeing doctors or to hospitalization. He was last hospitalized about one year ago, and after several days of enemas and laxatives given through a nasogastric (NG) tube, he was relieved of about ten pounds of stool. During that hospitalization he was also found to have significant iron-deficiency anemia, still unexplained. He thereafter took mineral oil with adequate results, but he stopped several weeks ago, and has not had a bowel movement for at least one month. His parents have been arguing (daily) with him about getting treatment, and he has refused, promising to go in a few days.

Yesterday his older brother and a friend carried him to the car (with him fighting, knocking over furniture). He was taken to the pediatrics clinic and admitted with obstipation[10] and severe anemia. He had an NG tube inserted repeatedly (about seven times) to administer laxatives, and he removed it each time. Last evening it took three security guards holding him down to reinsert it. Having had no results, he was transferred to the pediatric intensive care unit for sedation and further treatment. He refuses it and insists on going home. His parents and grandmother insist that he be treated against his will and are willing to sign a written request saying so, if needed. His parents describe him as otherwise a cooperative adolescent.

On examination, he sat in bed with abdominal distension the size of a full-term pregnancy. He moved with obvious discomfort. He was disdainful and refused to answer questions while his family was present. After they were asked to leave, he spoke a bit and said he didn't want treatment because it was uncomfortable. He recognizes the need for treatment but insists on going home to try enemas. He said he would return in twenty-four hours if he had no results.

X-rays of his abdomen show massive dilation of his colon. While his condition is not immediately life-threatening, his physicians believe further delay in treatment might lead to major complications, including perforation of his bowel.

DISCUSSION

Adults with **decision-making capacity** are allowed to refuse even lifesaving treatment. It may rarely be ethically justifiable to paternalistically override the treatment refusal of a seemingly competent adult when (1) the patient appears to have some defect in reasoning, and (2) serious harm is likely without intervention, and (3) the probable benefit from the intervention is greater than the harm of nonintervention.

Physicians routinely act paternalistically toward children at the request of loving parents seeking their **best interests**. This is routine for the infant and young child, but becomes more ethically problematic as the child reaches adolescence. While legal majority in this state occurs at midnight on the eighteenth birthday, valid decision-making capacity is gradu-

---

10. Total lack of bowel function.

ally developed over a period of several years. It would be ethically troublesome to force elective treatment on an unwilling adolescent, even at the insistence of well-meaning parents. It becomes easier to justify such action as the potential for harm increases, and as the irrationality[11] of the adolescent's choice increases.

In this case, criterion 3 is met; that is, recommended treatment is effective and without major risk. Criterion 1 is uncertain; he seems to recognize the seriousness of the situation but irrationally expects home treatment to be effective when his history and clinical condition clearly show that it will not work. One could question whether his severe anemia is interfering with his mental capacity; however, this is doubtful since his current decision is consistent with his past behavior. The primary question is whether criterion 2 is met. Will serious harm result if he is not treated urgently? This is a matter of clinical judgment, unfortunately without good predictive measures.

RECOMMENDATIONS

1. Efforts at persuasion should continue. More moral authority to exert pressure on unwilling patients is given to family members than is allowed for professionals.
2. If persuasion does not lead to consent, it would be ethically permissible to force treatment on this unwilling adolescent only if his physicians believe that to not do so puts him at significantly increased risk. If that is not the case, it would be ethically preferable to discharge him until he is willing to have the recommended treatment.

FOLLOW-UP

The patient was persuaded to take sedation while nasogastric and rectal tubes were inserted. In three days his bowels began to move, and after several days his abdomen became flat and soft. It was learned that he stopped taking his bowel medication at home after having a fight with his girlfriend. He was seen by the psychiatry service, found to be depressed, and started on an antidepressant.

11. An irrational choice is one that is not consistent with the patient's goals. For example, a patient with gangrene who says he wants to live but refuses amputation, the only therapy that will allow survival.

COMMENT

This fifteen-year-old, though forced to deal with a chronic bowel problem, had not developed the maturity to make an adult decision. He did not want to die, but he clearly did not appreciate the significant risk he was taking by not taking adequate treatment for his obstipated bowels. It was therefore ethically permissible to override his irrational request to treat himself at home.

Case 11.11

QUESTION

Is it ethically permissible to respect this sixteen-year-old patient's desire not to be tested for a genetic disease (muscular dystrophy) when her mother specifically requests the test?

STORY

Roxanne is a sixteen-year-old girl on her first visit to the pediatric neurology clinic. Her eighteen-year-old brother was diagnosed with facio-scapulohumeral (FSH) muscular dystrophy[12] three years ago. The patient feels fine other than injuring her knee slightly in a fall in dance lessons two weeks ago, but her mother wants her blood tested to see if she has this genetic disease. The patient's father, who also has FSH, told Roxanne that he knew he had the disease already when he was her age. The patient doesn't feel weak (although on exam, the **neurologist** found that she is a little weak), and though she could accept the possibility that she might develop symptoms in the future, she presently seems convinced that she doesn't have muscular dystrophy. When it was explained to her what testing her blood could reveal — the result could show that she will develop the disease for sure or that "maybe" she won't (if the test is negative) — she said she was not interested in having it done.

Roxanne's mother wants her tested because knowledge of whether her

12. This genetic condition is inherited as a dominant trait. People can live a full life with some limitations with this condition, but it's hard to say who might require a wheelchair in their forties, fifties, or sixties. There is no effective treatment.

daughter has FSH dystrophy will help her and her doctors interpret whether any musculoskeletal symptoms she might develop are due to that disease. There might also be implications for future governmental disability support for the patient and her family. At present, though, testing would be presymptomatic, and there would be no treatment or other immediate clinical implication (such as restriction of physical activity) for a positive test.

The physician did not tell the girl of her mild weakness on physical exam, nor of his suspicion that she does in fact have FSH muscular dystrophy. The physician simply said, "I'd like to see you again in a year." The patient voiced her appreciation for the physician respecting her opinion in not wanting the test, saying, "No doctor has ever taken my side of things that way before."

DISCUSSION

One of the foundational principles of medical ethics is autonomy, which the courts have said means every adult of sound mind has the right to determine what shall be done with his or her own body. Common law presumes that minors have the same right to bodily integrity as adults, but only their parents are allowed to exercise this right. According to the U.S. Supreme Court, "the law's concept of the family rests on a presumption that parents possess what a child lacks in maturity, experience, and capacity for judgment required for making life's difficult decisions."[13]

Much of the literature on decision making for minors has focused on situations where parents cannot or will not give their permission for a certain procedure.[14] In this case, though, the patient's mother is offering her permission but the patient is withholding her assent. Given the clinical context, the American Academy of Pediatrics (AAP) position statement places great importance on the assent of the patient: "There are clinical situations in which a persistent refusal to assent (i.e., dissent) may be ethically binding. . . . A patient's reluctance or refusal to assent should also carry considerable weight when the proposed intervention is not essential to his or her welfare and/or can be deferred without substantial risk."[15]

13. U.S. Supreme Court, *Parham v. J.R.* (1979).

14. The four classic exceptions to the requirement of parental permission (i.e., emergency exception, medical neglect, minor treatment statutes, and emancipated minor status) are predicated on this situation.

15. Committee on Bioethics, "Informed Consent," p. 316.

The age of the child is also relevant. For while this state has no formal "mature minor statute," there is a growing consensus within common law that a minor who can understand and appreciate the nature and consequences of a medical treatment and its alternatives can give valid legal consent. Thus the AAP encourages physicians to obtain the informed consent of adolescent and pediatric patients, in most instances. Such patients frequently have **decision-making capacity** and the legal authority to accept or reject interventions, and, in that event, no additional requirement to obtain parental permission exists. However, the Academy encourages parental involvement in such cases, as appropriate.

In this case, the patient has communicated her wish to continue to live a normal life (i.e., unaware of the likelihood of a serious diagnosis), which constitutes, in ethics terminology, a waiver of information. There is no medical harm in keeping one's suspicions to oneself, since the evaluation is presymptomatic and no beneficial interventions may be offered at this time. And the physician was clear that he did not tell the patient that she was weak (respecting the patient's wish not to know), which is fundamentally different from telling the patient she wasn't weak (which would be untrue). The patient's positive response to the physician's approach bodes well for their future therapeutic alliance, which may well be critical if the patient does indeed have FSH muscular dystrophy.

RECOMMENDATION

It was ethically permissible for the physician to refrain from testing the patient for FSH muscular dystrophy, and from informing the patient of his suspicions, based on the patient's waiver of information and dissent from the proposed procedure.

FOLLOW-UP

This mother was upset with this recommendation to honor adolescent autonomy, and I suspect other parents would likewise be unhappy with such a decision. However, this decision supports the adolescent's developing adulthood, and in this case, the result of the physician's decision will not adversely affect her health.

COMMENT

If there existed beneficial treatment for this condition, and if that treatment could extend life or prevent major complications, the recommendation would probably have been different — to try to persuade, and perhaps overrule, the adolescent if the consequences would be sufficiently detrimental.

Case 11.12

QUESTION

What is our professional responsibility to this adolescent who is endangering her life and well-being by poor compliance in treatment for her diabetes?

STORY

Paula is seventeen and three-quarters years old and was diagnosed with diabetes four years ago. She has been hospitalized several times with dangerously out-of-control blood sugar and ketoacidosis,[16] three times in the past month, because she failed to follow her diet and insulin regimen. She is angry about her diagnosis and just wants to be normal. Her mother reports that she knows enough about her disease and her condition to seek treatment when it becomes necessary. She has resisted or declined education, diabetic camp, and counseling on multiple occasions. She was admitted again four days ago with diabetic ketoacidosis, discharged for twenty-four hours, and readmitted yesterday, back in acidosis, and was found to also have a recurrence of pancreatitis. She is now improved, and her caregivers expect she will insist on discharge soon. Her mother claims she is an "emancipated minor." However, investigation determined that she has had no judicial declaration of emancipation.

The endocrinology consultant feels Paula should be treated as a child (i.e., treated over her objection) because she is displaying childlike behavior, but her pediatrician is reluctant to do this, even though she is making irresponsible decisions.

---

16. Diabetic ketoacidosis is a life-threatening complication of uncontrolled diabetes.

I spoke briefly with Paula, but she became angry with my questions, said it was none of my business, and walked out of the room. Her mother reports that she did not finish high school and works two jobs (at a flower shop and at Burger King), often fifty to sixty hours a week. Her parents have followed a style in rearing their children of allowing them to assume responsibility for themselves, and they have become frustrated with Paula's irresponsible behavior.

DISCUSSION

An adolescent is considered a legal adult at age eighteen in this state, or when officially emancipated by a judge. However, it is clear that the development of the moral capacity to make treatment decisions is a gradual process that may be completed as early as age twelve, or sometimes not until many years after legal adulthood. The clinical concept of a "mature minor" applies to one who has demonstrated adult **decision-making capacity**, irrespective of age. This capacity entails understanding the condition, the options, the consequences of the various options, and the ability to give reasons for one's decision. However, both adults and mature minors often demonstrate irresponsibility and make decisions that are counter to their well-being. It is almost never ethically justifiable for medical professionals to treat such patients by force, even when death or disability is likely.

This patient appears to have decision-making capacity but often becomes reckless and makes irresponsible decisions. When her well-being is in imminent danger, she becomes temporarily compliant until the crisis has passed. Her caregivers feel obligated to allow her personal autonomy, but at the same time they feel obligated to protect her from reckless behavior and irresponsible choices.

RECOMMENDATIONS

1. When Paula's condition has stabilized sufficiently that she is no longer in danger of death or disability, it would be ethically troublesome to continue to treat her over her objection.
2. Efforts at education and persuasion should continue. Offers of counseling for her and for her parents would be appropriate.
3. It would be ethically impermissible to try to manipulate or coerce the patient by threatening to withhold future professional services be-

cause of her behavior or noncompliance. Her professional caregivers are obligated to continue to treat her when crises arise, and to provide or arrange for ongoing care.

COMMENT

On the surface, this case seems similar to Case 11.10 — a late adolescent making poor decisions with potentially very serious consequences. Why were we willing to force treatment on the fifteen-year-old in that case but unwilling to force treatment here? In the first place, this patient would recognize when she was in danger and would submit to treatment to save her life, whereas the fifteen-year-old did not seem to appreciate his danger. Of course, there is always the danger that this patient may wait too long or become unconscious in a situation where help is not immediately available. That is a true risk in this patient, a risk that should be underlined in bold print for her. But in the second place, treatment to overcome the crisis in Case 11.10 was short term, so restraints were less problematic for this limited duration of time. In the current case, the primary period of irresponsibility is the time between life-threatening episodes. There is no practical way to enforce unwanted therapy or supervision several times a day for an indefinite period of time.

Case 11.13

QUESTION

Is it ethically permissible to allow the father of this almost eighteen-year-old young woman to refuse potentially lifesaving therapy?

STORY

Laura is seventeen years old, just two weeks from her eighteenth birthday. She was diagnosed with aplastic anemia[17] two months ago and was evaluated for bone marrow transplant (BMT). When no family or banked-

---

17. A disease, most common in adolescents and young adults, in which there is failure to generate all cellular elements of the blood, leading to anemia and susceptibility to infection and hemorrhage.

marrow match was immediately found, standard chemotherapy was recommended six weeks ago. Her father decided she should leave the medical center **AMA**, and he took her to Mexico where she received nonproven therapy three weeks ago. She was admitted here eleven days ago with infection and without improvement in her underlying condition. After being informed again of the standard therapy options, her father again refused to consider potentially lifesaving chemotherapy. He says he is considering consultation at another medical center to inquire about stem-cell (cord-blood) therapy. Laura's parents are divorced, and she has little contact with her mother.

Without chemotherapy or BMT, Laura has a less than 50 percent chance of survival for six months from the time of diagnosis. With either of these therapies, she has a 50-70 percent chance of five-year survival, better if instituted early after diagnosis. Cord-blood therapy has achieved some success in small children, but very poor results in adults.

The oncologist caring for Laura describes her as quite passive and dependent upon her father for decision making, even though Laura is nearly a legal adult. She has been informed, outside of her father's presence, of the standard therapy options and possible outcomes, and she seems to accept her father's decision without resistance or question.

DISCUSSION

Parents are the appropriate **surrogates** expected to make medical decisions for their children. In this capacity parents are given some discretion and are allowed to choose from a range of medically acceptable options, even to choose less than ideal therapy in some situations. However, if parents make a decision that is felt to be clearly not in the child's **best interests**, the child's physicians are expected to challenge that decision and seek judicial intervention.

While eighteen is the legal age of majority in this state, it is well accepted by physicians and by the legal system that many adolescents have the intellectual and psychological ability to participate in medical decision making.

If this patient were less than twelve years old, most physicians would feel compelled to report her to child protective services as a "medically neglected" child. If she were over eighteen and making this decision on her own, most would try to persuade her but would reluctantly accept her refusal if she clearly understood the situation and the consequences of refusal.

RECOMMENDATIONS

1. Someone should speak again with the patient alone to ensure that she clearly understands the treatment options and the possible outcomes.
2. If she clearly understands the risks of refusing standard therapy, and understands that she is able to consent to treatment herself, it is ethically permissible to accept her informed refusal.

FOLLOW-UP

The oncologist asked that I speak with Laura alone. She seemed to understand the treatment options and the possible outcomes. She said she and her father already had an appointment at another medical center to discuss cord-blood infusion. She said they had not been aware of its lack of efficacy in adults, but would still like more information. In addition, she planned to have outpatient follow-up with the oncologist at our medical center, and if her anemia had not improved in the time that the alternative treatment she received in Mexico was supposed to have worked (six to eight weeks from the time of administration), she and her father would consent to standard therapy. She also said she was aware that this standard therapy had less chance of working if its initiation were delayed.

COMMENT

Many untested alternative therapies seem to provide some benefit to patients, and many patients report improvement from using them. When such therapies are used to treat symptoms or conditions that have no effective standard therapy, it is often appropriate to support patients' decisions to pursue such modalities. When patients choose such therapies for life-threatening conditions for which there is no good treatment, it is easy to understand their decision to grasp at straws. However, when dealing with life-threatening conditions for which there is effective therapy, it is very frustrating for physicians when adult patients insist on trying alternative therapies, especially when that means forgoing or delaying standard therapy.

The frustration turns to anxiety when a parent makes such a choice for a child, and to confusion when that child is approaching adulthood.

*   *   *

Other Cases Involving Ethical Dilemmas in Pediatric Patients

All cases in chapter 10, "Ethical Issues in the Neonatal Period"
Cases 5.04, 9.05, 9.09, 9.10, 9.11, 14.04, 14.05, 14.08, 14.09

Reference on Pediatric Issues

Frankel, L. R., A. Goldworth, M. V. Rorty, and W. A. Silverman. *Ethical Dilemmas in Pediatrics: Cases and Commentaries.* Cambridge: Cambridge University Press, 2005.

CHAPTER 12

Ethical Issues in the Use of Reproductive Technology

Assisted reproductive technologies have been developed and can be used to help an infertile couple conceive and bear children. They can also be used to help a couple select for or against specific characteristics in their offspring.

Infertility has been and often continues to be viewed as "a curse." The Hebrew Scriptures report that Sarah, Rebekah, Rachel, Manoah's wife, and Hannah were devastated by barrenness. It is recorded that "In bitterness of soul Hannah wept much and prayed to the LORD."[1] By divine grace these women all eventually bore sons. One can only wonder how many other barren women did not.

Today, infertility affects 10-15 percent of all couples who wish to conceive. Several social factors contribute to this near epidemic, including sexually transmitted diseases, the widespread use of contraception to delay childbirth, and multiple (or serial) sexual partners. Infertility may be even more of a curse today than it was a generation ago for two reasons. First, since abortion became common, fewer babies are put up for adoption, so this alternative is less available for the infertile couple. And second, ironically, because of the availability of technological assistance to facilitate conception, those unable or unwilling to utilize these services, whether for financial or moral reasons, may feel doubly cursed.

A large number of reproductive technologies are available to help a couple conceive, including artificial insemination (using either husband's sperm or donor sperm), in vitro fertilization (using both sperm and egg from the couple; using donor eggs; using donor sperm; using both donor

---

1. 1 Samuel 1:10 NIV.

egg and donor sperm), **gestational** motherhood, surrogate motherhood,[2] and others.

Treatment of infertility using artificial reproductive technology raises many ethical questions. First, there are some basic questions: Is infertility a disease? Does a woman or a couple have a basic right to conceive? to deliver a baby? to raise a child? What is a family? What is the moral status of the **gametes** (sperm and egg) prior to fertilization? of the preimplantation **zygote**? of the embryo? of the fetus? of the father? How do these questions and technologies fit with the divine plan for humankind? How does stewardship fit into this picture?

In addition, there are specific questions about the sources and methods of obtaining the gametes, about storage, selection, and distribution of the gametes; and societal questions about who pays for these expensive technologies and about resolution of contested parentage. What should be done with "spare embryos" that remain in the freezer after efforts have been successful or abandoned? And of course, health-care professionals have questions about who they should be willing to help. May they limit their assistance to married couples? What about the same-sex couple who want to have a child using alternative methods?

As alluded to above, some couples are not infertile but request assistance with reproductive technology for different reasons. Such technologies can be used to help a couple select the sex of their child or even to help them bear a child with specific genetic characteristics. There is near universal condemnation of pursuing such "designer babies" among people of faith. However, there may be circumstances where serious consideration is given to such efforts. For example, should such technologies be used to help a couple avoid having a child with a genetic disease? If so, does it have to be a fatal or dreadful disease (e.g., Tay-Sachs disease),[3] or might it be permissible for a disease that is less severe

---

2. For some, there is a significant moral difference between gestational motherhood and surrogate motherhood. In surrogate motherhood, either husband's or donor's sperm is used to impregnate the woman who serves as surrogate mother; that is, the egg comes from the surrogate. In gestational motherhood, the woman who carries the pregnancy makes no genetic contribution because the egg is from either the wife or a donor; likewise, the sperm may be from the husband or a donor.

3. Tay-Sachs disease is an inherited (recessive) condition in which lack of an enzyme allows accumulation of an abnormal chemical in the brain. This causes severe neurologic symptoms (seizures, retardation, paralysis) and leads to early death, usually before age five.

or where it is difficult or impossible to predict the severity (e.g., cystic fibrosis)?[4]

In this realm of ethical discussion, some would condone diagnostic efforts in early pregnancy with subsequent abortion of affected fetuses (see chapter 13). Others would support using assisted reproductive technologies to select embryos for implantation that are not affected with a particular malady. Do these efforts come under the umbrella of allowed stewardship? Is the *imago Dei* present in these affected embryos?

Faith traditions have drawn boundaries in various places for the use of artificial reproductive technologies. Some condone only assistance that allows a married couple to conceive through coitus. Others support the use of various technologies as long as both gametes come from the married couple. Still others are willing to allow the use of donor gametes to help a married couple have a child. A few support assistance for unmarried or same-sex couples.

Our discussion here will not be of these very important generic policy questions. For a more thorough discussion of these issues, the reader is referred to the resources at the end of the chapter. Instead, let's look at some specific cases where the use of reproductive technologies raised specific ethical dilemmas.

Case 12.01

QUESTION

Is it ethically permissible and appropriate to use a gestational carrier for this woman who is unable to carry a pregnancy?

STORY

Sharon is a thirty-one-year-old woman who has never had any menstrual periods. She was found at age fourteen to have no uterus but intact ovaries and vagina. She has been married for ten years to Richard, a high school

---

4. Cystic fibrosis is an inherited disease of glandular function, affecting primarily the gastrointestinal and respiratory tracts. It has a range of severity, and may lead to early death (teens or early adult years) from chronic lung disease, or may allow a nearly normal life span.

history teacher. He has an adequate sperm count but has never fathered a child. Their marriage is stable and strong.

Richard's sister, Elizabeth, is a close friend of the patient. She has offered to be a **gestational** carrier, that is, to carry a baby conceived by in vitro fertilization using Sharon's eggs and Richard's sperm. She has had two uncomplicated and successful pregnancies and is an ideal obstetrical candidate. All four adults involved have had counseling, have been fully informed of the risks and benefits of the procedure, and have signed both a consent form and a gestational contract, including the stipulation that Elizabeth has the ultimate decision-making authority for all obstetrical decisions. Sharon and Richard will pay for all procedures needed to achieve pregnancy and for Elizabeth's pregnancy-related expenses, but Elizabeth will donate her gestational services without financial compensation.

DISCUSSION

There is quite a spectrum of belief among various faith traditions about the use of artificial reproductive technology. Some forbid any technologies that achieve pregnancy without sexual intercourse. Others limit the use of artificial reproductive technology to married couples, or even to married couples using both of their own **gametes**. Still others are willing to allow the use of donor gametes.

When professionals and patients are ethically comfortable using gestational surrogacy, as proposed in this case, several criteria still need to be met. Such matters include the source of the gametes; the identity or privacy of the gestational **surrogate**; who has authority over obstetrical decisions (e.g., whether the pregnancy should be terminated for either maternal or fetal problems); ultimate parentage of the offspring; and financial arrangements.

In this case, it appears that many of the clinical, social, and legal issues have been addressed.

RECOMMENDATIONS

1. An inquiry should be made of the prospective parents and the surrogate whether they have considered religious restrictions within their own faith traditions.
2. The gestational contract should be reviewed by clinic legal counsel to ensure that all criteria have been met.
3. If there are no religious or legal constraints, it is ethically permissible

and not inappropriate to use the gestational carrier technique to help this couple produce a child biologically related to both of them.

FOLLOW-UP

No follow-up is available.

COMMENT

In this case, the gametes originate from the two individuals who will be the parents of the resulting child; that is, the biological parents and the social parents are one and the same. This procedure avoids the significant complexities introduced by the use of donor gametes in many types of artificial reproductive technologies. However, several clinical and legal issues must be addressed before moving forward. In addition, gestational surrogacy still uses techniques that are problematic in some faith traditions.

Case 12.02

QUESTION

Is it ethically permissible to deny this man's request to freeze his semen before he undergoes sex-change surgery?

STORY

A man in his thirties recently called the male infertility specialist in the infertility clinic asking if he could have his semen frozen. He was about to begin the hormonal and subsequent surgical process of gender reassignment and wanted to preserve the option of having a genetically related child using a surrogate mother or **gestational** carrier at some later date.

The infertility clinic operates a small nonprofit sperm bank with very limited space. They provide this service for medical reasons. Most of their requests are from men with life-threatening conditions who will be undergoing chemotherapy or surgery that will likely leave them infertile. The clinic routinely turns down requests from men who will be undergoing vasectomies.

The physician practice group at the clinic has asked for an opinion on the ethical permissibility of their preference to decline this request.

DISCUSSION

The patient-physician relationship has been conceptualized in several ways, including professional, covenantal, contractual, fiduciary, and others. There is consensus that both parties in this relationship are autonomous individuals who are free to participate or not. However, the professional does have some inherent obligations that preclude him or her from avoiding or severing a particular relationship (e.g., providing emergency care, not abandoning an established patient, not discriminating among patients). Freedom from this obligation is more evident in "elective" situations, and less so as the medical need or urgency increases. There is also a growing recognition of a professional's right of conscience that allows discretion when the professional's reluctance is based on moral qualms (e.g., abortion services, withdrawal of life-sustaining therapy).

Some individuals consider elective services provided by physicians such as cosmetic surgery outside the realm of traditional medicine. Some would include assisted reproductive technology services in this list, but the majority of individuals in the profession and in society consider infertility a treatable disorder. Discussion of these questions will likely increase as available or proposed services are extended to include such things as surrogate motherhood, cloning, etc.

In this case, this man is requesting a service that is not within the established limited scope of this professional practice group. This is clearly within the realm of professional discretion based on space availability. It is probably also discretionary when considering scope of services, comparable to previous decisions made by this clinic to not provide sperm banking for men about to have an elective vasectomy. Assistance with infertility is sufficiently elective that a practice group should be able to determine what services they will or will not provide based on their capabilities and professional or moral comfort.

An argument could be made that a disorder of gender identity is a medical condition that is outside the control of the individual, and thus a medical need could be postulated for its treatment (i.e., with hormones, surgery). However, even if this were established, this line of reasoning would not obligate infertility professionals to assist with subsequent non-traditional reproduction unless it were also established that there is a fundamental right to reproduce.

RECOMMENDATIONS

1. It is ethically permissible for the infertility clinic to establish limits in the provision of services.
2. Their refusal to provide services and space for semen freezing and storage to men prior to vasectomy has already set a precedent.

FOLLOW-UP

No follow-up information is available.

COMMENT

Individuals from several faith traditions are troubled by "gender reassignment procedures" and would make a moral argument against this request. Since this is an elective procedure, professionals who adopt this moral stance could legitimately say, "We don't do that here," based on a professional right of conscience. However, in a secular environment, especially one in which advocacy for gay-lesbian-bisexual-transsexual "rights" is so dominant, it is perhaps more prudent to base the denial of this request on space and clinic policies in comparable situations, perhaps avoiding claims of discrimination.

Case 12.03

QUESTION

Should we deny assisted reproductive technology services to this HIV positive couple because their child may become an orphan?

STORY

Betsy is a thirty-eight-year-old woman who has two healthy children. She and her husband, Charlie, came to this infertility clinic four years ago for assistance in achieving a third pregnancy because she had infrequent and irregular menstrual periods and he had poor sperm quality. Charlie was known to be HIV positive (human immunodeficiency virus, the cause of AIDS) at that time. The clinic physicians expressed some reluctance to assist with conception, and the couple decided to go elsewhere for infertility assistance. However, Betsy conceived spontaneously. She took anti-HIV medication during the pregnancy, and the little girl she bore remains HIV negative.

Betsy recently returned to this clinic for assistance in achieving a fourth pregnancy, but now she too is HIV positive. She has been treated with multidrug therapy in the recent past and is now off therapy. Her viral load is undetectable (a measure of how active the HIV is), and she feels well. Her primary physician believes her survival potential is good, perhaps even normal. Though it is known that Charlie is also HIV positive, his current clinical status is not known by the infertility clinic staff. It is also not known if Betsy and Charlie have made plans for the care of their children should they both die.

The infertility specialist believes she could help this couple achieve pregnancy fairly simply by medically inducing Betsy's menstrual cycles and inseminating her using Charlie's washed sperm (which would also reduce somewhat the risk of viral transmission). If that failed, they could consider in vitro fertilization. They are paying for the reproductive services themselves.

While the vertical transmission rate (from mother to infant) of HIV in pregnancy is greater than 25 percent without antiretroviral treatment, at the time of this consultation it could be reduced to about 8 percent with the use of one medication from twenty-eight weeks' **gestation** until delivery, and to 2-3 percent by using a three-drug regimen. It may be possible to reduce this risk even further by avoiding vaginal birth (i.e., using Cesarean delivery).

The infertility clinic has no policy on, and has not practiced, denial of artificial reproductive technology services to women (or couples) with serious medical or genetic problems. They do, however, decline to provide services in some circumstances; for example, they have an upper maternal age limit (fifty-one, the average age of menopause), and they have denied services to some couples with a history of child abuse or drug abuse.

DISCUSSION

Health-care professionals have an ethical obligation to be good stewards of their services and society's resources. They also have some degree of professional discretion in what elective services they will provide for which patients. At the same time, they have ethical and legal obligations to justly allocate all their services, including elective medical services.

It is ethically permissible for a physician to decline to provide a requested service that is not medically indicated (e.g., a request for an appendectomy in a patient with viral gastroenteritis). It is also deemed ethically permissible to decline to offer or provide services that are physiologically **futile** (e.g., **cardiopulmonary resuscitation** for a patient with overwhelming infection and **multi-organ system failure**). However, since there is almost always some degree of uncertainty, most physicians will reluctantly provide requested services that they deem "inappropriate" if not truly physiologically "futile."

It is less clear if it is ethically permissible to decline to provide a requested treatment that the physician believes is not a good idea. It would be ethically and professionally permissible to have a policy that declines a requested treatment to all patients who meet certain criteria if there is a well-reasoned justification. Thus the age restriction, if based on risks and success rates, is justifiable. It would, however, be ethically problematic to decline treatment for a specific individual while providing the same treatment for others who are "morally equivalent." It would be even more problematic to decline treatment for a specific individual based on a potential, but unpredictable, "harm" or "risk" to another party.

This patient would appear to be "morally equivalent" to someone with known medical or genetic problems that place her prospective child at some risk of disease. There is a small risk that a child resulting from the proposed pregnancy will develop HIV, and an unknown risk of potential harm to the child if he or she should become an orphan. It is possible for the parents to make contingency plans that would satisfy their parental stewardship obligations in the event of their deaths.

RECOMMENDATIONS

1. It would be ethically problematic to decline artificial reproductive technology services for this couple based on the potential welfare of the prospective child.

2. It would not seem unreasonable, and could be viewed as good medical stewardship, to first require the parents to confirm that they have taken adequate steps to ensure the ongoing care of their children if they should both die. However, if they have not done so and decline to do so, this is probably not adequate justification to decline providing reproductive assistance.

3. If any member of the infertility clinic team feels sufficiently strongly that this couple should be denied reproductive assistance because they are exhibiting irresponsible behavior, they should be excused from participation in the care of this couple.

FOLLOW-UP

No follow-up information is available.

COMMENT

It might be tempting to some to deny services to this couple based on an assumption that being HIV positive demonstrates irresponsible (or even sinful) behavior on the part of this man. This may or may not be true of the man's past behavior (he might have become infected from a blood transfusion) but should not be used to predict his future behavior. People of faith in particular recognize the possibility of redemption and changed behavior. Thus denial of services based purely on his HIV positivity could be viewed as discriminatory.

An appreciation of the facts about HIV transmission to a fetus places this dilemma closer to other situations faced by infertility specialists, for example, whether to provide assistance to a couple with a known potential to transmit genetic disease to offspring. There are no firm rules or guidelines here; each case must be judged on its own merits.

Case 12.04 ——————————————————————————

QUESTION

Is it ethically permissible to either decline or place stipulations on assistance with infertility treatment for this woman with anorexia nervosa?

STORY

Barbara is in her late thirties and has a twenty-year history of anorexia nervosa[5] and consequent lack of menstrual periods. She has had three psychiatric hospitalizations in the past fifteen years. Her weight has been stable (seventy pounds, on a five feet one inch frame) for several years; she consumes 1,200 calories per day and rides her stationary bicycle for sixty minutes each day. She has been married to Rod for twelve years and they want to have a biologic child, but she has been unable to get pregnant because she lacks a menstrual cycle. Barbara sought reproductive assistance from another clinic about one year ago and was told she would need to gain forty pounds (to ideal body weight) before pregnancy and another twenty pounds during pregnancy. She has gained no weight, but is now being evaluated in our infertility clinic with the same request. Her infertility could be treated with drugs that would induce ovulation with a predicted 40 percent success rate and a 15-20 percent chance of multiple pregnancy. Her physician is concerned about risk to her both during pregnancy (cardiac failure, fractures due to osteoporosis, malnutrition with possible life-threatening complications) and postpartum (depression, exacerbation of the anorexia), as well as risk to the fetus (intrauterine growth retardation, prematurity, cerebral palsy). A literature search has revealed no published data on natural or assisted pregnancy in anorexia. The infertility specialist who requested this consultation has cared for two less severely anorectic women who achieved pregnancy; one had a successful twin pregnancy, the other had a significant postpartum depression.

Rod is reported to be quiet and noncommittal about pregnancy. Barbara's primary physician supports her request and believes she would be a good mother. The psychologist in the infertility clinic finds her to be highly functional, pleasant, and free of other psychopathology, though she finds that the patient does have obsessive-compulsive tendencies. She would be supportive of reproductive assistance under stipulations agreed to beforehand. Dr. Barcus, an obstetrician who specializes in caring for women with high-risk pregnancies, is willing to provide obstetrical care for Barbara if she agrees to several stipulations (daily caloric intake, weekly weight checks, etc.). However, he is fearful for the life and well-being of the patient and her child if she should not comply with those stipulations. He

---

5. Anorexia nervosa is an eating disorder of unclear origin that is characterized by a distorted body image, a morbid fear of obesity, a refusal to maintain a minimally normal body weight, and, in women, lack of menstrual periods.

reports that he would be very reluctant to seek a court order to force-feed Barbara under those circumstances.

DISCUSSION

Patient autonomy is very important in assessing a patient's right to refuse or request treatment. It is important to distinguish negative rights (i.e., the right to be left alone, the right to refuse treatment recommendations) from positive rights (i.e., an entitlement, or a right to demand specific treatments). Negative rights clearly have more moral weight than positive rights because professionals also have autonomy, including the right, or perhaps even the obligation, to decline to provide treatments or services that they believe would not be in the **best interests** of a patient. This is particularly true in assisted reproductive technology because assistance in overcoming infertility is elective and thus somewhat different from treatment of disease that could have clearly adverse physical consequences if left untreated.

In this case, the physician has the difficult responsibility of assessing the risks and benefits for this patient without adequate data. While the risk to the child cannot be ignored, it would appear to be secondary to the risks to the patient as long as plans are in place to care for the child in the event of her death or disability.

RECOMMENDATIONS

1. The theoretical risk of pregnancy in Barbara's current condition seems sufficient that it would be ethically problematic to provide reproductive assistance for her without stipulations.
2. The theoretical risk also seems sufficient that it would be within the accepted bounds of professional autonomy to decline to provide the requested assistance even with stipulations and contingency plans.
3. If stipulations and contingencies can be agreed upon that the professional caregivers believe would adequately assess or address these risks to this woman, it would likewise be ethically permissible to provide the requested assistance. If this course is followed, contingency plans should include how a situation would be managed if the patient declines to follow the agreed-upon plan after pregnancy has been achieved.
4. Before pursuing this option with its attendant risks, it would be pru-

403

dent for this couple to consider alternative plans for having a child (adoption, surrogate **gestation**) while avoiding the risk to patient and child.

FOLLOW-UP

No follow-up information is available.

COMMENT

This case raises questions about professional stewardship of elective procedures. It would go against the teachings of most faith traditions as well as those of the profession of medicine to provide assisted reproductive technology services merely because they were requested. At the same time, infertility has very real impact on a couple, and compassion requires that professionals not reject this request out of hand. Proceeding with reproductive assistance after contractual agreement on stipulations seems like a reasonable middle ground. But even that compromise should not move forward until there is agreement on the very difficult question of what to do if pregnancy is achieved but the stipulations are not followed.

Case 12.05

QUESTION

Is it ethically permissible to retrieve sperm from the corpse of this man at the request of his parents?

STORY

A man in his late twenties died late yesterday from a self-inflicted gunshot wound. His parents have requested that semen or tissue be retrieved and preserved so that he might have a posthumous genetic child. Dr. Barclay, a urologist, was asked by the mortician to retrieve sperm about eighteen hours after the man died. He was uncertain of the appropriateness of doing this, and requested an ethics opinion before proceeding.

The man's parents report that he had been married for five years. He and his wife had no children; his parents do not know if this was voluntary or not. The couple had recently separated, but his wife was coming back for reconciliation when he took his own life. His wife is not immediately available for discussion. It is not known if he left any **advance directive** or other written instruction about organ or tissue donation.

Viable sperm can be retrieved up to twenty-four hours (perhaps even longer) after death, by electroejaculation (a procedure that induces release of semen from its place of storage in the epididymis) or more commonly by surgical excision of the testes or epididymis, with the tissue then frozen for later usage. Using a fertilization technique called intracytoplasmic sperm injection,[6] only a small number of sperm need be retrieved as opposed to the several cubic centimeters of semen required by the older procedure of artificial insemination.

DISCUSSION

Voluntary posthumous conception has been done for many years, for example, for a man who requests that his semen be frozen prior to his death for use after his death. Only recently has this general concept been expanded to posthumous sperm retrieval. This significantly different procedure raises at least three ethical issues: respectful treatment of the dead body, consent for the procedure, and the welfare of the potential child.

Western society forbids desecration of corpses. However, it is considered socially acceptable to do invasive procedures on a corpse for the benefit of society (e.g., autopsy to determine cause of death) or other individuals (e.g., the retrieval of organs or tissues for transplantation). Authorization for such bodily invasions is granted by the deceased before his or her death, or by next of kin, or it is mandated by the state (e.g., medical examiners' cases). While posthumous sperm retrieval could likewise be seen as a potentially beneficial invasion of the body, it is significantly different in that the benefit will likely accrue to the person from whom permission is sought, that is, it might be considered less altruistic and more selfish than organ donation, highlighting the importance of consent.

When consent must be obtained for a procedure on a living patient who has lost **decision-making capacity**, we try to use **substituted judgment**, that is, to do what the patient would want if the patient were able to

6. A microscopic technique that selects a single sperm, often from a small sample, and injects it directly into an egg.

tell us. When we don't know the patient's wishes, we drop to a lower **best interests** standard. After a person has died, we should use similar standards in making decisions about the deceased's body (autopsy, organ donation, cremation versus burial, etc.). It is the rare young man who will express his wishes about having a posthumous child either in writing or verbally. Such a desire might be inferred when a couple have been trying to conceive, perhaps even more pointedly if they have been seeking help for infertility. However, even then we cannot be certain that a man who wants a child while living would want his widow (or surrogate) to have his child after he's gone. Thus the issue of consent will almost always be an insurmountable barrier to the ethical permissibility for such a procedure. However, the issue of best interests of the potential child must also be considered.

The best interests of the potential child are very difficult to assess. Some would argue against assistance to achieve single motherhood, believing health-care professionals have an obligation to not use technology if the outcome could be potentially harmful to the child. Others would argue that single motherhood is increasingly common and is not necessarily detrimental to the child. They might go on to argue that the benefit of having a child who is genetically her late husband's could be a great solace to the widow and could outweigh the potential harm to the child of being raised by a single parent.

In this case, we have no indication of the wishes of the deceased about having any children, more specifically no information about whether he would want either his widow or a surrogate to bear his child after his death.

RECOMMENDATIONS

1. It would be ethically problematic to retrieve and use sperm from this man without a clear understanding of his wishes about posthumous childbearing.
2. Because of the time constraints, it might be justifiable to obtain and freeze the requested sample, with the understanding that it will be released for use only if his wife (or others) could give credible evidence of his wishes. However, the very small likelihood of such evidence becoming available, along with the difficulty of refusing to release an already-obtained sample, makes the wisdom of this course of action questionable.

FOLLOW-UP

Sperm retrieval was not done in this case.

COMMENT

One can identify with the anguish of a couple dealing with the suicide of their son. And I can imagine them wanting to ensure the potential for carrying on his (and their) genetic line. However, even this strong emotional tug cannot overcome the firm foundational issue of consent as discussed above.

More difficult is the situation where the young man dies of accident or illness, still childless, perhaps even seeking artificial reproductive technology services for infertility. Retrieval of sperm in such a case could allow genetic offspring for the widow without the use of donor sperm, thus avoiding one major objection to artificial reproductive technology by some people of faith. However, even such an unusual case would have to be looked at very closely to try to understand the wishes of the dead donor about pregnancy for his (now widowed) former wife.

*   *   *

References on Infertility and Assisted Reproductive Technology

Glahn, S. L., and W. R. Cutrer. *The Infertility Companion: Hope and Help for Couples Facing Infertility.* Grand Rapids: Zondervan, 2004.

Kilner, J. F., P. C. Cunningham, and W. D. Hager, eds. *The Reproductive Revolution: A Christian Appraisal of Sexuality, Reproductive Technologies, and the Family.* Grand Rapids: Eerdmans, 2000.

President's Council on Bioethics. *Reproduction and Responsibility.* Washington, D.C., 2004.

CHAPTER 13

Ethical Issues in Pregnancy

Pregnancy is unique because it entails one human individual physically located within the body of another. Ethical questions must deal with this anatomic fact, and must consider the well-being and rights of both individuals. Most, but not all, of the ethical issues that arise during pregnancy have to do with whether the pregnancy may or even should be interrupted. Others raise questions about how the pregnancy should be managed.

Abortion was the primary spark that ignited early discussions of medical ethics. Advocates for legalizing abortion in the United States focused on the plight of women who were pregnant as a result of rape or incest and those carrying fetuses with severe anomalies. Recognizing that this was primarily a ruse to permit abortion on demand, many people of faith were quick to condemn the proposal. In the process, they were perceived as being cold and uncaring, condemning all women seeking abortion. Not until several years after the 1973 U.S. Supreme Court decision[1] did those opposed to abortion recognize their obligation to assist the woman with a troubling pregnancy to find alternatives.[2]

Most abortions are currently done for women who are pregnant with a presumably normal fetus but do not want to be pregnant, at least not at the time. It is rare that ethics consultation is requested in these cases, and we will not address this situation.

Individuals who hold a high regard for prenatal life are very troubled by the abortion of fetuses who would grow into normal babies if left un-

---

1. *Roe v Wade,* 410 US 113 (1973).

2. F. Schaeffer and C. E. Koop, *Whatever Happened to the Human Race?* Westchester, Ill.: Crossway, 1983.

disturbed. However, even those most fervently opposed to abortion are willing to make an exception when the pregnancy threatens the woman's life. In cases where the woman cannot survive the pregnancy, the baby is doomed, even if it appears to be normal, and even if it is wanted. In the not too distant past, the physiologic stresses of pregnancy might have seriously aggravated underlying severe heart or kidney disease. But medical advances have eliminated most of these life-threatening situations. Still, occasional cases lead to ethics consultation where a pregnancy with a presumably normal fetus threatens the woman's life or adversely affects her physical health, for example, malignancy in the pregnant woman. We will discuss a few cases where maternal health is the primary concern in the consultation (see Cases 13.01, 13.02, and 13.07).

Most ethics consultations for pregnant women, however, involve women who want a child but find they are carrying an abnormal fetus. This represents perhaps 2 percent of the women considering or seeking abortion. In some cases the abnormality will be lethal for the fetus (see Cases 13.06 and 13.10). In some the abnormality is quite consistent with a full life (see Case 13.03). Most are somewhere between these two extremes.

Ethical analysis of such cases requires an understanding of the process of pregnancy (often called **gestation** in medical discussions) and the neonatal period. Normal pregnancy lasts about forty weeks, measured from the first day of a woman's last menstrual period to the day of delivery. Babies born after twenty-five weeks have a very good chance of survival, though they may require intensive care for a time.[3] Such intensive care is very expensive and may cause some suffering for the infant. Occasionally, such infants later show developmental abnormalities resulting from the prematurity itself or even from their intensive treatment. Babies born between twenty-two and twenty-five weeks' gestation have a lower survival rate and a higher incidence of developmental anomalies if they do survive. Those born before twenty-two weeks rarely survive.

Fetal anomalies may involve abnormalities of the chromosomes (e.g., **Down syndrome**), other genetic conditions that do not visibly affect the chromosomes (e.g., cystic fibrosis), or structural anomalies that do not have a recognized genetic pattern (e.g., congenital heart disease, **anencephaly**).

Chromosomal anomalies may be diagnosed prenatally through am-

---

3. M. C. Allen, P. K. Donohue, and A. E. Dusman, "The Limit of Viability — Neonatal Outcome of Infants Born at 22 to 25 Weeks' Gestation," *New England Journal of Medicine* 329, no. 22 (November 25, 1993): 1597-1601.

niocentesis, a procedure in which a needle is inserted through the abdominal wall of the woman and into her uterus to remove some of the **amniotic fluid**. Fetal cells floating in the amniotic fluid can be retrieved and fetal chromosomes can be analyzed. This procedure is most commonly done when there is suspicion of chromosomal anomalies based on family history, maternal age, the results of screening blood tests, or ultrasound imaging of the developing fetus. Amniocentesis cannot be done until the uterus has grown enough to have risen out of the bony pelvis so it can be approached through the mother's abdominal wall, usually at sixteen to eighteen weeks' gestation. Analysis of fetal cells retrieved in this way takes several days, so the results are often not available until nearly the midpoint in pregnancy, even sometimes after the point of viability. The amniocentesis procedure carries about a 0.1–0.5 percent risk of inducing pregnancy loss by spontaneous miscarriage.

Fetal chromosomal anomalies can be diagnosed earlier using a different procedure called chorionic villus sampling. This procedure can be done as early as eight to eleven weeks. It involves a vaginal examination in which a biopsy needle is inserted through the woman's cervix and into the uterus to obtain fetal tissue from the placenta. It carries a 0.5–2.0 percent risk of fetal loss.

But most prenatally diagnosed anomalies of the fetus are not caused by abnormalities of the chromosomes. Most fetal anomalies found prenatally are discovered by ultrasound imaging of the developing fetus, sometimes early in pregnancy, but more often later. This procedure is now being done on a nearly routine basis and carries no known risk to baby or mother.

Some people of faith draw a firm line in the sand and maintain that abortion is always immoral and is only justified to preserve the life of the pregnant woman. This position is clear, easy to understand, and fairly easy to interpret, though it is sometimes difficult to predict whether the medical problem might take the woman's life.

Some would move the line a bit and allow abortion for the woman carrying a fetus who cannot live outside the uterus, for example, the fetus with anencephaly, or one with absent kidneys. The rationale is that this woman may be aware of the diagnosis and prognosis by twenty weeks' gestation but have another twenty weeks during which she knows the baby cannot live. During this time she must not only deal with her own thoughts and feelings, but also strangers will come up to her in the supermarket to "ooh and aah" over the pregnancy. A compassionate understanding of the psychological burden on the woman moves some to not prohibit or condemn abortion in such a case. Alternatively, many women in this situation choose to carry the baby to term and give birth. They often experience an irreplaceable opportunity for bonding and describe a sad peace by cuddling the infant during the minutes, hours, or days before he or she dies.

Still other people of faith would give the woman more moral leeway, permitting her to opt for abortion of any abnormal fetus. Most believe this moves dangerously close to the position of accepting only a "normal" baby. And I concur that there is a valid concern about a "slippery slope" here. An assessment of the "acceptability" of a particular anomaly is subjective and value-laden. Quite a spectrum of anomalies can be diagnosed prenatally. Some are life-threatening in the first minutes or days of life. Some might allow the child to live a short time but with painful conditions (e.g., the most severe form of osteogenesis imperfecta).[4] And of course, others are quite compatible with prolonged life with one or more disabilities, some of which are fully or partially correctable.

Regardless of where one falls on this spectrum of belief, it is very important to realize the limits of prenatal diagnosis. The morally important questions are: How certain are we of the diagnosis, and how certain are we of the prognosis? Sometimes we are virtually 100 percent certain that a fetus has a condition that is incompatible with extrauterine life. When either the diagnosis or prognosis is less than certain, I believe the moral obligation of both mother and physician to the fetus is raised to such a level that abortion is morally troublesome.

One further consideration is our continuing moral obligation to the doomed fetus. When a woman decides to terminate her pregnancy, regardless of whether our own boundaries consider her choice to be morally permitted or not, we (and she) have ongoing moral obligations to the fetus. I believe there is a significant moral difference between early induction of labor resulting in the death of a very premature infant and a procedure to intentionally dismember and destroy a still-living fetus. Even when we are not involved in the decision, do not approve of the decision, and are not involved in the procedure, I believe we have an obligation to speak up for the fetus.

---

4. Osteogenesis imperfecta, also known as "brittle bone disease," is a genetic disorder of connective tissue, most notably in the bones. The disease has quite a broad spectrum of severity. In its most severe form, it is lethal in the neonatal period, and it involves multiple fractures of the long bones, beginning prior to birth.

Let's now look at some specific cases that challenge our moral boundaries, trying to balance our obligations to both mother and fetus. These cases are arranged in order of gestational age.

Case 13.01

QUESTION

What are the ethically permissible treatment options for this pregnant woman (sixteen to seventeen weeks' gestation) with severe thyroid problems?

STORY

Kristen is a thirty-year-old librarian who has two healthy children and has had one spontaneous miscarriage. She developed severe thyrotoxicosis (overactivity of her thyroid gland) just before the beginning of her last pregnancy two years ago. This caused persistent vomiting for the entire pregnancy, such that she was unable to adequately retain her thyroid-suppressing medication. She had two life-threatening "thyroid storms" (abrupt worsening of the condition with anxiety, agitation, sweating, nausea, palpitations, and many other symptoms), each lasting a few hours during the pregnancy. During those episodes she felt awful and was certain she was going to die. She delivered six weeks early; she stopped vomiting; her thyroid condition was controlled with medication; and she felt quite well for several months. The plan was to treat her thyrotoxicosis with radioactive iodine once the thyroid symptoms were controlled (radioactive iodine cannot be used during pregnancy). However, she became pregnant again before this transpired, in spite of faithful use of oral contraceptives. Although she had tried to avoid pregnancy because of the thyroid problem, she was not upset with the prospect and does hope to have at least one more child.

She is now sixteen-to-seventeen weeks pregnant and has been even more ill than with the last pregnancy. This is her second admission for dehydration. The endocrinologist who has been treating her thyroid disorder since the original diagnosis has told her that her options now are: (1) continued attempts at medical control throughout pregnancy with definitive treatment after delivery, (2) medical control of the thyrotoxicosis followed by surgical removal of the thyroid during pregnancy, (3) termination of pregnancy followed by definitive treatment with radioactive iodine.

While thyrotoxicosis successfully treated in pregnancy is compatible with good maternal and fetal outcomes, continued thyrotoxicosis, in spite of treatment, places the patient at risk of thyroid storm, heart failure, and toxemia of pregnancy, each of which carries some risk of maternal death. Because of how awful she felt during her thyroid storms, she finds the prospect of continuing the pregnancy with further attempts at medical control to be unacceptable. She has been fearful of thyroid surgery during pregnancy because of potential complications, including damage to her vocal cords, inadvertent loss of her parathyroid glands, and transient precipitation of thyroid storms.

At present Kristen is inclined toward termination of her pregnancy to enable definitive thyroid therapy. Her husband, family, and friends are supportive of her and have encouraged her to terminate the pregnancy. She has never considered abortion to be morally acceptable and says she has never known anyone who had an abortion. Her greatest reluctance is her fear of God's judgment if she chooses this option. She and her husband are Baptists, though not currently active in a church. She states that this is the hardest decision she has ever had to make.

DISCUSSION

Of the many reasons offered to justify abortion in any specific case, threat to the pregnant woman's health or life has the greatest support among people of various moral persuasions. However, when a woman faces the prospect of terminating a pregnancy for medical reasons, societal and political consensus is less important than her own beliefs and moral reasoning.

In this case, any of the three medically acceptable options are also ethically permissible. Her rejection of medical management in order to complete the pregnancy is understandable because of her experience with this during her last pregnancy, and this should be supported. While many pro-life individuals would encourage her to choose surgery in order to continue the pregnancy, her considerable anxiety regarding this option is morally relevant and should not be discounted.

RECOMMENDATION

The patient and her husband should be encouraged to weigh the pros and cons of the two remaining options and make the choice they find less objectionable, on which they will be able to look back without regret. They should be encouraged to talk with family and clergy, but ultimately the decision should be theirs and should be supported by her health-care team.

FOLLOW-UP

Because of her long-standing belief that abortion is morally wrong, I encouraged Kristen to consider the surgical option. She was truly fearful of this, and said her only reluctance in choosing to terminate the pregnancy was her fear of God's judgment. I tried to balance this by speaking of God's compassion and forgiveness. I encouraged her to speak with a hospital chaplain since she had not identified any personal clergy. She did not do this. The patient and her husband decided to terminate the pregnancy to avoid the anticipated major difficulties during pregnancy and to obtain definitive thyroid therapy. This was done by inducing premature labor using prostaglandin suppositories. The infant was stillborn.

COMMENT

From a fetal standpoint, the moral high ground would have been for Kristen to accept thyroid surgery during pregnancy. Its risks are relatively small, but they are not insignificant. Assessment of risk is a very personal matter, and professionals should not impose their assessment on the patient faced with a difficult decision.

Case 13.02

QUESTION

What are the ethically permissible treatment options for this woman in early pregnancy (eighteen weeks' gestation) who has a noncurable malignancy?

STORY

Maria is thirty-four, pregnant, and has three healthy children. She was admitted to the hospital one month ago with a newly diagnosed tumor in the right temporal lobe of her brain, a tumor with a very poor prognosis. Only part of the aggressive tumor was removed in surgery, leaving her with permanent paralysis on her left side. Six weeks of radiation therapy was begun three weeks ago and she is now on the rehabilitation service, receiving continued radiation and obstetrical management from the consulting high-risk obstetrics service. Ultrasound confirms the pregnancy to be at approximately eighteen weeks' **gestation**. Different members of her care team have discussed options ranging from termination of pregnancy to aggressive maternal maintenance (to allow gestational maturation) if the patient should rapidly deteriorate, and an ethics consultation was requested to help sort out the options.

Maria and her husband have been active members of their Assemblies of God church for several years. They maintain a strong faith and have strong family values. Their three children are two, six, and nine years of age. Although this pregnancy was not specifically planned, it was accepted joyfully. The patient is an architect and her husband is a business executive.

The patient is clearly cognizant, demonstrates clear understanding, and answers direct questions slowly but articulately. However, her husband does most of the talking, and she nods agreement. Their understanding is that the tumor has been incompletely removed and radiation is being done to slow the tumor growth, not to cure it. They have heard prognoses ranging from six months to twenty-four months. It is their understanding that chemotherapy has not been recommended because it might harm the baby and would offer her only marginal advantage. While they have discussed termination of the pregnancy, they agree that this would be considered only if there were a high likelihood that this would be to her medical advantage. Their agreed-upon first priority is her health, and the baby's welfare is a very close second. They also place a high priority on getting home as soon as possible to be with her children. The patient clearly states that her husband should be her **surrogate** if she should lose **decision-making capacity**.

DISCUSSION

When a patient with decision-making capacity is faced with difficult treatment decisions, the patient should be given as much prognostic information as possible along with professional recommendations about a preferred course of treatment. The patient's decision, as long as it is within the bounds of acceptable medical practice, should almost always be followed.

When a pregnant patient faces such complex decisions, it is important that she be given as much information as possible about both her own prognosis and that of the fetus. It is also important to identify her choice of surrogate for both her and the fetus.

Termination of pregnancy at eighteen weeks is legally permitted in most jurisdictions in the United States. There is a spectrum of belief about the morality of continuing or terminating pregnancy when a pregnant woman is found to have a life-threatening condition. Many would recommend termination of the pregnancy to allow an undisturbed focus on her life and health. Others would recommend termination if continuation of the pregnancy would adversely restrict treatment choices for her malignancy. All, however, would recommend that the woman be fully informed about the options and consequences, and that her voluntary decision be honored.

RECOMMENDATIONS

1. It would be worthwhile to hold a multidisciplinary conference to include the patient and her husband, their pastor, and representatives from the departments of rehabilitation medicine, high-risk obstetrics, radiation oncology, and perhaps neurosurgery.
2. Since the patient has named her husband as her surrogate, it might be appropriate to discuss obstetrical management options if she should irreversibly deteriorate before the fetus has achieved viability. If that is deemed a significant likelihood, this discussion should occur soon in order to include her, but if it is not very likely, it would be permissible to discuss this only with him if it should come to pass.

FOLLOW-UP

After the recommended conference was held, Maria and her husband chose to continue the pregnancy. Her neurological condition slowly deteriorated. Delivery of a small but apparently healthy baby girl (named Maria) was carried out by Cesarean section at thirty-six weeks' gestation, based on consent from her husband. Maria lived for seven months after her daughter was delivered.

COMMENT

This pregnant woman with an incurable tumor had decision-making capacity. She had expressed the desire to pursue life-prolonging measures and also indicated a high value for fetal protection. While it would have been understandable for her to choose to terminate the pregnancy so that she could focus on her own health, prolonging her life, and experiencing fully her three children, her decision to continue the pregnancy was noble and demonstrated her high regard for fetal life.

Case 13.03 ───

QUESTION

Is it ethically permissible to terminate this pregnancy (twenty weeks' gestation) because the fetus has Down syndrome and will thus have developmental delay?

STORY

Jessie is a thirty-nine-year-old woman with two teenage children who is now at about twenty weeks' **gestation**. She had an amniocentesis four weeks ago, the report from which showed that the fetus has **Down syndrome**. The patient and her husband were counseled about their options but were uncertain what they wanted to do. The patient was concerned about a possible lab mix-up, so the amniocentesis was repeated and the fluid sent to a different lab. The result came back five days ago confirming the diagnosis. She was again counseled at length and was still uncertain of what she wanted. However, she did know that if she chose termination, she did not want a destructive procedure done on the fetus. She and her husband subsequently were in contact with a Down syndrome support group, and they talked with parents of a child with the condition. The patient called yesterday requesting termination of her pregnancy.

There has been some discrepancy between her menstrual dates and the gestational age suggested by three ultrasound studies. The best consensus on dating is that she is just over twenty weeks.

Jessie was a stay-at-home mom for several years, but she returned to teaching elementary school when her two children reached their teens. Her husband is manager of an auto parts store. They were married in a Methodist church but have not been observant in recent years.

DISCUSSION

From an ethics standpoint, there is a wide range of opinions about justifiable reasons for termination of pregnancy. (a) Some believe that length of gestation is irrelevant, and any reason given by the patient is justification for termination. (b) Some believe that duration of gestation is of moral significance, so that requests for termination in later gestation (e.g., especially after viability) require greater justification. (c) Others believe that the underlying reason for the request is the factor of moral significance, rather than the duration of gestation, so that some reasons for the request might be justifiable while others would not be. Many who hold this position would find a certain diagnosis of mental retardation, but of unpredictable severity, to be insufficient justification. (d) Still others believe that the only justifiable reason for termination of pregnancy of any duration is to save the life of the mother.

With no societal consensus on moral justification for termination of pregnancy, we often use the arbitrary legal limits (gestational limit, maternal request, physician agreement) as our default guideline. Elective termination of pregnancy up to twenty weeks is a legal option in this state, and may be done at the request of the patient for any reason.

RECOMMENDATIONS

1. If there is professional consensus that this pregnancy is no longer than twenty weeks, her request for termination is legally permissible.
2. There is a spectrum of ethical opinion about whether it is permissible to terminate a twenty-week pregnancy for reasons of mental retardation in the fetus. It is my personal opinion that this is inadequate justification.
3. Regardless of the patient's decision, and regardless of individual professionals' personal opinions about her choice, she and her husband should be given ongoing support through this difficult situation.

FOLLOW-UP

After several hours of induced labor, a 279 gram (nine- to ten-ounce) baby was born alive and pronounced dead sixteen minutes later. Nurses reported that the father examined the baby closely and said, "I thought he was going to be abnormal."

COMMENT

As an ethics consultant, I try to educate patients and professionals about the boundaries of currently acceptable practice as established by the profession and by society, including legal precedents. Only rarely do I express my personal moral opinion when there is a spectrum of belief across society. I have been criticized by some people of faith, who contend that I should serve as a moral policeman. I think that might be justified if I were working within a faith-based institution, but I do not believe it is in the secular sphere. Sometimes, however, as in this case, I am unable to remain silent when people are asking for guidance. I believe the father's sad comment after delivery of this baby with Down syndrome highlights the tragic paradox that has developed in our society — advocacy for the rights of the disabled on the one hand with nearly unfettered protection of a woman's "right to choose" the outcome of her pregnancy on the other.

Case 13.04

QUESTION

Please assist in evaluating the ethical appropriateness and the proper professional response to this patient's request for termination of this pregnancy (twenty-one weeks' gestation) when the fetus has hydrocephalus.

STORY

Marjorie, age twenty-six, has one child, has had two spontaneous miscarriages, and is now at about twenty-two weeks in her fourth pregnancy. An ultrasound at approximately nineteen weeks revealed possible brain abnormalities of the female fetus, and follow-up studies showed significant hydrocephalus.[5]

When Dr. Foster informed Marjorie, he also explained that infant prognosis and outcome are difficult to predict for this type of hydrocephalus. The degree of infant cognitive function, retardation, or other disability, or even the ability to survive, is unknown. However, a significant proportion of infants born with this condition alone (without other underlying or accompanying anomalies) have had good outcomes, while others in the same group, especially males, have had profound retardation and disability.

After giving it some thought, three days ago Marjorie requested termination of this pregnancy, expressing fear of a bad outcome for this baby.

DISCUSSION

Our institutional policy limits abortions to first- and early-second-trimester cases in which the fetus is highly compromised and unlikely to have consciousness, or in which continuation of pregnancy is a threat to the life and health of the mother. This case does not meet those criteria since there remains a distinct possibility that this fetus will have normal mental development.

However, the chance of a poor outcome is significant enough that some would consider Marjorie's request for termination "within the bounds of a reasonable request," despite falling outside the bounds of institutional policy. This raises the question of how much information and assistance regarding the option of abortion we owe to the patient. Though legal abortion at this gestational age is not available in this state, clinics in other states are willing to do an abortion procedure beyond twenty weeks' **gestation**.

RECOMMENDATIONS

1. Termination of this pregnancy falls outside of current institutional policy and should not be done here at the patient's request.
2. The primary obstetrician or perinatal team should ask the mother to consider the unborn child's **best interests**. Such attempts at moral

---

5. Hydrocephalus is a dilation of the normal fluid-filled spaces within the brain, usually caused by an obstruction of outflow of the fluid. In this case, there was dilation of the first and second (lateral) ventricles without evidence of dilation of the third and fourth, leading to a presumed diagnosis of aqueductal stenosis.

suasion should not be coercive, but may help the mother to make a more informed choice and would help achieve a better ethical balance between the mother's free autonomous choice and our beneficence-based obligations to consider the best interests of the fetus.

3. If the patient remains steadfast in her request, we should give her the information and assistance necessary to pursue pregnancy termination out of state.

FOLLOW-UP

No information is available.

COMMENT

It is tempting sometimes to "just say no" when requests for abortion fall outside our own ethical boundaries. Doing this, however, would fly in the face of our society's acceptance of the predominance of patient autonomy, and specifically of a woman's "right to choose" whether to continue a pregnancy or not.

Case 13.05

QUESTION

Is it ethically permissible to terminate this woman's pregnancy (twenty-three weeks' gestation) at her request when the fetus has hypoplastic left heart syndrome?

STORY

Juanita is a twenty-year-old woman at twenty-three weeks' **gestation** in her first pregnancy. She is a college student and her husband is employed by a large retail store. They are delighted with this pregnancy and eagerly looking forward to the birth of their first child. Unfortunately, three days ago an ultrasound examination showed that the fetus has a life-threatening condition, hypoplastic left heart syndrome (HLHS), an anomaly of heart structure in which the left side of the heart, the main pumping chamber, is underdeveloped. Untreated, this congenital condition is incompatible with life for more than several days or weeks after delivery.

A multistage surgical treatment (Norwood procedure) has been developed to allow the child's life to continue for several years. In this approach, the first of four operations must be done very soon after birth, and further corrective surgical steps are done over the subsequent months and years as the heart grows. More recently, heart transplant has been the treatment of choice in most pediatric cardiac centers. The downside of this is that not enough hearts are available, so about 25 percent of the newborns put on the transplant waiting list die before a heart becomes available.

Yesterday Juanita and her mother met with a pediatric cardiologist who explained the condition and offered four options: (1) placing the baby on a waiting list for neonatal cardiac transplantation with a risk of death while waiting for a heart to become available; (2) doing the first stage of the Norwood procedure soon after birth (to be followed by three later surgical steps), which might allow the baby to live for several years; (3) delivery with comfort care and no plans for surgical intervention; or (4) termination of pregnancy. Juanita has chosen to terminate the pregnancy, saying that carrying the pregnancy to term and experiencing a neonatal cardiac death would be too difficult for her.

Other morally relevant facts or assumptions:

- The diagnosis of HLHS can be made prenatally with a very high degree of certainty.
- Neonatal cardiac transplantation for HLHS currently (i.e., at the time of the consultation) has an 80 percent one-year survival and a 75 percent five-year survival with unknown long-term survival. Palliation with multistage surgery has a comparable rate of early survival with a life expectancy into childhood. Both entail significant morbidity and burden (painful surgery, frequent invasive testing, as well as chronic immunosuppressive therapy after transplantation).
- Comfort care of an infant with HLHS usually results in death in hours or days; rarely does such an infant survive for a few weeks. The dying infant experiences heart failure with shortness of breath, which may be moderated with medication, and he or she is pale or **cyanotic**, which is often distressing to family and caregivers.
- Induced labor at twenty-three or twenty-four weeks would be of comparable duration to labor at forty weeks, but possibly of higher intensity. The life of an infant with HLHS of twenty-three or twenty-four

weeks would likely be shorter than that of a full-term infant with the same condition.

- It is impossible to predict and difficult to compare parental grief after death from termination of pregnancy with that after a neonatal death.

DISCUSSION

When fetal anomalies are discovered that require management decisions, well-informed and caring parents are given almost complete decision-making authority. Only when they are acting hastily or do not appear to be acting in the fetus's **best interests** do we consider overriding their choices. Ethically permissible options are determined by assessing the certainty of the diagnosis and the certainty of the consequences of each choice.

When a prenatal diagnosis is made late in gestation with a high degree of certainty that the fetus has a condition that either is incompatible with survival outside the womb or will result in cognitive underdevelopment, it is considered by most to be ethically permissible to offer: (a) induction of early delivery with comfort care for the dying premature infant, (b) non-aggressive obstetrical management and neonatal comfort care, or (c) aggressive obstetrical management aimed at survival for as long as possible.

When the diagnosed condition is correctable, however, the ethical assessment is not as clear. Federal regulations mandate that lifesaving treatment not be withheld from handicapped newborns except in three narrowly defined situations.[6] HLHS does not fit any of these three "Baby Doe" exceptions. However, offering the options outlined above continues to be the accepted pediatric standard of practice because of the scarcity of transplantable hearts, and it would be unseemly to force transplantation and the consequent chronic illness on to one family when other children are dying while waiting for a heart. In addition, the multistage surgical procedures are a difficult burden to the patient with a questionable long-term outlook.

In this case, there is a very high degree of certainty of both the diagnosis and the lethal prognosis without treatment. After being counseled by a cardiologist and perinatologist, the mother has quickly made a choice, not

---

6. Federal regulations require that treatment that would be given to a healthy newborn not be withheld from a handicapped newborn unless (1) the infant is permanently unconscious, (2) treatment would be futile, or (3) treatment would be virtually futile and inhumane. See chapter 10 for further discussion of these "Baby Doe Regulations."

only against surgical interventions to prolong life, but also to terminate the pregnancy. From a maternal standpoint, the choice is quite understandable. It is, however, imperative that such an irreversible decision not be made hastily, but after adequate reflection.

From a fetal standpoint, an argument might be made that if survival is no longer a goal, then term delivery with subsequent comfort care would be morally preferable to termination of the pregnancy since that option would allow a short extrauterine period and thus show greater respect for the fetus's right to life. However, the counterargument that termination of pregnancy at twenty-four weeks would lessen the infant's postdelivery suffering is also morally significant. In sum, these considerations would not preclude, from a moral standpoint, early termination of pregnancy as long as fetal suffering was not increased by the termination (i.e., no destructive procedure on the fetus).

RECOMMENDATIONS

1. Termination of pregnancy for prenatally diagnosed HLHS is not ethically precluded.
2. A woman making such a choice should be given adequate time for reflection and confirmation of that decision.

FOLLOW-UP

Upon further reflection, the patient decided to continue the pregnancy until term. She also said she would like to give more thought to the choice of surgical intervention versus comfort care.

COMMENT

This case highlights the importance of time and reflection when confronting life-and-death decisions. In addition, it raises other issues. It is tempting to opine that babies with HLHS should not be allowed to die without treatment, but rather that the professionals involved (or even the courts) should intervene to protect these lives by insisting on surgical intervention. However, this understandable position must take into consideration the whole picture, as discussed above.

It is not clear why the physician offered termination of pregnancy to Juanita. Standard practice when HLHS is diagnosed prenatally is to offer the other three options but not the option of termination. If neither of the surgical options is available or chosen by the pregnant woman, I guess the fetus could be considered "doomed," and early induction of labor might be considered, much as it is when **anencephaly** is found.

Case 13.06

QUESTION

Is it ethically permissible to terminate this pregnancy (twenty-four weeks) at the mother's request since the fetus has a lethal condition (Potter's syndrome: the failure of any kidney tissue to develop)?

STORY

Rosa, a twenty-four-year-old woman with one healthy child, is now at twenty-four weeks' **gestation**. This second pregnancy was uncomplicated until an ultrasound done a few days ago showed markedly diminished amount of **amniotic fluid**. Further evaluation shows in addition that the fetus has no stomach, no bladder, no kidneys, and a very small chest. The diagnosis of Potter's syndrome has been made with a very high degree of certainty, and carries with it the certainty of intrauterine or neonatal death. The patient and her husband were offered the options of continuation of pregnancy or termination of the pregnancy by early induction of labor. Rosa was initially ambivalent, but her husband favored termination of the pregnancy. She subsequently agreed that this was the best option for them.

DISCUSSION

There is a consensus among physicians and ethicists that when it is clear that a fetus cannot survive outside the uterus because of uncorrectable anomalies, it is ethically permissible to terminate the pregnancy if the patient feels that the psychic stress of carrying the pregnancy to term is too burdensome. However, the prenatal diagnosis of a fetal anomaly that is not compatible with life outside the womb should not automatically imply that termination of pregnancy is the only, or even the preferred, option.

From a fetal perspective, continuation of the pregnancy demonstrates a greater respect for prenatal life. It also offers the possibility of neonatal cuddling, whether live-born or stillborn, either of which may be of great meaning. It is thus preferable to offer the pregnant woman both options of continuation or termination, as was done in this case.

RECOMMENDATION

It is ethically permissible to induce premature labor in this twenty-four-week pregnancy at the patient's request.

FOLLOW-UP

At the time of admission for induction of labor two days after the consultation, the patient and her husband argued about the plan. Paradoxically, he said, "You're killing the baby!" After further counseling, they decided not to terminate the pregnancy, but to carry the baby to term. She went into spontaneous labor at thirty-eight weeks and delivered a baby with minimal signs of life. No resuscitative measures were used. Both parents cuddled the little girl until she died about three hours after delivery.

COMMENT

While the initial decision of this couple was felt to be ethically justifiable, this case illustrates that initial decisions (even initial opinions) can change with reflection. Ambivalence or differences of opinion between husband and wife should encourage the professionals involved to allow a bit more time and to offer further counseling.

Some people of faith would disagree with the consensus that abortion of a fetus who cannot survive outside the uterus is justifiable for maternal psychological reasons. They would assert that the moral obligation to continue fetal life as long as possible outweighs the consequential argument that allows the distressed psychological state of the mother to trump this moral rule. People of faith who support the consensus would counter that this is one of the uncommon situations where compassion for the woman may be determinative.

426

Case 13.07 ───

QUESTION

What are the ethically permissible treatment options for this pregnant woman (twenty-seven and a half weeks' gestation) who has been found to have a potentially curable pelvic malignancy?

STORY

Vicki, age twenty-two, is at twenty-seven and a half weeks' **gestation** in her first pregnancy. She had some vaginal bleeding at eighteen weeks, felt to be from a low-lying placenta. She was admitted to the hospital one week ago because she was unable to empty her bladder. It has now been determined that the urinary obstruction is caused by a rare type of malignant muscle tumor (alveolar rhabdomyosarcoma) on the left side of her vagina and vulva. Testing is under way to determine the extent of the tumor and to assist in the development of management plans for the patient and her baby. The estimated weight of this female fetus is 1,000 grams (about two and a quarter pounds).

The patient has said she would like the baby to survive if possible, but her first priority is her own life and health. She is not a religious person. She feels abortion is generally wrong, but may be justified in some cases. She has been married to Jack for two years. He and Vicki's extended family are supportive of her and of her choice.

The oncology consultant reports that this malignancy has a cure rate of 70-80 percent if detected early. Its location, and the fact that the patient has had frequent recent vaginal exams, suggests that this tumor is early and thus curable. Standard treatment in the nonpregnant patient would be surgery first, followed by chemotherapy, then radiation, and finally more chemotherapy. Because she is pregnant, it is an acceptable alternative to postpone the surgery. The chemotherapeutic agents required are not known to cause fetal anomalies when used in the third trimester of pregnancy. There is, however, about a 5 percent chance that they might be carcinogenic for the baby, inducing malignancy at some time in the future.

The tumor occupies space in her pelvis, so she will have to have a Cesarean section delivery. The neonatology consultant reports that delivery by Cesarean section at this gestation gives the baby a greater than 90 percent chance of survival. The baby will need a long stay in the neonatal intensive care unit on a **ventilator** and has about a one-in-three chance of having some significant residual lung problems. Survival statistics would not improve much with one or two more weeks' gestation, but the extra time might decrease how long the baby would have to stay on the ventilator.

DISCUSSION

An obstetrician should try to achieve a pregnancy outcome that is in the **best interests** of both the mother and the baby, and at the same time should allow the adequately informed mother to make choices between professionally and legally acceptable treatment options. In some situations, there is irresolvable tension between these goals. Fortunately, that does not appear to be the case here.

Since either immediate or delayed delivery is professionally acceptable, and since there is more than one sequence of treatments for the maternal malignancy, the information this mother needs to help her plan her treatment includes:

- Will her survival chances vary depending on the sequence of her treatments? If yes, by how much?
- How long could delivery be postponed if chemotherapy is begun now? How much would this change the baby's chances of survival, duration of hospitalization, chances of long-term lung problems?
- Is it known how much exposure to chemotherapy would cause a significant risk of future malignancy in the baby?

RECOMMENDATIONS

1. Once this patient has been adequately informed, she is free to make a final decision about her management plans. Jack may have valuable input and support, but if they do not agree, the final decision should be hers if only her health is at stake. If alternative treatment plans will not affect her physical outcome or emotional state but might make a significant difference to the baby, both parents should be asked to make the choice. Should they have irresolvable conflict in such a situation, the mother's desires should be honored.

2. If one management plan is clearly superior to others from a medical standpoint, her physicians should make a clear recommendation in that direction. She is, however, free to ignore that recommendation if

her values differ and she can make a rational argument for an alternative plan that is also professionally acceptable.

FOLLOW-UP

No information is available.

COMMENT

As opposed to the situation in Case 13.01, this woman has a viable fetus at the time of her malignant diagnosis and a good chance for cure of her malignancy. Thus she would have a more difficult time justifying a request for termination of this pregnancy. The father of the child has a significant role to play in making decisions for the baby, as outlined above.

Case 13.08

QUESTION

Is it ethically permissible to honor this patient's request that her unborn baby (twenty-eight and a half weeks' gestation) be given preference if a life-versus-life situation arises? Should we honor her request for postpartum sterilization if she lives but her baby does not survive?

STORY

Brenda is a single thirty-one-year-old woman at twenty-eight and a half weeks' **gestation** in her third pregnancy (one living child, one induced abortion). She was found collapsed in a bus station eight days ago and was admitted with dehydration. She was rehydrated, gaining fifteen to twenty pounds, and was transferred to the obstetrical unit two days ago because of preterm labor. She has been treated with medications to stop her labor and to speed maturity of the fetal lungs. Her labor has diminished and the fetus is stable, though in the breech position, which will likely require Cesarean delivery. The patient developed severe shortness of breath yesterday and was transferred to the intensive care unit (ICU). In the subsequent twenty-four hours her pulmonary situation has progressed to respiratory failure (cause as yet unknown) requiring the insertion of a tube into her airway and attachment to a **ventilator** just two hours ago.

At the time of transfer to the ICU, Brenda said she was certain she was going to die, and she initiated discussion with four individuals (nurse, social worker, two physicians) saying if it came to a choice between her life and the baby's, she wanted the baby to live. She gave no reason for this choice. All four professionals report that she was emphatic and mentally clear, though very anxious. She asked the social worker to complete a written statement to this effect, which she signed, and she named her mother as her health-care proxy. She also emphatically said she wanted to be sterilized if she lives, even if her baby does not survive.

Brenda has a history of hepatitis and intravenous drug abuse in the past, and recent alcohol abuse. She also has had multiple psychiatric hospitalizations for treatment of psychosis and for suicide attempts. A psychiatric consultant was unable to evaluate her for depression because of the severity of her medical condition. Her eight-year-old daughter lives with relatives out of state. The father of this child is reported to have been abusive to the patient.

DISCUSSION

Treatment choices should ideally be made by fully informed patients who have **decision-making capacity** and are free of coercion. If they lose capacity, we should make a **substituted judgment**, that is, we should make the decision they would make if they could, based on their written wishes, their previous statement, or an understanding of their values. Valid questions can be raised about the decision-making capacity of a patient who is critically ill or has a history of chronic mental illness. However, neither of these situations automatically renders the patient incapacitated; those caring for the patient must make that judgment.

In this case, a critically ill pregnant patient with a history of depression, suicide attempts, and disordered thinking, emphatically verbalized a choice that may be contrary to what most pregnant women would choose, though not categorically so. Those to whom she made her emphatic request felt she fully understood her situation and the implications of her request. It is unclear if her request is based on maternal altruism, or might be a manifestation of depression.

RECOMMENDATIONS

1. It is ethically appropriate to continue aggressive treatment with the goal of survival of both mother and baby. If delivery is required because of fetal distress, this should be done while efforts continue to preserve the mother's life. If, however, delivery is forced because of irreversible maternal deterioration, it would then be ethically permissible to give priority to fetal salvage over (unlikely) maternal survival based on her clear and repeated statements.

2. Honoring the patient's request for surgical sterilization at the time of Cesarean delivery is less clear. If the baby's condition seems good, this request should probably be honored. However, if the baby's condition is poor or uncertain, it would seem prudent to postpone such an irreversible move. Though doing the sterilization procedure at the time of Cesarean delivery might avoid a second surgery (if she should insist on sterilization at a later date), the potential burden of repeat surgery seems to be outweighed by the potential good of preserving her reproductive potential in case she desires to retain that when her condition has stabilized.

FOLLOW-UP

This patient's pulmonary situation remained critical and unstable for about three weeks, and then slowly improved. She went into spontaneous labor while still on the ventilator at nearly thirty-two weeks' gestation and delivered by Cesarean section. The baby appeared healthy; surgical sterilization was done at the time of delivery. The premature baby girl stayed in the neonatal ICU for four weeks. It was subsequently determined that the respiratory failure was probably a rare side effect of the medication used to slow her labor. The mother improved very slowly and was discharged to her parents' home two months after admission, with plans for ongoing psychiatric care.

COMMENT

Sometimes the chaotic social situation of a patient expands the ethical dilemmas and may restrict the available options. In this case, the patient was verbalizing a choice that might suggest a person with a religious background. It was not known at the time of consultation if she had a recent or remote pathway of faith, but her history and lifestyle choices should not be used to judge that she did not. It is possible she was making this seemingly paradoxical choice as an attempt at atonement. On the other hand, she might have been looking at this life-threatening situation and making a choice that seemed to go against her own well-being as a substitute for suicide. Regardless of her (unknown and probably unknowable) motivation, resolution of the ethics questions must rely on the precepts of clinical medicine and ethics as they could be best applied to what was known of her situation.

Case 13.09

QUESTION

Please help the obstetricians and neonatologists discuss management options for a Jehovah's Witness patient who is bleeding in late pregnancy.

STORY

Hilary is a twenty-six-year-old Jehovah's Witness at thirty weeks' **gestation** in her third pregnancy (two healthy children at home). Two days ago she experienced short-lived, painless, brisk vaginal bleeding. An ultrasound showed a central placenta previa; in this the placenta is abnormally positioned in the uterus and partially or completely covers the outlet. It can lead to massive bleeding before labor or during labor and delivery. This condition can be life-threatening to the baby and also to the mother, especially when the placenta is lying in the central position, as it is in this case. Standard treatment is blood replacement and Cesarean delivery.

Hilary is currently having minimal spotting, her blood pressure is stable, and her blood count is satisfactory (hemoglobin = 10.7 grams/deciliter). The ultrasound confirms a thirty- to thirty-one-week pregnancy, with an estimated fetal weight of 1,630 grams (three and one-half pounds). The patient is cooperative and appreciative, but is clear in her demand to not receive blood products. She has been a Jehovah's Witness since age twelve. She understands that her choice might lead to her death, and she accepts this risk. Her husband, Jeff, has been a Jehovah's Witness for several years and supports her position.

The obstetrical team at this teaching hospital maintains a high regard for maternal autonomy and most would be averse to seeking a court order to transfuse this woman. It is their considered opinion that, should she resume heavy bleeding that endangers either her or the baby, they would be able to do an emergency Cesarean section quickly enough to salvage the baby in good condition. This might involve a decision to operate earlier than they might in a non–Jehovah's Witness patient (i.e., they might wait longer with another patient to see if her bleeding would slow, hoping to give the baby more intrauterine time), and this might result in some unnecessary prematurity for the baby. One member of the obstetrical team says he would seek a court order or even transfuse her without a court order in order to protect her life and health.

If this baby were delivered now, it would have a 90 percent chance for survival, and standard practice would be to obtain a court order to give it blood if medically indicated. The neonatal team also respects parental discretion and would use slightly different standards in determining need for transfusion for this baby than they would for the child of a non–Jehovah's Witness. The **neonatologists** present also expressed an obligation to protect this currently healthy child from reckless exposure to risk, and they might encourage court-ordered transfusion of Hilary if the baby's life were endangered by her hemorrhage.

DISCUSSION

Jehovah's Witness patients generally desire the best possible medical care for themselves and their children short of the receipt of blood products, which they consider an abomination to Jehovah with eternal consequences to them. They are thus exercising a negative right of refusal of therapy but at the same time demanding a positive right to alternative medical care. When only their own life and health are at stake, the medical profession should honor such demands.

When a second party is also endangered (such as a fetus), the problem is more complex. If the alternative requested is a reasonable medical option, it is generally felt to be justified to honor that refusal or request, even if it entails some increased risk to the second party. If the alternative is not a reasonable medical option, and by following it the second party would be doomed, it may be justified to override the refusal.

RECOMMENDATIONS

1. Emergency Cesarean section at the first sign of dangerous bleeding in this patient would appear to be a reasonable medical alternative, and the increased risk of prematurity for the baby would appear to be acceptable.

2. Since the gestation is sufficient that the risk of premature birth would not preclude an emergency Cesarean, and because the surgery could likely be performed more quickly than could initiation of a transfusion, it seems unnecessary to be concerned about overriding the patient's refusal of transfusion for herself in order to protect the baby.

3. The proposed neonatal management of this child is standard practice.

4. The issue of intra-operative transfusion of this patient should her life be in danger needs thorough discussion since so many professionals are potentially involved in this teaching hospital environment. Such discussions should include the patient, the obstetrical attending physicians, the obstetrical residents, the department of anesthesiology, and possibly the hospital attorney. No one on the care team should be forced into a situation in which he or she feels morally or professionally compromised (right of conscience). At the same time, if there is significant likelihood that the patient might be transfused against her wishes, she should be so informed so that she can consider continuing her care elsewhere. I would strongly encourage the care team to accept the limitation she requests, and to do all alternative therapies that might preserve her life and health (including availability of the Cell-Saver, equipment to retrieve and reuse her lost blood, if she finds this morally acceptable).

FOLLOW-UP

I was subsequently asked to speak with Hilary and Jeff. I gave them a copy of my consultation report. They had seriously considered transferring to a smaller hospital where she would be under the care of a single obstetrician instead of a teaching team in an attempt to assure a higher degree of certainty that their wishes would be followed. They have decided against this because of the (admittedly small) risk of bleeding during transport and because of their high regard for the medical care rendered here. In light of this decision, it would seem best to try to make available those individuals on the team most compatible and comfortable with their wishes, if possible, when surgery is needed.

The patient remained in the hospital. Bleeding resumed two and one-half weeks later, but was initially fairly light. When it continued for two hours without letup, Cesarean section was done with an estimated blood loss of 1,000 cubic centimeters. Mother and baby did well.

COMMENT

Religious beliefs are a vital component of treatment decisions for many patients (see chapter 9). Health-care professionals should seek out such beliefs and try to honor them if at all possible, even if that means a less ideal outcome. When the potential for an adverse outcome involves another individual, the ethical analysis becomes more complex.

Case 13.10

QUESTION

Is it ethically permissible to induce premature labor in this woman who is carrying a fetus (thirty-one weeks' gestation) with a lethal condition (thanatophoric dwarfism)?

STORY

Jennifer is twenty-six and is now at thirty-one weeks' **gestation** in her second pregnancy (the first was a spontaneous miscarriage). A recent ultrasound was found to be abnormal. Further testing showed marked excess of **amniotic fluid**, shortening of the long bones of all four extremities, deceased size of the fetal thorax, short ribs, and a deformity of the normal-sized skull. This constellation of findings is most consistent with the diagnosis of thanatophoric dysplasia (or thanatophoric dwarfism); it shows all the expected findings and no unexpected findings. This condition is virtually 100 percent lethal; most infants die within minutes, hours, or days of birth because of immature lungs in a very small chest. Aggressive pulmonary measures in the neonatal period may allow survival for a few weeks or months.

A specialist in high-risk obstetrics discussed these findings with Jennifer, her husband, Tom, and her parents and recommended nonaggressive obstetrical management (i.e., no emergency procedures during the remainder of the pregnancy or during labor and delivery to preserve the life of the baby). They displayed appropriate grief, and the patient asked if she had to go on with the pregnancy since the baby was going to die anyway.

DISCUSSION

Questions often arise about ethically permissible obstetrical and neonatal options when major fetal anomalies are discovered in late gestation. Decisions about which options are permissible and which are ethically justifiable turn on the two questions of degree of certainty of the diagnosis and degree of certainty of lethality. When both are certain (e.g., with **anencephaly**), most agree that the mother and the professionals have minimal moral obligations to preserve the life of the fetus, and management decisions can be based primarily on the wishes of the mother and her assessment of the psychological burden of knowing she is carrying a "doomed fetus." However, the obligation to the fetus increases as the degree of certainty decreases.

In this case we have a high degree of certainty of both diagnosis and prognosis, but not complete certainty of either alone. The consulting **neonatologists** believe the degree of chest development of this fetus is insufficient to permit survival, even if the overall diagnosis is incorrect. Thus, even though we are less than 100 percent certain of the diagnosis, and even though not all infants born with thanatophoric dysplasia die immediately, in this case the degree of certainty of lethality approaches 100 percent. This then raises the moral weight of the psychological burden that the mother might experience.

RECOMMENDATIONS

1. The ethical high ground in this case would be to offer either (a) normal obstetrical care or (b) nonaggressive obstetrical management. The latter would include continuation of pregnancy awaiting spontaneous labor without using prenatal or intrapartum fetal salvage interventions, and then providing comfort care to the neonate if he or she indeed appears to be imminently dying.

2. Because the degree of certainty of lethality for this particular fetus approaches 100 percent, it would also be ethically permissible to honor the mother's request for early induction of labor to reduce her psycho-

logical burden, as long as she understands the small degree of remaining uncertainty.

3. It would not be ethically permissible to utilize a destructive procedure on this fetus to terminate the pregnancy.

FOLLOW-UP

A joint decision was made to induce premature labor at thirty-six weeks (giving the fetal chest more time to grow) and to give the newborn only comfort care if the initial exam was consistent with the prenatal diagnoses. However, she was admitted at thirty-four weeks with premature labor. A four-pound boy was born after a few hours of labor, and the diagnoses were confirmed by two consultants. Jennifer and Tom named him Peter and cuddled him for five hours before he died.

COMMENT

Some people of faith would strongly urge this woman to continue the pregnancy until natural labor ensued. In fact, she and the professionals caring for her took what they felt was the moral high ground of continuing the pregnancy to give the baby the best possible chance to survive. However, if she had been insistent that the psychological burden of carrying a "doomed fetus" was overwhelming for her, most in ethics and medicine would not have been uncomfortable acceding to her request.

Case 13.11

QUESTION

What are the appropriate management options for this pregnant woman (thirty-two weeks' gestation) who has premature rupture of her membranes, is carrying a child with lethal anomalies, and wants "everything done"?

STORY

Geri, a nineteen-year-old woman in advanced pregnancy, had no prenatal care until she arrived at the emergency department two days ago for evaluation of a gush of fluid from the vagina followed by a persistent slow leak of fluid. Ultrasound showed the pregnancy to be at approximately thirty-two weeks' **gestation** and the fetus to have multiple anomalies. Geri has no fever and is not currently having contractions. She has been treated with steroids to enhance maturity of the fetal lungs.

The ultrasound shows a single female fetus in a breech presentation with multiple anomalies suggestive of limb-body-wall defects. She has mild hydrocephalus, severe curvature of the spine, marked chest deformity, and possibly an abdominal wall defect. The ultrasonographer states that although the diagnosis is less than certain, the severity of the chest wall deformity makes it quite certain that the child cannot survive. The consulting **neonatologist** concurs, and believes that the child cannot survive for more than a few minutes after birth.

The mother is homeless, has used multiple street drugs, and was released from jail (in for robbery) a few months ago. She has been told of the severity of the fetal anomalies and the likelihood of immediate perinatal demise. However, she insists that everything be done to ensure survival, because someone has suggested to her that ultrasound is not always accurate.

The high-risk obstetrics team wanted to discuss management of labor (should the fetus be monitored? should interventions be undertaken if there is evidence of fetal distress?) and delivery (should a Cesarean section be done because of the breech position? if vaginal delivery is pursued, what should be done if there is arrest of the after-coming head?). They further wanted guidance if the mother should change her mind and request induction of labor.

DISCUSSION

Management of pregnancy, labor, and delivery when severe fetal anomalies are discovered in the third trimester depends in large part on the degree of certainty of the diagnosis and the prognosis. With a very high degree of certainty of lethality, moral obligations shift from fetal to maternal beneficence. If, however, there is any significant possibility that the fetus could survive, even for a few days or weeks, the mother should be allowed to choose the degree of risk and burden she wants to bear.

RECOMMENDATIONS

1. With a very high degree of certainty of lethality, if the mother were to change her mind and request induction and nonresuscitation, that would be ethically permissible.

2. With her request that "everything" be done, it is appropriate to await labor; however, it would then be appropriate to intervene only for her protection since there is certainty that the fetus cannot survive. Most would assess the increased maternal risks and burdens of Cesarean delivery to be inappropriate if it is certain that the child cannot survive for more than a few minutes.

3. If she delivers vaginally and the after-coming head becomes trapped, expectant management would also be appropriate rather than operative intervention. A destructive procedure on the fetus would be justified only if postponement of vaginal delivery would endanger the mother.

FOLLOW-UP

Spontaneous labor began five days after the ethics consultation (seven days after admission). The baby died during labor, prior to delivery. No fetal interventions were used.

COMMENT

It is difficult or impossible to know if this woman's request for fully aggressive treatment was based only on her skepticism about the accuracy of ultrasound testing or if other factors affected her request. If there truly were any doubts about the fetal outcome, her request should have been honored. In this case, the virtual certainty of fetal death precluded interventions that increased her burden or risk.

Case 13.12

QUESTION

What are the ethically permissible obstetrical and neonatal management options for this patient (thirty-six weeks' gestation) who is carrying a baby with a life-threatening genetic abnormality (spinal muscular atrophy)?

STORY

Susan is a twenty-eight-year-old woman whose first child, Reggie, born two years ago, has spinal muscular atrophy. He appeared normal at birth, but this genetic disorder was diagnosed at six weeks of age when he developed respiratory failure. He has since been cared for at home, on full-time **ventilator** support, with twenty-four-hour nursing assistance.

Susan is now at thirty-six weeks' **gestation** in her second pregnancy. She had genetic testing done (via chorionic villus sampling) prior to twelve weeks' gestation that showed that this fetus has the same condition. She and her husband chose to continue the pregnancy. Her pregnancy has otherwise been uncomplicated except that she is now showing some elevation of her blood pressure. Dr. Gokey, the obstetrician caring for her, has asked for guidance in making plans for the remainder of her pregnancy, her labor, and her delivery.

Patients with spinal muscular atrophy lose motor ability but have normal cognitive development. There is a spectrum of severity, with early onset indicating more profound neurologic impairment. The most severe variety becomes manifest in early infancy and usually leads to early death (infancy or under two years). It is believed that affected siblings usually follow a similar course.

DISCUSSION

When choosing ethically permissible *obstetrical options,* a woman carrying an unhealthy fetus must take into consideration the degree of certainty of the diagnosis and the degree of certainty of the prognosis for survival and cognitive development.

In this case, the diagnosis is highly certain, but a spectrum of severity exists within which survival in and beyond the neonatal period is possible, though this might require some degree of artificial support at some time. Thus our ethical obligation to this fetus is only slightly less than for a normal fetus. If the parents, after thorough discussion, requested noninvasive obstetrical management, this might be ethically justifiable if they felt that the burden of emergency surgical delivery for the mother outweighed the benefit of shortened neonatal life, which entailed significant burden for the baby.

Legally and ethically permissible *neonatal options* for an infant with anomalies are somewhat restricted. The "Baby Doe Regulations" prohibit the withholding or withdrawing of lifesaving treatment from a handicapped newborn except under three conditions: (a) if the infant will be permanently unconscious; (b) if full treatment would be futile; or (c) if full treatment would be virtually futile and inhumane. Professional recommendations are somewhat more flexible; the American Academy of Pediatrics allows parental discretion about the use or nonuse of full therapy when it is not clear if that therapy would be beneficial to the infant.

In this infant, specific treatment decisions must await neonatal assessment. The presumption should be for treatment unless the infant's condition indicates that full treatment would not work or might work but would cause the infant disproportionate suffering that cannot be ameliorated.

RECOMMENDATIONS

1. Susan and her husband should be fully informed about obstetrical and neonatal management options.
2. The presumption should be for routine obstetrical management unless the parents believe the maternal burden of such management would outweigh the expected shortened life of this handicapped infant.
3. The presumption should be for routine neonatal management unless the professionals believe full therapy would not work or would cause the infant disproportionate suffering.
4. Whether to use long-term vent support if this baby develops respiratory failure is another major decision-point in clinical ethics. Ethics consultants should be called on to meet with the parents and their professional caregivers to discuss this if they wish.

FOLLOW-UP

The parents were relieved at the recommendations of this consultation. Dr. Gokey raised the questions in the first place because of his concern for the mother, but also because of his perspective on the cost of medical treatment. When this was balanced against the ethical precepts put forward here, he was less uncomfortable proceeding with our recommendations.

COMMENT

Some might be critical of this couple for having a second child when the care of their first occupies so much of their time and is so burdensome to him and expensive for society. We don't know, however, if their faith tradition forbids sterilization or contraception. We do know that they made a morally sound choice to continue the pregnancy in spite of the same diagnosis.

*   *   *

Other Cases Involving Ethical Issues during Pregnancy

Cases 7.11, 10.01

References on Ethical Issues in Pregnancy

American Association on Mental Retardation. *Before Their Time: Fetuses and Infants at Risk.* Washington, D.C.: AAMR, 1990.
Goldworth, A., W. Silverman, W. Stevenson, E. W. D. Young, and R. Rivers, eds. *Ethics and Perinatology.* New York: Oxford University Press, 1995.
McCullough, L. B., and F. A. Chervenak. *Ethics in Obstetrics and Gynecology.* New York: Oxford University Press, 1994.

CHAPTER 14

Ethical Issues in Organ Transplantation

As with the introduction of any new technology, developments in transplantation in the last half of the twentieth century raised many new questions about application, allocation, and cost. However, some of the questions surrounding transplantation are different from those dealing with other new technologies because organs available for transplantation are very scarce. It would be possible to manufacture as many **ventilators** as might be needed, but we can't manufacture new lungs, hearts, or livers.

The transplantation endeavor in medicine has become, ironically, a victim of its own success. If kidney transplantation were not as directly beneficial to patients, we would not be facing a long waiting list for kidneys. And, as mentioned in chapter 5, the list is particularly long because we have an effective artificial kidney that can keep people with kidney failure alive for an extended period while awaiting the preferred real kidney. But when hearts, livers, and lungs fail, people can be kept alive for only a limited time, and if the needed organ does not become available, they will die. In the United States, several thousand people die each year while their names are on the waiting list for an organ transplant.

Many of the ethical issues surrounding transplantation are issues of medical ethics, that is, they are focused on policy matters. For example, where do we get organs for transplantation — from cadavers, from living donors, from animals? What about taking organs from patients in the **persistent vegetative state**, or from people who die a cardiac death after disconnection from ventilator support, or from executed prisoners? What criteria should be used to "list"[1] a patient? How is the list to be prioritized? Does celebrity count?

1. Listing is the process of determining who is eligible to receive an organ transplant,

Should we transplant organs into patients with developmental delay or **dementia**? Should prisoners sentenced to die be eligible for transplantation? Should we give a new liver to a person who has ruined his own by abusing alcohol? Should we give a second liver to a patient who has rejected the first transplant? How should the available organs be allocated? Should ability to pay be a factor? How does geography factor in? And the list of issues goes on.

The American Medical Association has concluded that, as a general rule, the following factors should be considered in allocation of organs: (a) likelihood of benefit to the specific patient; (b) impact on the patient's quality of life; (c) duration of benefit; (d) urgency of the patient's condition; and (e) the resources required for successful treatment. Many people of faith balk at such a purely utilitarian calculation where the goal is to achieve the greatest good for the greatest number. However, even though we may support the sanctity of human life and the inherent equality of all persons, when dealing with an absolutely scarce resource, most believe that such utilitarian reasoning is ethically justified.

As interesting and challenging as these policy questions are, we will not directly look at them since we want to focus on specific dilemmas. But even as we look at specific cases of listing or distribution, we must realize that our ethical analysis here is a bit different from other case analyses. This is because here we must be more aware of justice issues.

If patient X is at the top of the waiting list and is given an organ, even though he is in very poor condition and has a high chance of dying with or without the transplant, will this allocation decision lead to the death of patient Y, who will not get that organ even though he has a greater chance of survival after a transplant? Should this be part of our consideration in caring for patient X? Clearly, we have a primary goal of serving the needs of the patient sitting right in front of us, but in transplantation issues, it is vitally important not to overlook issues of justice.

And what if patient X ruined his own liver by drinking too much alcohol (see Case 14.06)? How does that factor into the allocation decision? Or what if patient X has some degree of mental retardation (see Cases 14.02 and 14.09)? How does the patient's social situation (see Case 14.03) or cultural beliefs (see Case 14.04) affect our decision?

---

including classification by urgency. This is done by the hospital or team that will be performing the transplant. The criteria used are fairly uniform, so individual patients waiting on the list at different transplant centers are presumably on a par, but these criteria are subject to some local interpretation.

Let's look at some specific cases that led to requests for clinical ethics consultation.

Case 14.01

QUESTION

Is it ethically permissible to retrieve organs from this man who meets the clinical criteria for brain death but may still have some sedation (pentobarbital) in his system?

STORY

Norman is a forty-two-year-old man who lives with his parents and has a history of diabetes and chronic paranoid schizophrenia. Four days ago he was found unresponsive with seizure activity. A head **CT scan** showed massive **intraventricular hemorrhage** and **subarachnoid hemorrhage**. He was admitted, **intubated**, and treated aggressively. The day after admission he was put into a pentobarbital coma, a therapeutic effort that uses a sedating drug that can also reduce brain swelling in an effort to preserve brain tissue and function. Just eight hours later, however, progressive neurologic deterioration led to a decision to withdraw support. The pentobarbital was stopped. His parents requested organ retrieval because Norman had said on several occasions that he wanted to help others in this way. At that time, his clinical exam was consistent with death by neurologic criteria, but he still had electrical activity on an **electroencephalogram**. He has now been thirty-eight hours without pentobarbital; his repeat clinical exam shows no brain activity; and a cerebral blood flow shows no flow. The retrieval team is ready to proceed with apnea testing[2] and organ retrieval, but wants to ensure that the recent use of pentobarbital is no longer an issue that should preclude retrieval.

Serum pentobarbital levels cannot be measured at this hospital, so

2. The apnea test is the final step in declaration of death by neurologic criteria (brain death), used after all other criteria have been met. It involves disconnecting the ventilator and close observation for ten minutes to see if the patient makes any effort at breathing. No effort (apnea) confirms absence of brain function; any respiratory effort indicates that some brain tissue retains function and the patient is not brain dead.

there is no objective way to know if it has cleared from his system or is still present in sufficient amount to confound the clinical determination of death by neurological criteria. The clinical pharmacologist in the intensive care unit has calculated (using information about drug half-life, the patient's age, liver function, etc.) that this patient's pentobarbital level is now almost certainly less than 50 percent of the therapeutic level needed to maintain coma. In addition, she is convinced that whatever residual pentobarbital is present would not be sufficient to cause total lack of cerebral flow.

DISCUSSION

Declaration of death by neurologic criteria is a clinical determination that requires two clinical exams separated in time; there must be a known proximate cause of death that is known to be irreversible; and there must be no confounding medical condition or drug intoxication. Confirmatory exams (electroencephalography, cerebral blood flow, angiography)[3] are optional. The clinical exam must demonstrate complete absence of cortical function, complete absence of brain stem function, and complete lack of respiratory effort (apnea).

This patient has a known and irreversible cause of brain failure; he meets the clinical criteria for brain death except that an apnea test has not yet been done; however, he recently received pentobarbital, which could confound the clinical determination. Though any residual pentobarbital could theoretically confound a declaration of death using neurologic criteria, the fact that he has no cerebral blood flow assures us that he has no viable brain tissue. The understanding that this lack of flow is not the result of pentobarbital eliminates concern about any residual drug since a brain without flow is a permanently nonfunctional brain.

RECOMMENDATION

It is ethically permissible to proceed with standard organ retrieval from this patient if he demonstrates apnea.

---

3. Electroencephalography is the measurement of electrical activity of the brain; cerebral blood flow is the measurement of the amount of blood flow in major arteries supplying the brain; and angiography consists of X-rays taken after the injection of dye into the arteries supplying the brain.

FOLLOW-UP

At organ retrieval, he was found to have multiple nodules in his lungs suspicious for tuberculosis, so organs were not retrieved.

COMMENT

Some patients/families are highly motivated to donate organs for transplant. Health-care professionals are usually well motivated also, and want to do all they can to facilitate the process, for the sake of both the donor's family and the recipients. However, it is critical that the professionals maintain accepted medical standards and not bend the rules. In this case, there was some question whether a drug used in treatment of the dying young man might make it difficult to determine that he was actually dead using neurologic criteria. Since he was clearly dying, it might have been tempting to proceed in order to retrieve organs. But retrieval before certainty of death would not only be morally problematic, it could also lead to distrust of medical professionals if others became aware that the rules were not strictly observed.

Case 14.02

QUESTION

Is it ethically appropriate to consider this child with moderate developmental delay for renal transplantation?

STORY

Curt is a nine-year-old boy who was born with **Down syndrome** and congenital obstruction of his urinary tract. The urinary obstruction was not recognized in infancy, and he eventually developed kidney failure. He has been on dialysis three times per week for two or three years, and his father has asked about listing him for transplantation. Dr. Stewart, the pediatric **nephrologist** caring for him, expects that transplantation would significantly improve Curt's quality of life. In addition, intravenous access for continued dialysis may soon become difficult or impossible to maintain so that Curt might die if continued on dialysis.

Past medical history shows that Curt has had a tonsillectomy for recurrent ear infections, and he has had just two hospitalizations for infections in his dialysis lines.

He is cared for at home in a rural community about one hour from the medical center by his father, who is a retired laborer, and his mother, who has a seizure disorder. He has two healthy siblings. He is able to walk but is reported to be essentially nonverbal. He goes to a school for handicapped children.

On examination, he sits happily in his crib, playing with good hand-eye coordination, smiling and eager to interact. He can speak at least a few words — he pointed to a steam engine on the TV screen and said, "Toot, toot," and when I left the room, he spontaneously said, "Bye-bye."

DISCUSSION

In allocating scarce medical resources, several groups of criteria are often discussed, including medical criteria (need, likelihood of benefit, length of benefit, quality of benefit), socio-medical criteria (age, psychological ability, supportive environment), personal criteria (willingness, funding), and social criteria (social value, favored group, special responsibilities).

Two guiding principles should be considered in this case. First is the inherent worth of each individual human life, and second is justice, the principle that patients should be treated without discrimination. Most who comment on such issues believe it preferable to consider social criteria last, and then only when there is urgent competition for a single resource. Even then, the decision is often reframed in terminology to suggest that the developmentally delayed individual could appreciate less benefit than the cognitively intact person. In a medical situation where there is a temporizing modality (such as dialysis for end-stage renal disease), most believe that social criteria should not be used at all.

RECOMMENDATION

It is my opinion that this child should be evaluated in the same manner as any other nine-year-old child. If he meets the medical criteria and has adequate environmental support and funding, he should be listed for kidney transplantation.

FOLLOW-UP

Curt was listed for transplantation, and an organ became available in about eighteen months. His surgery was uncomplicated, and he did very well at home with careful follow-up by his primary physician and nephrologist.

COMMENT

These sentiments of inherent worth and justice mirror the federal guidelines for treatment of newborns — medical care should not be withheld because of handicaps. This black-and-white rule sounds easy and precise, but requires some wisdom and latitude in implementation. It would seem unreasonable to consider transplanting an expensive and scarce resource (e.g., a heart) in a severely handicapped infant who would never have awareness (e.g., an infant with **anencephaly**) or in another with limited life expectancy from another congenital problem. Although such an infant would gain some medical benefit from the procedure in the form of life prolongation, he or she would still have a dismal prognosis precisely because of the handicap. Others with no handicaps or less severe handicaps could benefit more from the scarce resource. This would seem to be an instance when utilitarian reasoning (the greatest good for the greatest number) would justify withholding the scarce resource from a severely handicapped individual.

Case 14.03 ———————————————————————————————

QUESTION

Should we provide transplantation for this infant son of undocumented foreign national parents?

STORY

Eduardo was born two weeks ago at a small community hospital in the southern United States, near the Mexican border. Soon after birth it was determined that he had congenital heart disease. He was transferred to a large children's hospital to be evaluated for possible corrective surgery or trans-

449

plantation. Workup has shown that he has complicated congenital heart disease. Pediatric cardiology and cardiothoracic surgery consultants believe he has insufficient residual tissue to do palliative surgery; they expect such an attempt would have greater than 50 percent operative mortality and, if he survived, major morbidity that would require close subspecialty follow-up. They believe heart transplantation offers a significant chance of long-term survival. Without this, he will likely die within a few weeks. Options of transplantation and comfort care have been discussed with his parents. Medical evaluation for transplantation is under way.

His parents are from Mexico and are living temporarily in the United States. They do not have green cards, and they plan to return to Mexico in the near future. Their major family support is in a small mountain village in Mexico. They have talked extensively with children's hospital physicians and social workers, and have given the impression that they are seeking the child's **best interests**, but they are not medically sophisticated and do not seem to comprehend the logistic requirements for transplantation (the need to live locally, the undetermined wait for an available heart, etc.) and the need for intensive and close follow-up. They did offer to relocate to a community on the Mexican side of the border, but it is over three hours away from the children's hospital, not close enough for adequate follow-up. The hospital social worker and legal counsel are in conversation with the U.S. and Mexican consulates.

DISCUSSION

When dealing with an absolutely scarce resource, patient selection criteria include medical, social, and personal factors. While medical need and medical benefit tend to (appropriately) dominate the discussion, it would be poor stewardship to ignore such social factors as the presence of a supportive environment and such personal factors as ability and willingness to provide adequate follow-up. It is difficult to decline to list a potential recipient for a solid organ for social or personal reasons, but it is necessary in order to maximize the benefit from available organs.

In this case, the social factors appear to be nearly insurmountable. However, placing the infant in guardianship, in foster care, or even up for adoption might allow him to receive the benefit of transplantation with the required close medical follow-up.

Because it is difficult to not list any given patient, it is tempting to treat all reasons as "medical" and merely say to the parents that the patient is "not a transplant candidate." If, however, even a small possibility exists that a given patient could benefit from a transplant, it would be deceptive to disguise or withhold the true reasons.

RECOMMENDATIONS

1. Conversation with immigration authorities should continue to see if there is any way to accommodate this family's medical needs.
2. It would be paternalistic and thus unethical to presume that the parents would not be willing to make (or allow) alternative living arrangements for this child and thus to not offer transplantation at all. It may not be morally obligatory that the parents be offered the explicit options of guardianship, etc., but they should be told why transplantation is not recommended and what would be required for it to be considered. If they suggest other workable living arrangements or make further inquiries, it would clearly be in the infant's best interests to explore other options.
3. If alternative arrangements cannot be made, it would be ethically permissible to make a professional recommendation to the parents of this infant for comfort care.

FOLLOW-UP

Further discussion determined that relatives in the United States, the only option they would consider for adoption, were also undocumented. Comfort care at home was recommended since transplantation was not feasible. They seemed content with this and took the baby home.

COMMENT

Health-care professionals are obligated to seek what is in the best interests of the patients under their care. There is little question that a heart transplant would be in the best interest of Eduardo. However, professionals are increasingly being asked to act as stewards of expensive or scarce resources. This is a legitimate social function, but it can distort one's professional judgment, and often results in a conflict of interest. Given the huge social barriers that weigh against successful transplantation in Eduardo, it is (regrettably) justifiable to allow the stewardship factor to trump the patient obligation factor in this case.

451

Case 14.04

QUESTION

Is it ethically permissible to allow this child's parents to decline a potentially lifesaving heart transplantation?

STORY

Lai Lee is a five-year-old Hmong girl who emigrated from Laos to the United States with her parents soon after her birth. She had previously been healthy, but six weeks ago she was admitted with progressive shortness of breath. It was determined that she had a serious viral infection of her heart muscle. She was given standard therapy but did not improve. She is now critically ill, and her cardiology physicians believe that her only chance of survival is a heart transplant.

Her parents are not medically sophisticated, but when first told of the option of transplantation they appeared to be willing to proceed so that their daughter might survive. They were told that Lai Lee had a 90 percent chance of dying without a transplant, but with a transplant she had an 80 percent chance of one-year survival and a 75 percent chance of five-year survival. After more detailed discussion, however, they have declined consent for surgery and want to take her home.

Lai Lee's nurses have become very attached to her, want what is best for her, and cannot understand her parents' unwillingness to consent to surgery. They requested ethics consultation.

I spoke with her professional caregivers and with her parents. Her father told me that where Lai Lee dies is very important. If they take her home, they expect her to die, and her spirit would then be in their home and they would know how to properly care for it. If she has surgery, however, there is a significant chance she would die in the hospital, and we would not know how to care for Lai Lee's spirit. So it is their belief that it would be in her **best interests** to go home and die.

DISCUSSION

Differing cultural beliefs may lead different individuals to make different assessments of health and illness, life and death, and even life after death. Such different beliefs may lead to dramatically different decisions in similar situations. In this case, a belief about the place of death and care for the spirit of a departed loved one outweighed the agreed-upon good of continued life.

In Western culture, overriding parental refusal of potentially lifesaving treatment for a child is generally thought to be justifiable, even when the refusal is based on cultural or religious belief (e.g., court-ordered transfusion of children in Jehovah's Witness families). However, when the therapy in question is so scarce, such as organs for transplantation, it is generally not felt prudent to force such treatment on an unwilling family when other families face the prospect of a child's death due to a lack of an available organ for transplantation.

RECOMMENDATION

It is ethically permissible to accept parental refusal of heart transplantation for this child. It is, however, important that they fully understand the options and consequences, presented to them in their own language, before authorities accept this refusal.

FOLLOW-UP

After another full discussion with the parents, using a professional translator, the parents again requested that they be allowed to take their daughter home. She was discharged, and no further follow-up information is available.

COMMENT

Lai Lee's nurses and doctors were sad to see her go home without potentially lifesaving surgery, but were able to reluctantly accept the cultural basis for her parents' decision.

Case 14.05

QUESTION

Should this adolescent be denied a lifesaving heart transplant because she has not been compliant with therapy?

STORY

Johanna is a fourteen-year-old girl who became ill five months ago and was hospitalized for six weeks. She was found to have a severe dilated cardiomyopathy,[4] which did not respond to standard therapy with steroids and immunosuppressants. It was not definitely determined if her illness was of viral origin or was caused by substance abuse.

She has a history of at least one year of daily amphetamine use and has also used other illicit drugs. She has a tragic history of sexual abuse beginning in early childhood, and it is reported that her mother sold her into prostitution. Her mother was banned from visiting her here at the hospital because of verbal and physical abuse. The family was referred to child protective services.

While in hospital, it is known that Johanna has used illicit substances. She went out on passes on at least two occasions with specific proscription against drug use and sexual activity, but returned with urine tests positive for drug metabolites and sperm.

Two months ago it was determined that her only effective therapy would be cardiac transplantation. She was referred to Metropolitan Children's Hospital because her funding source (Medicaid) has a transplantation contract with that institution for patients of her age, and does not contract with our hospital. Metropolitan has subsequently determined that she is medically a candidate, but they have declined to list her for transplantation because of her noncompliance with treatment. Prior to making this decision, they apparently made several attempts to change her behavior, including separation from her family and having her sign a behavioral contract that she kept for only five days. She is currently out of hospital in a protected and supervised home.

---

4. Cardiomyopathy is a life-threatening dysfunction of the heart muscle in which the muscle itself is weak and unable to contract sufficiently to pump the blood as it should, resulting in a large, floppy heart. In young people, it is usually caused by viral infections or toxins.

Recently Johanna's psychiatrist, Dr. Fuller, called the transplant team at our hospital asking them to reconsider listing this patient. He believes that Metropolitan has unfairly excluded her. He feels she will be compliant if separation from her family is maintained. He strongly believes that she is salvageable, and he says he will guarantee compliance. It is not clear how he would do this.

DISCUSSION

Of the many selection criteria used in choosing which patients should receive absolutely scarce medical resources, we tend to be most comfortable implementing medical criteria (likelihood of benefit, length of benefit, quality of survival) and least comfortable with psychosocial criteria (age, supportive environment, psychological ability). Exclusion on psychological grounds is particularly troublesome because it rests on the prediction of human behavior. Although troublesome, it may be ethically justifiable to exclude some patients from organ transplantation because of their inability to adhere to the complicated chronic regimen, since to include them would necessarily mean that others with greater likelihood of compliance (and thus benefit) would not receive the transplant.

In the five months of this adolescent's illness, she has repeatedly been noncompliant. The likelihood that her behavior pattern is attributable to her tragic past social circumstances makes it tempting to say that she is not to blame and should therefore not be punished. This laudable social sensitivity does not, unfortunately, change the present situation of a noncompliant patient who is much less likely to benefit from transplantation than other patients who do not have the burden of antisocial behavior. The focus of discussion should not therefore be on the past, but on her present and future. The pivotal questions are: Are her tragic circumstances insurmountable? Has she been given adequate opportunity to change her behavior?

RECOMMENDATIONS

1. If the evaluation team at this hospital believes this patient has been given adequate support and resources to change her pattern and has failed, it is ethically justifiable to not place her name on our transplant waiting list.
2. Since she has such an unusually strong advocate in Dr. Fuller, he should be given a full hearing to see if there is sufficient reason to be-

lieve she has not been given adequate opportunity or has been treated unfairly.

3. Even if Dr. Fuller is able to convince our transplant team that Johanna is transformable, financial and logistic factors (which would similarly exclude others) may preclude listing her here. If this is the case, her advocate should be encouraged to re-petition the transplant team at Metropolitan using the same information.

FOLLOW-UP

No information is available.

COMMENT

Some might be tempted to say that Johanna does not deserve a transplant because she has not done her part. This is understandable human reasoning, but it becomes more difficult when one puts these thoughts into theological terms. From a Christian perspective, our eternal reward is not predicated on our contribution, but on divine mercy and grace. Should our assessment of another's temporal reward be similar?

If the treatment modality in question were something else, something perhaps expensive but readily available like the use of a **ventilator** in an intensive care unit, I believe it would be unethical to withhold it from a patient because of noncompliance. However, stewardship not only gives us some flexibility here, but also a moral responsibility to ensure that the resources at our disposal are put to the best possible use.

Case 14.06

QUESTION

Should this man with severe alcoholic liver disease be considered for liver transplantation?

STORY

Everett is a sixty-two-year-old business executive with a forty-year history of daily moderate to heavy alcohol use. He has no history of violence, blackouts, or legal or work problems because of his drinking. It is reported that his wife has been a problem drinker all during this time, and his two adult daughters are moderate to heavy drinkers.

Rather suddenly nine months ago, he suffered liver decompensation.[5] He was stabilized, he (reluctantly) stopped drinking, and he was referred to our liver transplant program. Part of the prelisting evaluation for patients with liver failure caused by substance abuse involves a one-week stay on the inpatient psychiatric unit, to see if any psychiatric, psychological, or characterological problems would make the patient a poor candidate. This evaluation was completed two months ago, and it was the consensus of the evaluation team that, although he did not exhibit those problems, he was not then a good candidate because of continued denial of his alcoholism and an attitude that he had a liver problem, not a drinking problem. Because he was stable at that time, it was recommended that both he and his wife enroll in an alcohol recovery program and that he be reevaluated upon completion.

He reluctantly agreed to enroll in a recovery program if that was the only way he could get a transplant. He was slow in enrolling, attended one meeting, then unfortunately had further liver decompensation without known noncompliance regarding medications, diet or alcohol, and his hepatic **encephalopathy**[6] has precluded further participation in the recovery program. He has thus moved to a more urgent transplantation status, and again the question has been asked about his psychological suitability for liver transplantation. In addition, his insurance company is willing to fund the procedure only if he has been psychiatrically cleared.

Although he has now been abstinent for nine months, the psychiatric evaluation team still has reservations about his acceptance of the underlying alcohol problem. His retort that "I have learned my lesson and will never drink again" has not been persuasive for them. At the same time, however, his family has proven to be very supportive. His wife has removed all alcohol from the house and has stopped drinking herself, and the two daughters visit regularly and will not drink in his presence. All seem committed to helping him stay abstinent.

---

5. Decompensation is the tipping point whereby an organ that has been slowly losing function is overwhelmed and slips into organ failure, perhaps by addition of a new stress (e.g., infection), or perhaps merely by an inability to keep up with normal demand.

6. Delirium, caused in this case by liver dysfunction, manifested by confusion and somnolence.

DISCUSSION

There is a growing consensus that it is discriminatory to categorically exclude people with alcoholism from liver transplantation on the basis of either a willful contribution to their condition or a presumption of recidivism. However, because of the absolute scarcity of livers, many believe it is ethically justifiable to give alcoholics a lower priority, after patients with liver failure from other causes, and in addition to require some assessment of their risk of recidivism. The reasoning is that alcoholism, although a disease and not purely a moral failing, is treatable. Once it is diagnosed, the patient has some moral responsibility to seek treatment. Research data suggests that transplanted alcoholic patients who had a shorter period of abstinence (fewer than six months) had a higher rate of recidivism and a higher mortality rate.

This patient has not had any alcohol for nine months. However, since he has been too ill to go out and get any alcohol on his own, it is not clear if this absence of alcohol could be considered voluntary abstinence. If he was not aware of his alcoholism until his precipitous liver decompensation, he could not be accused of failing to seek treatment. However, his denial of the root problem, and his agreement to seek treatment only when coerced by the idea of nontransplantation and inevitable death, do raise legitimate concerns about his candidacy in a system that gives priority to nonalcoholics or alcoholics who are truly remorseful and have shown evidence of a willingness to seek treatment.

RECOMMENDATION

It is ethically appropriate for the psychiatric team to assess that the patient has no psychiatric, psychological, or characterological problems that preclude his candidacy for transplantation, but at the same time to raise their legitimate concerns about his insight, motivation, and potential for recidivism.

FOLLOW-UP

The patient was denied insurance coverage for liver transplantation based on the psychiatric report; that decision was appealed. The company agreed to reconsider the patient after he completed an alcohol rehabilitation program. However, the patient had clinical deterioration and died of liver failure.

COMMENT

When liver transplantation first became available, it was generally not offered to patients with liver failure from alcoholism. The reasoning was twofold: they had already ruined their original liver (so didn't deserve a new one), and they were likely to resume drinking after surgery and ruin the new one. The latter was a bit tenuous since it might take several years of drinking to have the same deleterious effect on the new liver; however, alcohol abuse might interfere with medication and follow-up. Then again, it might not. Transplant surgeons were wont to say, "Transplantation is a very sobering experience," suggesting that someone who goes through this process is better motivated to avoid alcohol than are other patients with an alcohol problem. Data subsequently showed that people with liver failure from alcoholism had good results from transplantation if they admitted they had an alcohol problem, completed an alcohol rehabilitation program, and were abstinent for at least six months.

Everett fell between the cracks. He was reluctant to admit his underlying problem. He was abstinent, but not purely on a voluntary basis. And he had not completed the rehabilitation program. When he had further deterioration making his surgery more urgent, it was very difficult to know which way to go. In this case, those doing his evaluation allowed stewardship to trump the patient's **best interests**. We could still debate whether this was the right decision.

Case 14.07

QUESTION

Is it ethically permissible to do a living-related kidney transplant that is outside the standard of care when the outcome is uncertain but clearly compromised?

STORY

Myrna is a forty-three-year-old woman who developed renal failure from a genetic cystic disease of her kidneys nineteen years ago. She had a transplant at that time, but it failed almost immediately, and she then began

459

hemodialysis. She has been on the kidney transplant waiting list for nearly fifteen years, and at the top of the list for a long time. She has not received a transplant because she has multiple antibodies in her blood that have made tissue matching impossible, most likely the result of her earlier transplant and rejection. The patient is developing joint problems that are not uncommon in patients on long-term dialysis, and she recognizes the diminished life span for patients on long-term dialysis. Thus she very much wants a transplant.

The patient's sister, who does not have cystic kidneys, is willing to donate a kidney, but they are a serious tissue mismatch. This increases the chance of rejection fivefold, though rejection episodes are treatable, so the survival curve is not a lot different from a perfect match. Transplantation between individuals with a cross-match incompatibility is outside the standard of care.

The patient underwent therapy for the past three months with immunoglobulins in an attempt to reduce her antibody level. Unfortunately, her titers did not drop significantly.

Dr. Gaskins, the renal transplant surgeon, has been discussing the possibility of transplant with the patient and her sister for nearly a year. He has been open with them about the risks, stating that graft survival is unpredictable but is almost certainly less than the ten- to fourteen-year average; it could even fail immediately. Based on her past experience of treatment for graft failure, Myrna says she becomes hesitant if there is more than a 50 percent chance of failure, and grows more hesitant as the risk increases. She says her sister is willing to proceed even with a 98 percent risk of failure.

The patient has no obvious alternatives to continued dialysis or this risky innovative transplantation. The surgical morbidity and mortality risk to the donor and recipient are quite small. If the graft were to fail immediately, the additional risk to the recipient would likewise be relatively small. Failure later, however, would place her at some increased risk because of the need for aggressive immunosuppression.

Because renal transplants between tissue-incompatible individuals have not been reported, quantification of success versus failure is impossible. Dr. Gaskins has told the patient that his estimate of the chance of graft survival is 50 percent. All other specialists with whom I spoke agreed that, while it is not impossible that this proposal could work, the chances of success were quite small (one estimated a 5-10 percent chance of graft survival for three months).

DISCUSSION

There is nothing inherently unethical about doing innovative or experimental treatment. However, ethical research depends on (a) scientific background, that is, that there is a reasonable chance it will work, based on the best available evidence from bench, animal, or human research, and (b) the investigator having adequate experience.[7] Even then, it is ethically imperative that all parties give informed consent after fully understanding the burdens, risks, potential benefits, and alternatives. The standard for informed consent for innovative therapy is generally felt to be more stringent than for standard therapy.

In this case, most professionals in the renal transplant field recognize that the proposed transplant might work, though most agree that the chances are relatively small. The renal transplant team clearly has adequate experience in the surgical procedure; however, the research question is not about the surgery, but rather about transplants between persons who have tissue incompatibility.

RECOMMENDATIONS

1. Before considering this innovative procedure, a second opinion should be sought from other centers experienced in the management of tissue incompatibility.
2. If one or more other centers support the proposal for this innovative transplantation, the team and the patient should decide whether the procedure is done here or at a center with more experience in this particular problem.
3. If a decision is made to proceed, either here or elsewhere, the patient, her husband, and the donor need to be fully informed about the following: the risks and burdens of surgery to both donor and recipient; the risk of increased illness for the recipient from rejection and its treatment; whether insurance will pay for this innovative treatment; and the range of (speculated) success from those most knowledgeable in the field.
4. If no other center supports the proposal, it would not necessarily be ethically impermissible to proceed with transplantation here. How-

7. F. Moore, "Three Ethical Revolutions: Ancient Assumptions Remodeled under Pressure of Transplantation," *Transplantation Proceedings* 20 (1988): 1061-67.

ever, prudence would dictate extreme caution, repeated detailed discussion, and full documentation of the reason for the decision from both the treatment team and the research subjects.

FOLLOW-UP

The patient sought a second opinion at a transplant center with more experience in caring for patients with severe tissue incompatibility. After further treatment, that referral center did the kidney transplant from her sister. The donor, the recipient, and the kidney were all doing very well one year after the transplant.

COMMENT

When contemplating treatment options, patients and professionals must consider many things, including benefits, risks, and burdens. This can be difficult enough for standard procedures, but becomes even more difficult when trying to decide for or against innovative therapies when little outcome data exists. In such situations, it becomes imperative to seek out the best available information and opinions from those most knowledgeable. The goal is to avoid an unwise decision based on either patient desperation or physician enthusiasm.

Case 14.08

QUESTION

Is it permissible to offer cardiac transplantation with attempted avoidance of use of blood products to this adolescent daughter of a Jehovah's Witness mother?

STORY

Juanita is a fourteen-year-old girl who was born with congenital heart disease.[8] She has had two surgical procedures (at five months and at twelve

---

8. Transposition of the great vessels and a ventriculo-septal defect.

years of age) and insertion of a pacemaker for symptomatic intermittent slow pulse. She has been under the care of Dr. Lincoln, a pediatric cardiologist, for several years and has had progressive tricuspid valve insufficiency and dysfunction of the heart muscle. Apart from limited exercise tolerance, she was relatively asymptomatic until the recent onset of life-threatening **arrhythmias** for which her pacemaker was replaced with a device that is also a defibrillator. It can automatically shock her heart if it resumes a life-threatening rhythm. Because of this deterioration, consideration has been given to transplantation.

The patient's mother has been an active member of a Jehovah's Witness congregation for six years, and she requested second opinions about the feasibility of transplantation without the use of blood products. Appointments have been made to discuss this at two other institutions, but a recent second episode of **ventricular fibrillation** (with firing of her implanted pacemaker) has caused the patient significant anxiety, prompting her to request listing now. The patient also has been attending Kingdom Hall regularly and has gone out on home visitation, but she has not yet become an "unbaptized publisher," the first step toward membership. She would prefer to avoid blood products, but her stated reason is fear of AIDS and other diseases. Specifically she reported minimal concern and displayed little understanding of the Jehovah's Witness beliefs regarding the spiritual consequences of blood transfusion. Her father is not a Jehovah's Witness. He wants Juanita to have the transplant, and he does not want to delay listing to complete the consultations about bloodless surgery. The transplant team has indicated their willingness to do the transplant while trying to avoid the use of blood products, though with her history of previous surgery, they expect the procedure to be more lengthy and they recognize that they may not be able to avoid using blood.

DISCUSSION

Medical treatment decisions for children are generally made by the parents. As children enter adolescence, they may participate in such decisions to the extent of their understanding. Many fourteen-year-olds, especially those with a history of chronic illness, are able to fully participate and may ethically be treated as adults. In this case, the patient appears to have a good understanding of her condition, the treatment options, and the likely consequences.

Professionals caring for a child of Jehovah's Witness parents are obligated to seek the patient's **best interests**, and often seek a court order to allow the use of lifesaving blood products over the objection of parents. From an ethics perspective, adolescent members of the Jehovah's Witness faith are often treated as adults vis-à-vis the use of blood, much as they are allowed to make other treatment decisions, but judicial review is usually sought before allowing them to refuse lifesaving blood products. In this case, the patient is not yet a member of the faith community. Though she has displayed significant interest in future membership, she currently values life preservation over avoidance of transfusion.

RECOMMENDATIONS

1. Since this relatively mature adolescent and her father both request listing for transplantation with the understanding that (a) efforts will be made to avoid blood products if possible, but that (b) her life and health will not be compromised in this effort, it is ethically permissible to accept their joint consent.
2. Since delaying listing for a few days would not likely alter the outcome, and since it might be a comfort to her mother to obtain at least one other opinion about bloodless transplantation, it would be ethically permissible to wait a few days to allow this. However, immediate listing may be justified because of the patient's level of anxiety or other issues of family dynamics.

FOLLOW-UP

Consultation with a "bloodless surgical team" led to a decision by Juanita and her parents to go on the transplant list. When a heart became available about five weeks later, Mom became upset "because she is doing so well" (and Juanita also expressed some reservations about proceeding), and she requested another echocardiogram. When Dr. Lincoln told them that such results would not change the long-term prognosis or the recommendation for urgent transplantation, they agreed to proceed with the understanding that the surgeons would try to avoid transfusion if possible. Transplantation was completed successfully, but blood transfusions were needed during and immediately after surgery.

COMMENT

As was discussed in chapter 11, the medical management of adolescents from Jehovah's Witness families can be challenging. The ultimate decision about the use or nonuse of blood products often depends on the level of maturity and understanding of the adolescent, but must always take into account the eternal seriousness of the decision in the eyes of the family. The goal of health-care professionals should be to offer the best possible care to the child while preserving family religious beliefs using a non-adversarial approach. Sometimes both cannot be accomplished, leading to wrenching decisions, often in court. Sometimes, as in this case, a patient or family will be willing to accept a professional recommendation that is accompanied by a sincere offer to avoid blood products if possible, but with the understanding that blood will be used to prevent death or disability.

Case 14.09

QUESTION

Are we ethically allowed (or perhaps obligated?) to do a second transplant on this child who is now cognitively impaired?

STORY

Kevin is nearly eleven years old now. He was found to have dilated cardiomyopathy at two months of age and received a heart transplant at this hospital five months later. He did well until a severe rejection episode at twenty-seven months caused an out-of-hospital cardiac arrest from which he was resuscitated. After a long hospitalization, it was clear that he had suffered severe brain damage from temporary lack of oxygen to his brain. His teenage single mother cared for him at home until two years ago, at which time he entered institutional care so she could work. He has been in his current home with very dedicated caregivers for nearly a year; he goes home every other weekend.

His development has been delayed and slow. He was able to sit by age four; now he can walk with assistance from two people. He drinks from a cup and can eat some finger foods, but mostly he requires full care. He assists minimally with dressing and is in diapers. He does not speak, but he tries to mimic sounds, and he loves to hum music. He can make known a few simple needs, and he uses a programmable electronic voice to give messages, usually appropriately.

Although Kevin is now a long-term transplant survivor, he is showing signs of two conditions that cause some concern about his future. His kidney function is significantly diminished, and his last annual coronary angiogram showed 50 percent narrowing of one coronary artery. These are being treated medically, but coronary narrowing in posttransplant patients typically progresses to generalized disease, at which time listing for retransplantation is considered as one option. I was asked to meet with this patient's mother and caregivers to discuss ethically permissible options.

DISCUSSION

Decisions about whether or not to use invasive and burdensome medical procedures on a child are value-laden and often difficult. This is especially true when the child's cognitive development has been compromised and he may not understand the nature of or purpose for painful procedures. We generally make such decisions by trying to balance the anticipated benefits and burdens. For example, if the proposed procedure is readily available, has a high degree of success, poses minimal burden, and without it the child is at risk of disability or death, the procedure is almost always recommended and almost always done. In fact, if parents refuse such interventions, medical professionals often go to court to challenge their parental authority.

On the other hand, if the procedure is difficult to obtain, is very burdensome to the patient, is risky in and of itself, or has a significant chance of not achieving its goals, it may not be recommended in the first place, or it may be declined by parents even if recommended. Such decisions are subject to the values of the parents.

In this case, the discussion is still theoretical in that it is not known if major interventions such as retransplantation or dialysis will ever be indicated.

MANAGEMENT CONFERENCE

I met with Kevin's mother, two of his daily caregivers, and three members of the transplantation team to discuss future management options. We tried to make it clear that we were not making any decisions about **limitation of treatment**. However, if his mother decides not to put him through another transplant because of its great burden and his limited capacity to understand, it would be ethically permissible to change treatment goals and methods. If such a decision is made, all treatment modalities except obligatory comfort measures become optional. For example, it would be permissible to forgo the transplant but continue to monitor for coronary disease and treat it medically; or to forgo monitoring as well; even to forgo medical efforts to forestall death from a coronary event. A similar range of options exists if his kidney disease were to progress.

His mother and caregivers asked appropriate questions and appeared to understand the issues and options. They were encouraged to call with further questions.

RECOMMENDATION

If this patient develops progressive disease that threatens his life, the use of invasive and burdensome procedures is optional; it would be ethically permissible to use or not use them. A decision for or against their use is a value decision to be made by his mother and will be supported by the transplant team.

FOLLOW-UP

No information is available.

COMMENT

It was clear from the discussion with the transplant team alone that they would prefer not to use another heart or a kidney for Kevin, based on their belief that other patients could achieve greater benefit from these organs than would he. However, they also understood the importance of parental choices, and of this particular mom's dedication to her son.

One other factor enters into discussion of such cases. The transplant team often feels an ongoing obligation to patients for whom they have pro-

vided services in the past, and might in some instances prefer to do a repeat transplant on their long-standing patient rather than a first transplant on a new patient. There are difficult trade-offs when dealing with
absolutely scarce resources.

*   *   *

Other Cases Involving Transplantation

Cases 3.05, 3.06, 4.01, 5.10, 11.02, 11.09, 11.13, 13.05

References on Ethical Issues in Transplantation

Arnold, R. M., S. J. Youngner, Renie Schapiro, and C. M. Spicer. *Procuring Or-
gans for Transplant.* Baltimore: Johns Hopkins University Press, 1995.
Shelton, W., and J. Balint, eds. *The Ethics of Organ Transplantation.* Greenwich,
Conn.: JAI Press, 2001.

PART V

CHAPTER 15

The Priesthood of Believers

Many of the cases presented in this book are quite straightforward. On the basis of the precepts of clinical medicine, or the principles of clinical ethics, or precedents established by case law or statute, it is often fairly easy to say, "The ethically permissible options are A, B, and C, but options D and E are outside the boundaries of accepted medical practice." Or sometimes even to say, "In this case, the patient's fiancé is the most appropriate surrogate." In such cases the clinician, the ethicist, or the spiritual adviser can offer ready assistance to the patient or family struggling with a difficult decision.

Sometimes, however, the choices do not separate out into neat black or white options. And the spectrum of shades of gray in a given case may be quite impressive. It is tempting to say in these gray cases, "There are no right or wrong answers here, so you can do whatever you think is best." But that is of little help. What advice can be given to patients or families in these cases?

At still other times the recommendations for permissible options, as determined by professional or legal standards, may conflict with accepted boundaries within the patient's faith tradition. One may be confronted with a situation where the recommendations include "It is professionally and legally permissible to terminate this nineteen-week pregnancy because the fetus has Down syndrome," but the distraught mother comes from a faith tradition that does not allow ending the life of a fetus because he or she will be developmentally delayed. What advice can be given by the clinician, ethicist, or clergy here?

In situations where there is not a clearly right or wrong answer, or where clinically permissible options conflict with the patient's belief system, the Protestant Christian tradition often relies on a precept called the priesthood of believers. I suspect people of faith from other traditions have similar precepts, though I have less experience with this outside my own Christian faith.

The precept of the priesthood of believers comes from Holy Scripture. In the Hebrew Bible, shortly after Moses led the children of Israel out of bondage, he recorded that Yahweh had said they would be his priestly kingdom (Exod. 19:4-6). The mission of God's people was to be priests to those around them and to each other. Certain individuals were anointed to perform some of the priestly tasks such as animal sacrifice and entering the Holy of Holies. These anointed priests took on the role of mediator between the people and God.

In the Christian Bible, it is recorded that at the time of Jesus' sacrificial death, the curtain separating the Holy of Holies from the remainder of the temple was torn in two, signifying the possibility of direct access to God for all believers (Matt. 27:51). At that moment the concept of priesthood changed. After his onetime sacrifice for sin, Jesus became the High Priest, and all believers in Jesus had direct access to the Divine. Peter later recorded, "As you come to him, the living Stone — rejected by men but chosen by God and precious to him — you also, like living stones, are being built into a spiritual house to be a holy priesthood, offering spiritual sacrifices acceptable to God through Jesus Christ. . . . But you are a chosen people, a royal priesthood, a holy nation, a people belonging to God, that you may declare the praises of him who called you out of darkness into his wonderful light" (1 Pet. 2:4-5, 9).[1] Not all believers are called to a priestly office, but all are given the gift of a priestly function. This concept of a universal priesthood of all believers, in contrast to a special priesthood of those ordained by the church, was rediscovered and emphasized by Martin Luther at the time of the Protestant Reformation. He taught that all believers have equal and direct access to God, and he thus encouraged all Christians to read Scripture on their own, to pray on their own, to exercise their direct access to God.

Thus, in both the Hebrew and Christian traditions, individuals are called to minister to each other. The Christian tradition expands this concept of ministry to include direct access to God. Many Christian denomi-

---

1. Non-Protestant Christians (i.e., Orthodox and Roman Catholic) traditionally believe that this verse gives responsibility to all believers for the preservation and propagation of the gospel and the church, as distinct from the liturgical and sacramental roles of the ordained priesthood. In spite of this, both Orthodox and Roman Catholic teachings encourage believers to have a personal relationship with God.

nations continue to distinguish between clergy and laity, but all encourage believers to pray and seek God's wisdom.

In a spiritual understanding of clinical ethics, the basic idea is that the individual who is facing a difficult dilemma is not alone. He or she can look to others for assistance. Those "others" include, first of all, clergy, who in most instances will have a better grasp of the precepts and boundaries. I think it is ideal for the patient's own clergyperson to be engaged in the discussion, since there is already an established relationship. But when this is not possible, hospital chaplains provide a valuable service. In addition, the clergyperson will be at least one step removed from the situation, so may be able to offer advice somewhat more dispassionately than those who are intimately involved.

But this concept includes more than clergy — it encompasses other individuals within the decision-maker's faith community, and in the Christian tradition, it even includes the person of the Holy Spirit.

Not to diminish advice gleaned from clergy or fellow travelers in the faith, but divine assistance from the Holy Spirit may be of more value than the assistance of other people. These other people are, after all, humans, and are thus subject to some degree of personal, psychological, or social bias. This does not mean, however, that the Christian seeking divine guidance may pray for "the answer" and then just sit back and await handwriting on the wall or some other clear pronouncement. In fact, when I pray with or for a patient or family member facing a difficult decision, I do not pray for "the answer." Instead, I pray for three things: guidance, wisdom, and peace.

I pray for guidance because I want God to help me (or the decision-maker) to be able to set aside personal, psychological, or social biases. I want the divine authority to take precedence in the reasoning process.

I then pray for wisdom. It is a truism that "good ethics begins with good facts." So collecting valid information is an extremely important part of the process. The facts in a given case should include an inquiry about the patient's own faith tradition and an exploration of documents, teachings, or precedents in that faith tradition that may bear on the situation at hand. But how one assesses all these medical and spiritual facts, how one balances competing interests, how one prioritizes the options — this requires wisdom. Some human wisdom, perhaps, but more importantly, divine wisdom.

And I pray for peace. This is my personal barometer. I want the divine Spirit to give me a feeling of "unpeace" or even turmoil if I am moving in the wrong direction with my human assessment. I hope for "the peace that passes all understanding" if I am working within acceptable faith boundaries.

Guidance, wisdom, and peace. Sounds simple, perhaps even simplistic. But as I look at the accepted standards, as I wrestle with the gray areas, and as I deal with conflicts, I find considerable comfort in these precepts that ensure that I am not alone.

*   *   *

References on the Priesthood of All Believers

Blevins, Carolyn D. "The Priesthood of All Believers." From the Baptist History and Heritage Society. Available at http://www.baptisthistory.org/priesthood.htm.

Haberer, Jack. "The Priesthood of Believers." In *What Presbyterians Believe.* Available at http://www.pcusa.org/today/believe/past/mar04/priesthood.htm.

Wollenburg, George. "The Priesthood of Believers and the Divine Service." Available at http://www.lcms.org/pages/internal.asp?NavID=841, originally published in *Lutheran Worship Notes,* issue 32 (1995).

Glossary

adult respiratory distress syndrome (ARDS)   A syndrome of respiratory insufficiency with low serum oxygen levels due to swelling of the microscopic tissues of the lungs; has many causes; usually requires assisted ventilation for an extended period.

advance directive   An advance declaration, usually in writing, constructed by an adult with decision-making capacity (called the principal), giving instructions about treatment wishes if he or she should lose the ability to participate in decisions; the instruction may involve (a) what he or she would want to have done or not have done, and/or (b) who the principal wants to endow with the authority to make treatment decisions (called the agent).

agent   The person named as surrogate decision-maker in an advance directive. *See also* Advance directive

AMA (against medical advice)   A phrase pertaining to a patient's decision to discontinue a treatment despite advice to the contrary from medical professionals, most commonly used when a patient leaves the hospital AMA.

amniotic fluid   The protective fluid in which a fetus is suspended throughout pregnancy; it is produced by the fetus and fetal membranes.

amyotrophic lateral sclerosis (ALS)   A degenerative disease of motor nerve cells that involves progressive weakness of muscles throughout the body; it does not affect cognition; it often leads to questions about the use or nonuse of feeding tubes or assisted ventilation; ALS most often begins in middle age and leads to death in two or three years; also known as Lou Gehrig's disease.

anencephaly   A developmental anomaly of the brain involving absence of all or most of the upper portions of the brain, usually with normal development of the brain stem and spinal cord; incompatible with life; can usually be diagnosed during pregnancy by ultrasound imaging.

anticoagulation   Treatment with drugs to reduce the ability of the blood to clot.

Apgar score   Evaluation of a newborn's physical condition, usually done at one minute and five minutes after delivery; based on a rating of five factors (pulse, respiratory effort, color, muscle tone, reflex irritability) that reflect the infant's ability to adjust to the extrauterine environment; each factor is given a score of 0, 1, or 2, so the Apgar score ranges from 0 to 10.

arrhythmia   Any variation of the normal rhythm of the heart; may involve abnormal rate, regularity, or origin of the heartbeat.

aspiration   When either food or fluid accidentally goes into the airway during swallowing; this can happen during a state of diminished consciousness (e.g., during general anesthesia or when inebriated) or with diminished muscle control (e.g., after a stroke).

asystole   Absence of a heartbeat; cardiac standstill or arrest ("systole" is the term used for contraction of the heart muscle).

best interests   The standard used to determine the appropriate course of action to follow for a patient who has never had decision-making capacity (i.e., a child or an adult with developmental delay) or for a patient who has lost decision-making capacity but for whom we have no knowledge about wishes or values; this is a broad and rather nebulous standard, but includes such matters as an assessment of benefits, risks, and burdens of the available options, and an estimate of how most individuals would weigh these factors.

bronchoscopy   A procedure involving the insertion of a tube into the large airways of the lungs (trachea, bronchi) to visualize structure and/or to retrieve samples of tissue or secretions.

cardiopulmonary resuscitation (CPR)   The artificial substitution of heart and lung action used by rescuers on a person who has experienced cardiac arrest or apparent sudden death; involves the use of artificial ventilation and closed chest cardiac massage.

congestive heart failure   Weakness of the heart muscle leading to "pump failure" such that blood and fluid back up in the lungs or peripheral circulation; may be sudden in onset or chronic in nature.

CT scan   Computer tomography; an X-ray method of imaging tissues in selected layers.

cyanosis   A bluish discoloration of skin or lips most often caused by lack of oxygen in the tissues.

decision-making capacity   The mental ability to receive and use information in the process of making a decision consistent with one's own values.

delirium   An acute reversible mental condition characterized by disorganized thinking and the reduced ability to maintain attention to external stimuli; may be caused by a large variety of conditions.

dementia   A chronic irreversible mental condition characterized by a general loss of intellectual abilities including memory and judgment; many possible causes; the most common type is Alzheimer's dementia, but dementia is also seen as part of Parkinson's disease, Huntington's disease, strokes, etc.

do-not-resuscitate order (**DNR order**)   Documentation in a patient's medical record or elsewhere that a decision has been made to not use cardiopulmonary resuscitative measures when the patient experiences a cardiac arrest.

Down syndrome   A congenital chromosomal disorder (trisomy 21) that results in multiple physical abnormalities and varying degrees of mental retardation.

electroencephalogram (EEG)   A recording of the electrical activity of brain cells; made by applying recording electrodes to various parts of the scalp.

encephalopathy   Abnormal function of the brain; multiple causes; may be reversible or irreversible.

endotracheal tube (ETT)   A plastic or rubber tube inserted through a patient's mouth and into his or her upper airway (trachea) so that breathing can be assisted, most often by attachment to a ventilator; insertion of the ETT is called intubation, and removal is called extubation.

extubation   Removal of a plastic or rubber tube that was inserted through a patient's mouth and into his or her upper airway (trachea) so that breathing can be assisted, most often by attachment to a ventilator.

full code status   The absence of a do-not-resuscitate order; the professional and societal presumption that all persons without a DNR order should be given full resuscitative efforts in the event of a cardiac arrest.

futility   Futile treatment is treatment that will not work for a given patient's condition; a clinical judgment made by professionals; ongoing discussion about the scope of futility; the term is sometimes misused in situations where the professional believes the treatment in question is "inappropriate" but perhaps not truly futile. See discussion in chapter 1.

gamete The name given to reproductive cells (egg or sperm) because these cells contain half the number of chromosomes present in all other cells.

gestation Pregnancy; the time from fertilization to birth.

herniation of the brain stem Occurs when increased pressure within the skull causes the base of the brain to protrude through the opening into the spinal canal; often the final event in any pathology inside the skull that elevates pressure; it is irreversible and leads to imminent death.

Huntington's disease An inherited disorder that causes progressive brain degeneration, beginning in one's thirties or forties, that leads to severe disability with behavioral, cognitive, and movement disorders and ultimately to death, usually within several years; a genetically transmitted (dominant inheritance) disease that can be detected by testing before the onset of symptoms.

hypoxia Deficient oxygenation of the blood from any cause, so that tissues and organs receive insufficient amounts of oxygen.

imago Dei The theological concept that each human being, regardless of physical or mental abilities, contains the image of the Divine.

intracerebral hemorrhage Hemorrhage inside the skull that involves the brain tissue itself; clinical manifestations and prognosis depend on size and location of the hemorrhage.

intracranial hemorrhage Hemorrhage inside the skull; may be into the brain tissue itself (intracerebral hemorrhage), into the ventricular space in the center of the brain (intraventricular hemorrhage), into the space between the brain and the skull (subarachnoid hemorrhage), or a combination; clinical manifestations and prognosis depend on size and location of the hemorrhage.

intracranial pressure Pressure inside the skull; likely to cause severe damage to the brain if it rises too high, and may result in death.

intraventricular hemorrhage Hemorrhage inside the skull that involves the ventricular space in the center of the brain; clinical manifestations and prognosis depend on size and location of the hemorrhage.

intubation Insertion of a plastic or rubber tube through a patient's mouth and into his or her upper airway (trachea) so that breathing can be assisted, most often by attachment to a ventilator. *See also* Endotracheal tube

ischemia/ischemic Deficiency of blood, usually due to constriction or obstruction of an artery.

J-tube A feeding tube placed into the stomach and extended beyond its outlet into the jejunum (the second part of the small intestine); these placements are more involved than a more simple gastric tube.

limitation of treatment A decision to use less than maximal treatment for a given patient. This may include written orders for no resuscitation (DNR), no intubation (DNI), or no transfer to a higher level of care (do not transfer to hospital or to ICU).

minimally conscious state (MCS) A state of severe brain dysfunction in which the patient has minimal awareness; see discussion in chapter 7.

MRI Magnetic resonance imaging; a method of visualizing internal structures that uses the inherent magnetic properties of substances rather than the application of external radiation as is done in X-rays and CT scans.

multi-organ system failure (MOSF) A critical condition involving failure of two or more physiologic systems (lungs, heart, kidneys, liver, bone marrow, etc.), often cascading from one organ system to others; very poor prognosis, especially if the MOSF continues for more than a few days.

neonatologist A physician who specializes in the care of newborns with medical problems.

nephrologist A physician who specializes in the care of patients with kidney problems.

neurologist A physician who specializes in the care of patients with problems of the nervous system (brain and peripheral nerves).

palliative care ". . . the active total care of patients whose disease is not responsive to curative treatment"; ". . . the control of pain, and other symptoms, and of psychological, social, and spiritual needs is paramount"; "The goal of palliative care is achievement of the best quality of life for patients and their families." World Health Organization, 1990.

PEG tube Percutaneous endoscopically-placed gastrostomy tube; a feeding tube inserted through the abdominal wall into the stomach using a relatively simple technique that does not involve major surgery or opening the abdomen.

persistent vegetative state (PVS) A condition of severe brain dysfunction in which the patient has signs of wakefulness but is completely unaware of his or her surroundings; see chapter 7.

pulmonologist A physician who specializes in care of patients with lung problems.

renal insufficiency A condition of inadequate function of the kidneys; may be partial or complete (renal failure), temporary or permanent.

sepsis   A critical condition of infection in the blood stream, usually beginning as a localized infection (e.g., in the lungs) that has broken down natural defenses and is spreading throughout the body.

slow code   An immoral pretense at doing cardiopulmonary resuscitation, when the participants know that their less than conscientious efforts will be ineffective.

subarachnoid hemorrhage   Hemorrhage inside the skull that involves the space between the brain and the skull; clinical manifestations and prognosis depend on size and location of the hemorrhage.

substituted judgment   A process of decision making for patients who have lost the capacity to participate in the decision; in this process, a surrogate is to use his or her understanding of the patient's wishes and values to arrive at a decision that the patient would make, if able.

surrogate   A substitute decision-maker.

total parenteral nutrition (**TPN**)   The administration of a nutritionally adequate solution of sugars, amino acids, fats, minerals, and vitamins, delivered into a large central vein; used when the gastrointestinal tract is unavailable for nutrition; an expensive modality of treatment that requires close monitoring and is subject to many potential complications.

tracheostomy   The surgical placement in the front of a patient's neck of a plastic or metal tube through a hole in the trachea, the main airway; some patients may breathe spontaneously through this "trach tube" and others require attachment to a ventilator to assist breathing; if a patient cannot be weaned from a ventilator after two or three weeks, a tracheostomy is used to prevent erosion of the lining of the trachea by the endotracheal tube.

ventilator   A machine used to instill air, usually enriched in oxygen content, into the patient's lungs; used to treat respiratory failure.

ventricular fibrillation   A cardiac arrhythmia characterized by uncoordinated ineffective rapid contractions of various parts of the ventricles; may respond to electrical shock to restore coordinated contractions.

weaning   The process of gradual withdrawal of ventilator support from a patient who has been dependent on the machine to breathe for him or her; the expectation is usually that the patient's inherent ability to breathe will return.

zygote   A fertilized egg; the cell resulting from the union of a sperm and an egg.

Case Index Cross-Reference

Advance Directives

Cases 3.07, 3.10, 4.01, 4.04, 4.05, 4.10, 6.03, 6.06, 6.08, 7.02, 7.09, 8.06, 9.13

Alternative/Complementary Treatments

Cases 9.04, 11.13

Autonomy

Cases 3.07, 3.08, 3.11, 4.01, 4.02, 4.05, 4.10, 4.11, 4.12, 4.14, 5.04, 5.05, 5.10, 5.11, 6.07, 6.08, 6.09, 6.10, 6.11, 7.04, 7.05, 7.09, 8.05, 8.06, 8.08, 8.11, 9.08, 9.09, 10.01, 11.12, 11.13, 12.02, 12.03, 12.04, 12.05, 13.01, 13.02, 13.03, 13.04, 13.05, 13.06, 13.07, 13.08, 13.09

Capacity/Competence

Cases 3.02, 4.04, 4.05, 4.08, 4.09, 4.10, 4.11, 4.12, 5.02, 5.08, 5.10, 5.12, 6.07, 6.09, 7.04, 7.05, 7.10, 8.01, 8.09, 13.02

Conflicts — between Family and Physician

Cases 3.01, 3.03, 3.04, 3.06, 4.03, 4.12, 4.13, 5.07, 6.02, 6.04, 6.06, 7.03, 7.04, 7.06, 7.09, 7.11, 8.06, 9.01, 9.02, 9.03, 9.04, 9.05, 9.06, 9.07, 9.10, 9.12, 9.13, 10.02, 10.04, 10.05, 10.06, 10.07, 10.08, 10.11, 11.05, 11.07, 11.08, 11.11, 11.13, 14.09

Conflicts — between Family Members

Cases 3.01, 4.06, 4.07, 5.01, 5.13, 7.03, 7.08, 7.10, 9.08, 10.08, 11.06, 13.06, 14.08

Conflicts — between Health-Care Professionals

Cases 3.09, 4.03, 4.09, 7.06, 9.04, 11.03, 11.06, 13.09, 14.01, 14.05, 14.06

Conflicts — between Patient and Doctor

Cases 3.05, 4.08, 4.12, 5.04, 5.06, 6.07, 6.10, 6.11, 7.04, 8.03, 8.04, 8.05, 8.08, 8.10, 10.01, 11.10, 11.12, 13.11

Conflicts — between Patient and Family

Cases 7.09, 11.10, 11.11, 11.12

Consent

Cases 5.10, 8.01, 8.09, 9.03, 10.03, 10.05, 12.01, 12.05, 13.02, 13.07, 13.08, 14.01, 14.07

Disclosure of Information (Right to Know)

Cases 9.03, 11.07, 11.11

Finances/Stewardship/Allocation of Resources

Cases 4.13, 5.03, 6.10, 7.06, 11.03, 11.04, 11.05, 12.03, 12.04, 13.12, 14.02, 14.03, 14.06

Futility

Cases 3.02, 3.05, 3.06, 4.03, 4.13, 5.06, 5.08, 6.05, 6.10, 7.06, 8.03, 9.05, 9.06, 9.07, 9.12, 10.03, 10.05, 11.03, 11.04, 13.10

Irrational Choices

Cases 5.04, 6.10, 6.11, 7.05, 8.05, 8.08, 11.12

Jehovah's Witness Refusal of Blood Products

Cases 9.09, 9.10, 13.09, 14.08

Physician Influence on Decisions

Case 11.04

Restraints

Cases 5.09, 6.01, 6.08, 6.11, 7.01, 7.04, 8.08, 11.10, 12.04

Right of Conscience

Cases 3.06, 4.03, 6.02, 6.04, 6.05, 8.04, 9.11, 9.13, 12.02, 12.03

Socially Isolated Patients (No Family, No Surrogate)

Cases 3.02, 5.06, 7.04

Suffering/Quality of Life

Cases 4.14, 5.05, 5.06, 5.09, 5.11, 6.01, 6.06, 6.10, 8.02, 9.05, 9.07, 10.05, 10.07, 10.09, 11.02, 11.03, 11.04, 11.08

Surrogacy/Substituted Judgment

Cases 3.02, 3.03, 3.04, 3.10, 4.01, 4.02, 4.05, 4.06, 4.07, 4.11, 5.01, 5.02, 5.04, 5.05, 5.08, 5.09, 5.13, 6.03, 6.04, 7.03, 7.06, 7.07, 7.09, 7.10, 8.01, 8.02, 8.06, 9.01, 9.08, 10.01, 10.02, 10.03, 10.04, 10.08, 11.02, 11.06, 11.08, 11.10, 11.11, 11.13, 12.05, 13.02

Uncertainty

Cases 3.02, 4.01, 4.04, 4.05, 4.07, 4.08, 4.09, 6.03, 6.04, 6.06, 7.04, 7.07, 8.02, 8.08, 10.01, 10.05, 10.06, 10.10, 11.01, 11.02, 11.03, 11.04, 11.06, 11.09, 13.05, 13.07

Withholding versus Withdrawing Treatment

Cases 3.08, 3.09, 4.11, 4.14, 6.05